T0229922

Medical and Scientific Writing in Late Medieval English

Medical and scientific writing in English has evolved over more than a millennium, from its genesis in the Anglo-Saxon era to its present-day position as the *lingua franca* of science. This volume focuses on its development as a register in late medieval English. During this period it emerged in the vernacular, as its Graeco-Roman conventions were modified in a new sociohistorical context. Seven experts discuss the various linguistic and textual processes involved in vernacularising science, and how they related to communicative practices and to the writers and readers of medical and scientific texts. Referring to authentic medieval texts, they show how discourse communities adopted scriptorial 'house-styles', how vocabulary and code-switching patterns reflect the multilingual context of the period, and how intertextuality featured between shared materials. Bringing together several perspectives on this new research area for the first time, this book will be welcomed by linguists and historians of science alike.

The idea of this book comes from the work done by the Scientific thought-styles project team in the Research Unit for Variation and Change in English at the University of Helsinki. Three of the contributors are members of the team and compilers of the electronic *Corpus of Middle English Medical Texts* (Taavitsainen, Pahta, and Mäkinen).

Medical and Scientific Writing in Late Medieval English

STUDIES IN ENGLISH LANGUAGE

The aim of this series is to provide a framework for original work on the English language. All are based securely on empirical research, and represent theoretical and descriptive contributions to our knowledge of notional varieties of English, both written and spoken. The series will cover a broad range of topics in English grammar, vocabulary, discourse, and pragmatics, and is aimed at an international readership.

Already published

Christian Mair
Infinitival complement clauses in English: a study of syntax in discourse

Charles F. Meyer
Apposition in contemporary English

Jan Firbas
Functional sentence perspective in written and spoken communication

Izchak M. Schlesinger
Cognitive space and linguistic case

Katie Wales
Personal pronouns in present-day English

Laura Wright
The development of standard English, 1300–1800: theories, descriptions, conflicts

Charles F. Meyer
English Corpus Linguistics: theory and practice

Stephen J. Nagle and Sara. L. Sanders (eds.)
English in the Southern United States

Anne Curzan
Gender Shifts in the History of English

Kingsley Bolton
Chinese Englishes

Forthcoming

Elizabeth Gordon *et al.*
New Zealand English: its origins and evolution

Raymond Hickey
Legacies of Colonial English

Medical and Scientific Writing in Late Medieval English

Edited by
IRMA TAAVITSAINEN
University of Helsinki
and
PÄIVI PAHTA
University of Helsinki

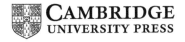

CAMBRIDGE UNIVERSITY PRESS

CAMBRIDGE UNIVERSITY PRESS
Cambridge, New York, Melbourne, Madrid, Cape Town,
Singapore, São Paulo, Delhi, Mexico City

Cambridge University Press
The Edinburgh Building, Cambridge CB2 8RU, UK

Published in the United States of America by Cambridge University Press, New York

www.cambridge.org
Information on this title: www.cambridge.org/9780521831338

© Cambridge University Press 2004

First published 2004

A catalogue record for this publication is available from the British Library

Library of Congress Cataloguing in Publication Data
Medical and scientific writing in late medieval English / edited by Irma Taavitsainen and
Päivi Pahta.
    p.   cm. – (Studies in English language)
Includes bibliographical references and index.
ISBN 0 521 83133 4
1. English language – Middle English, 1100–1500 – Medical English.   2. English prose
literature – Middle English, 1100–1500 – History and criticism.   3. English language – Middle
English, 1100–1500 – Technical English.   4. Scientific literature – England – History – To
1500.   5. Medical literature – England – History – To 1500.   6. Medicine, Medieval – England.
7. Science, Medieval.   I. Taavitsainen, Irma.   II. Pahta, Päivi.   III. Series
PE664.3.M44   2003
427′.02′02461 – dc21

ISBN 978-0-521-83133-8 Hardback
ISBN 978-0-521-11041-9 Paperback

Contents

Contributors

The idea of this book comes from the work done by the Scientific Thought-Styles project team in the Research Unit for Variation and Change in English at the University of Helsinki. Three of the contributors are members of the team and compilers of the electronic *Corpus of Middle English Medical Texts* and the *Corpus of Early English Medical Writing* (Taavitsainen, Pahta and Mäkinen).

RUTH CARROLL is a Senior Lecturer (Associate Professor) in linguistics in the Department of English Philology at the University of Turku, and was also a visiting scholar at the University of Helsinki when she began the work published here. Her previous publications include work on the lexical semantics of Middle English, as well as historical discourse linguistics.

CLAIRE JONES is Research Fellow at the Centre for Medieval Studies at the University of York. She has published in the fields of vernacular medical manuscripts and medieval literacy and is currently working on a large-scale database of medieval English urban manuscripts.

MARTTI MÄKINEN is a doctoral student at the Department of English, University of Helsinki. His research interests are manuscript and genre studies, corpus linguistics and historical pragmatics. His dissertation topic is intertextuality in medieval herbals.

JUHANI NORRI is Lecturer in English at the University of Tampere. He is the author of *Names of Sicknesses In English*, 1400–1550 (1992) and *Names of Body Parts In English*, 1400–1550 (1998). He is currently compiling a dictionary of medical vocabulary in English during the period 1375–1550.

PÄIVI PAHTA is Research Fellow in the multidisciplinary Helsinki Collegium for Advanced Studies and a member of the Research Unit for Variation and Change in English, both at the University of Helsinki. She is the author of *Medieval Embryology in the Vernacular: The Case of 'De spermate'* (Société Néophilologique, 1998) and a co-editor of *Writing in Nonstandard English* (Benjamins, 1999) and *Placing Middle English in Context* (Mouton de Gruyter, 2000).

IRMA TAAVITSAINEN is Professor of English Philology, Head of the Department of English and Deputy Director of the Research Unit of Variation and Change in English at the University of Helsinki. She has authored and co-edited several books, including *Diachronic Perspectives on Address Term Systems* (Benjamins, 2003), *Placing Middle English in Context* (Mouton de Gruyter, 2000), *Writing in Nonstandard English* (Benjamins, 1999) and *Index of Middle English Prose: A Handlist of Scandinavian Collections* (Boydell and Brewer, 1994). She is the co-editor of the *Journal of Historical Pragmatics* (Benjamins).

LINDA EHRSAM VOIGTS, Curators' Professor Emerita at the University of Missouri-Kansas City, publishes on Old and Middle English scientific and medical texts and is responsible, with Patricia Deery Kurtz, for the searchable database on more than 8,000 such texts: *Scientific and Medical Writings in Old and Middle English: An Electronic Reference*, CD-ROM (University of Michigan Press, 2000).

Illustrations

Figures and map

Tables

Preface

To understand the characteristics of present-day scientific writing, we need to know about the earlier stages of language use. This book deals with the early phases of the development that was to lead to the present situation where English has a global position as the *lingua franca* of science. The first steps of writing about medical and scientific matters in English were taken more than a millennium ago in the Anglo-Saxon era, and from the later Middle Ages there is an unbroken chain of texts covering more than six hundred years. Vernacular scientific writing in the late medieval and early modern periods is still an understudied area, though more attention has been attached to it recently. New data have been discovered, and new methods of linguistic research make new insights possible and enable researchers to pose questions that would have seemed unanswerable a generation ago. The evolution of scientific writing shows interesting shifts from more detached to more involved style and back again, and from an abundant use of foreign phrases and Latinate vocabulary to more native and plain style. Surprisingly, late medieval scientific writing has several features in common with characteristics of present-day scientific writing.

This book is an outcome of the research project 'Scientific thought-styles: The evolution of English medical writing' in the Research Unit for Variation and Change at the University of Helsinki, with invited chapters by international scholars working in the field. We wanted to contribute to the discussion on vernacularisation processes, and transfer and establishment of genre conventions and special languages; our future work will focus on developments in a diachronic perspective.

We wish to thank the Academy of Finland for granting us research funding for a three-year period 1999–2001 (project number 37930). Most of the work for this book has been carried out at the Research Unit for Variation and Change in English at the University of Helsinki, and our corpus work has partly been funded by the Research Unit. We are grateful for this support. We would like to thank our research assistants Carla Suhr and Turo Hiltunen for their unfailing spirit and help in editing this book. We are also grateful to the other members of our project team Alpo Honkapohja, Martti Mäkinen and Maura Ratia, and our former project members Paula Korhonen, Noora Leskinen and Minna Vihla for their help and collaboration. Irma Taavitsainen visited King's College Cambridge during the Michaelmas term 2001, which is gratefully acknowledged. We would also like to thank the scholarly libraries mentioned in this book for letting us consult the manuscripts. We are indebted to several people for inspiring discussion, advice and encouragement. Our special thanks are due to Peter Murray Jones, Teresa Tavormina, Michael Benskin, George Keiser, Linda Voigts, Ronald Waldron, and Kari Anne Rand Schmidt.

Helsinki, February 2003
Irma Taavitsainen, Päivi Pahta

Abbreviations

AN	Anglo-Norman
BL	British Library
CEEM	*Corpus of Early English Medical Writing*
CL	Classical Latin
DML	Latham and Howlett, *Dictionary of Medieval Latin from British Sources*
EMode	Early Modern English
eVK	Voigts and Kurtz, *Scientific and Medical Writings in Old and Middle English: An Electronic Reference*
Gr	Greek
IMEP	*The Index of Middle English Prose*
L	Latin
LALME	McIntosh *et al.*, *A Linguistic Atlas of Late Mediaeval English*
Mdu	Middle Dutch
ME	Middle English
MED	Kurath and Kuhn, *Middle English Dictionary*
MEMT	*Corpus of Middle English Medical Texts*
MF	Middle French
ML	Medieval Latin
MNW	Verwijs and Verdam, *Middernederlandsch woordenboek*
MS(S)	manuscript(s)
OE	Old English
OED	Murray *et al.*, *Oxford English Dictionary*
OF	Old French
OLD	Glare, *Oxford Latin Dictionary*
RMLW	Latham, *Revised Medieval Latin Word-List*
STC	Pollard and Redgrave, *A Short-Title Catalogue of Books Printed in England, Scotland, & Ireland and of English Books Printed Abroad 1475–1640*
TK	Thorndike and Kibre, *A Catalogue of Incipits of Mediaeval Scientific Writings in Latin*

1 Vernacularisation of scientific and medical writing in its sociohistorical context

PÄIVI PAHTA AND IRMA TAAVITSAINEN

1.1 Science and medicine in the medieval period

In the history of the English language, the register of scientific writing is one that shows almost unbroken continuity from the earliest periods to the present. However, the conception of what counts as science and scientific writing has undergone fundamental changes in the course of time. Medieval classifications of knowledge include fields like music, physiognomy, and areas that border on the occult and magic.[1] Distinctions between various branches of science were not made in the present way, for example astronomy was a main scientific interest of the scholastic age with astrology as its application; it also formed an integral part of medical theory and practice (see e.g. French 1994). The influences of the macrocosm projected on the microcosm of man, the centre of the universe. The heavens influenced all worldly conditions and affairs from health to appropriate times for performing various actions (see Plate 1).

The earliest layer of scientific writing in English dates from the Anglo-Saxon period. A continuous line of development can be traced from the end of the fourteenth century up to the present in the field of medicine, which provides us with the perspective of register and genre conventions vacillating and developing over seven centuries. The fourteenth and fifteenth centuries, i.e. the time when scientific texts started to appear on a larger scale in English, fall within the prime of scholasticism in England. Thus the vernacular tradition emerges from the background of already established conventions of scientific writing in Latin. The Latin tradition and its conventions also provide a point of comparison for the assessments of early vernacular scientific writings in the present volume.

One of the most distinctive characteristics of scholasticism has been said to be its unfailing persistence in examining its own progress (Jacquart 1998: 197). This feature is attested in the layered nature of learned texts of the period. Western science was initiated by ancient Greek scientists in their search for principles of nature and, at the same time, for principles of argumentation for presenting their ideas (Crombie 1995: 225). New generations of scientists based their studies on texts written by their predecessors, quoted and elaborated them or explicated

2 Päivi Pahta and Irma Taavitsainen

their sayings. Accordingly, references to authorities are perhaps the most conspicuous feature of the logocentricity of medieval science (see Demaitre 1976,
and Taavitsainen and Pahta 1997, 1998). Within this general frame there was,
however, room for innovation and progress. The attitudes to the 'new' and the
possibility of progress vary according to the epistemological levels and different genres, such as commentaries, compendia, and surgical or pharmacological
writings (Crisciani 1990: 120, 126).

Theoretical foundations of medicine were likewise derived from antiquity.
Learned Arab scholars emphasised and systematised the links between medicine
and philosophy already extant in the basic core. The development of medicine
towards its high peak of scholasticism took place in Italy from the twelfth century
onwards (Siraisi 1990: 11–13, 48). Unlike for example philosophy, medicine was
both a science and a craft, and combines both theory and practice (cf. Demaitre
1975; see also French 2001: 68–75). Moreover, the practical nature of medicine
was undoubtedly a major incentive for the social diffusion of academic knowledge
in the field, and through the process of vernacularisation, more people gained
access to learning and useful knowledge. Practical considerations were probably
not the only factors promoting vernacularisation. The process was also advanced
by ideas about the vernacular language and was tied to issues of nationalism
(cf. Evans et al. 1999; see also Taavitsainen 2001b).

1.2   The aim and approach of this volume

This volume describes the late medieval period of English scientific writing
from the late fourteenth to the sixteenth century. It tackles three core issues in
the vernacularisation of scientific and medical writing, illuminates them from
various angles, and shows how this field of writing developed. The emergence of
the scientific register in English is part of a larger pattern. Similar developments
took place in other vernaculars in Europe at the same time, and new discourse
communities were created alongside the pan-European discourse world in Latin.
Writings in the new medium, the English language, altered the scene as access
to knowledge became available for a wider readership. The new discourse world
was not created in a vacuum: what we have as the basis of our assessment is
texts, i.e. communicative exchanges, from the scientific discourse world of the
late medieval period. Historical information about the social basis of discourse
communities is scarce, but the sociohistorical context necessarily includes the
people who produced the texts and those who consumed them. The chapters
in the book take this into account and deal with linguistic processes without
forgetting language-external factors – the people who wrote and read these texts,
the conditions under which they worked, and the materials they had at hand.
This is the first unifying theme.

The second theme shifts the focus to the producers of texts and approaches
vernacularisation specifically from the point of view of people involved in the
processes of book and text production from the commentator, the compiler and
the translator to the scribe. The introduction of a new field of writing in English

posed several challenges to those in the vanguard as the means of expressing scientific ideas in the vernacular had to be invented. Writers developed various strategies to overcome the difficulties. Decisions were made at several levels, as will be demonstrated in the following chapters. The language form adopted for texts in the new register may also have involved conscious choices to ensure communication and enhance the national language. Strategies for rendering scientific texts into the vernacular, whether on the level of discourse forms, phrasal units, lexis, or dialectal forms and spelling variants, are the second focus of this volume.

The third theme is perhaps more abstract and less obvious, but it is nevertheless an important underlying influence in scientific writing of the Middle English period. The scientific register was created and its writing conventions established at a time when no national standard in language use existed. Models were adopted from foreign sources, though it is also possible that some practices arose within vernacular discourse communities. The influence of Latin traditions is conspicuous at every level: in the macroforms of discourse, how they became modified in the vernacular; in lexical patterns, how the vocabulary was formulated to express new concepts; in code-switching, what was rendered in the vernacular, what retained in Latin and why; the creation of text-type conventions and even the 'house-styles' of scriptoria reflect the tendency towards some kind of focused use and 'incipient standards'. Standardisation and foreign models are the third unifying theme. The difficulty here is that Latin traditions are to a large extent uncharted, but much can be done on the basis of our limited knowledge at present, nevertheless.

The book approaches vernacularisation of medical and scientific writing from a sociolinguistic and sociopragmatic point of view, combining modern methods of linguistic analysis with contextual assessment on the levels of culture, societal developments and textual evolution. Both the broad and the narrow contexts have been taken into account. All levels of written language from spelling forms to discourse structures are discussed in this volume. On the macrolevel, textual patterns were transferred and disseminated through various layers, and intertextuality is an important feature in the dissemination of knowledge. On the microlevel, the cotext, i.e. the surrounding text, with its lexical and collocational patterns, needs to be taken into account. The chapters of this book approach their topics with different methodologies, but all the authors try to use the most modern tool-kit suitable for their research tasks. We have tried to reconstruct some of the scene and discuss the pertinent questions of what, how, and why. We hope to provide new insights into these issues through new approaches to new data, and in this way encourage new studies.

1.3   Earlier studies – editorial activities, early surveys, linguistic studies

Early scholarly activity on English scientific writing in the late nineteenth and much of the twentieth century was directed towards editing. Non-literary practical and scientific prose was not, however, a major focus; the choice of materials for editing was biased towards religious treatises and literary works instead, in accordance with the value judgements of the times. In scientific writing, the earliest editions are from the nineteenth century, the first edition being *Reliquae antiquae* by T. Wright and J. O. Halliwell, in two volumes from 1841–43. It consists of eclectic passages of recipes and remedybook materials, selected for their curiosity. George Stephens published an edition of extracts from the materials of the Stockholm Royal Library in 1844 (see Taavitsainen 1994b). Similar texts are included in F. Heinrich's *Ein Mittelenglisches Medizinbuch*, published in 1896, and G. Henslow's collection of *Medical Works of the Fourteenth Century* from 1899. Some surgical treatises attracted early attention as well. R. von Fleischhacker's edition of Lanfranc's *Surgery* is from 1894, and D'Arcy Power's edition of John Arderne's *Fistula in Ano* from 1910. Early reviews of the field of scientific writing are found in manuscript catalogues, including Dorothea Waley Singer's 'Handlist of scientific manuscripts in the British Isles dating from before the sixteenth century' (1922), and in surveys by, for example, H. S. Bennett (1944) and R. H. Robbins (1970). Recent and on-going activities charting the underlying reality of extant manuscripts in various repositories have led to the discovery of abundant new materials. Some attempts have been made to balance the situation and make a wider and more systematic range of texts available to scholars. Editions of several vernacular versions of Chauliac's learned surgical writings by Björn Wallner from 1964 onwards and Margaret Ogden (1971) have broadened our views. Academic and technical scientific texts containing information on contemporary physiological theory and recommended practice in the vernacular have been edited more recently (Voigts and McVaugh 1984; Carrillo Linares 1993; Eldredge 1996; Pahta 1998; Tavormina forthcoming a; Voigts forthcoming). Astronomical and astrological materials have also received some attention (e.g. Mooney 1984; Taavitsainen 1987, 1988, 1994c). Alchemy is still a fairly unknown field of science, but work is being done in this area, too.[2] In general, only a fraction of the extant texts have been published in modern editions. This can be easily verified by comparing the number of editions with the most up-to-date information about texts extant in manuscripts: less than a hundred texts have been edited out of the approximately 10,000 extant items included in the recently published electronic catalogue of early English scientific and medical texts by Linda Voigts and Patricia Kurtz (see below).

Besides various surveys and editions of texts, towards the end of the twentieth century philological scholarship produced analyses that are relevant for our understanding of the language of medieval science and medicine. Analyses of translation techniques or lexical strategies in individual Middle English learned and technical translations are a case in point (e.g. Voigts and McVaugh 1984; Minnis 1987; Wallner 1987; P. M. Jones 1989; Pahta 1998). Some studies have applied theories and methods of modern linguistics to the analysis of medieval medical and scientific language, but these are still rare. The pioneering linguistic studies in the field are M. A. K. Halliday's diachronic study of the language of physical science (1988), using Chaucer's *Treatise on the Astrolabe* as evidence of medieval scientific writing; Juhani Norri's analysis of the lexical field of names of sicknesses in 1400–1550 (1992); Irma Taavitsainen's study of involvement features in different types of late Middle and Early Modern English scientific texts (1994a); and Linda Voigts's discussion of multilingualism in medieval scientific and medical writings (1996). These innovative studies are linked with recent developments in research tools that have made new approaches possible (see also section 1.6).

1.4   New reference tools and electronic databases

A new phase was reached in the last few decades of the twentieth century, with a number of important surveys outlining the field of scientific and utilitarian writing in more detail. Recent scholarly work in these areas has focused on improving bibliographical tools. Extensive research projects have been launched to chart extant manuscripts, and new electronic research tools have been created. The first landmark was the volume *Middle English Prose* (ed. Edwards) from 1984. It brings together articles that focus on various genres and registers of prose. The book provides an overview of the extent of knowledge and scholarship up to the early 1980s, including chapters on medical prose by Linda Voigts and on scientific and utilitarian prose by Laurel Braswell. Another useful work, *The Index of Printed Middle English Prose*, came out a year later in 1985, a survey of all editions up to that time. A comprehensive and up-to-date review of scientific writing in English is available in a recent volume by George Keiser in *A Manual of Writings in Middle English* (1998). It gives bibliographical details of both editions and background literature. The major international project of *The Index of Middle English Prose* (*IMEP*) was launched at the beginning of the 1980s. Its aim is to chart all extant Middle English prose in manuscript repositories all over the world; some thirty scholars are working on this project. *Handlists I–XVII* have now come out (by spring 2003). The volumes for the Ashmolean Collections (Eldredge 1992), Trinity College, Cambridge (Mooney 1995), and Gonville and Caius College, Cambridge (Rand Schmidt 2001) are of special importance to our knowledge of the nature and extent of scientific writing in this period. Other repositories contain scientific materials as well, for example the Royal Library of Copenhagen has a large number of alchemical texts (Taavitsainen 1994b). Revisions of *The Index of Middle English Verse* are in progress by A. S. G. Edwards, Julia Boffey, and Linne Mooney. This work is also relevant for our knowledge of the field, as medical texts were transmitted in verse form as well.

An indispensable research tool is provided by the recently published electronic catalogue of *Scientific and Medical Writings in Old and Middle English Writings: An Electronic Reference* compiled by Linda Voigts and Patricia Kurtz (2000; henceforth *eVK*). It gives us knowledge of the underlying manuscript reality and makes it possible to chart the extent of survival of vernacular texts in manuscripts in an easy and reliable way. The related field of medical texts in Anglo-Norman French has been most comprehensively studied by Tony Hunt (1990, 2000; Hunt and

Benskin 2001). A revised and supplemented edition of the bibliographical index of Latin scientific writings by Thorndike and Kibre (1963; *TK*) is under way, in electronic form, directed by Linda Voigts (*eTK*). Another valuable contribution to our knowledge of extant sources and their interrelations is provided by Monica Green's detailed charting of gynaecological and obstetrical writings in Latin, English and other vernacular languages (Green 1992, 1996, 1997, 2001). Scientific and medical illustration has been studied by John Murdoch (1984) and Peter Murray Jones (1984, 1998a).

Other new sources and research tools have become available. These include the four-volume *Linguistic Atlas of Late Mediaeval English* (*LALME*), which contains localisations of a large number of manuscripts and provides a basis for mapping further texts through regional patterns of linguistic features. The basis of the *LALME* method is the insight that the patterns of co-occurring language features at any one place are different from those which occur in other areas, so that it is possible to localise the dialect of a text with greater precision than before. The method has brought new accuracy to Middle English linguistic studies on regional variation, and it is possible to locate most texts written before the rise of the national standard fairly precisely with this method. Scribal language with its spelling variants and diverse morphological forms gives us valuable information about the patterns of the period covered by *LALME*; for the south of England the date 1430 is usually given as the deadline after which it is difficult to localise texts with accuracy. In addition to providing information about regional characteristics of language use, the method can be applied to a multitude of other subjects: to gain knowledge about scribes and scriptoria, multiple copies and textual histories, the circulation of texts, the dissemination of ideas, and the geography of writing.[3]

The new electronic dictionaries serve as reference tools for a broad range of studies. As a result, lexical developments can be accessed through them with new efficiency, precision, and coverage. Besides their traditional uses, they can be adopted for a number of other study purposes. The *Oxford English Dictionary* (*OED*) has been released on CD-ROM and as an Internet version, allowing complicated searches with the query language. The *Middle English Dictionary* (*MED*) is accessible on-line as part of the *Middle English Compendium*. The *Dictionary of Old English* is also available on-line. *A Historical Thesaurus of English* is being prepared at the University of Glasgow.

Other large-scale ongoing philological and linguistic research that in the near future will provide invaluable information on the language, texts, and discourse communities of the period is being carried out in the Linguistic Atlas of Early Middle English project in the Institute for Historical Dialectology at the University of Edinburgh, in the Middle English Grammar Project at the University of Glasgow, and in the Urban Manuscripts Database Project at the University of York. Our knowledge about book production and trade before the age of printing has also substantially increased through recent work by several scholars, notably C. Paul Christianson (1987, 1989a and b), and Linne Mooney's ongoing work on professional scribes' hands in multiple manuscripts will undoubtedly provide a fuller picture (see e.g. Mooney 2000).

The advent of electronic text collections has made the retrieval of data for linguistic studies on texts speedy and effective. With text corpora, the whole research paradigm in linguistics is changing: the focus of linguistic analysis has shifted to actual language in use instead of individual examples of structures that in reality may be rare. The more comprehensive databases yield new accuracy to linguistic studies and it is possible to find answers to new research questions. The pioneer in the field of historical corpora is the *Helsinki Corpus of English Texts*, a multipurpose, multigenre corpus, compiled in the 1980s by a research team at the University of Helsinki (see Rissanen *et al.* 1993). Over the past ten years it has become a standard tool in historical linguistics and proved useful in indicating new lines of research. However, its text selection and sample size have proved too limited for some more specific research questions raised by pilot studies (e.g. Taavitsainen 1994a). This in turn has sparked off a new trend in historical corpus compilation that aims towards larger databases of one register or one genre. This volume has benefited from modern techniques and medical text corpora. Jones's chapter on medical discourse communities draws on results of recent manuscript surveys, Norri's study of medical terms is based on his private electronic database (see below), and the studies by Mäkinen, Pahta and Taavitsainen rely on the corpus compiled for the purposes of the research project on 'Scientific thought-styles' (see section 1.6 below).

1.5   The *Corpus of Middle English Medical Texts*

The electronic *Corpus of Middle English Medical Texts* (*MEMT*, forthcoming 2004), used as material in some of the studies in this volume, consists of medical treatises from *c.* 1375 to *c.* 1500. The corpus contains more than half a million words of running text and comprises edited medical texts and early printed books from different traditions of writing. The range is from theoretical treatises transmitting specialised top-level knowledge through learned surgical and anatomical texts to simple recipes for practical use and miscellaneous collections bordering on household literature. When released for wider scholarly distribution on a CD-ROM, equipped with suitable Windows-compatible software developed specially in co-operation with Raymond Hickey (Essen University), the database will serve the needs of linguists as well as historians of science, philologists, and manuscript scholars. It will complement *eVK* by giving direct access to editions of texts listed in it. The two databases can be used simultaneously on a personal computer to create a new kind of interface. A flexible and readily available personal tool like this is valuable especially for researchers studying original manuscripts in library archives.[4]

1.6   Applications of corpus-based methodology

Larger electronic databases make empirical studies on the characteristics of early scientific writing possible. Our research project 'Scientific thought-styles: The evolution of early English medical writing' (University of Helsinki) approaches scientific writing from a new angle by examining in detail a large amount of data in this register in electronic format. We aim at describing linguistic changes in medical English in relation to the generic and sociolinguistic context in which texts were produced, including the changing scientific thought-styles, i.e. the underlying scientific concepts, objects of enquiry, methods, evaluations, and intellectual commitments, which are mediated to us through language. Different periods are traditionally connected with different styles of thinking and making decisions. Variability in language use is a key concept in our approach: changes in the underlying scientific ideology as well as the discourse community can be verified both on the microlevel of individual linguistic features and on the macrolevel of argumentative structures and textual organisation. Evidentiality and modality in language have proved important in our studies. Linguistic features reflecting the mode of knowing are crucial for analysing thought-styles as they change in the course of time (Taavitsainen 2001a). References to authors and prescriptive phrases are prominent in scholastic writing. Both the frequency and the specificity vary according to the tradition and genre of writing (Taavitsainen and Pahta 1998). So far our focus has been on writings of the scholastic period and on three aspects of the history of science: the underlying scientific paradigms, the transmission of scientific knowledge, and the dissemination of scientific knowledge across society (for an overview, see Taavitsainen et al. 2002). Some pilot studies have covered a longer time span in order to provide an idea of how changes in thought-styles proceed, and how these changes can be detected on the level of linguistic and textual structure. Pilot studies are helpful: the more we know about the texts, the easier it is to detect features for future studies, and lines of development gradually begin to emerge.

Several studies in this volume apply corpus-linguistic methods to new research questions and use *MEMT* as the database. Computer-searches of lexical items or longer strings have been used to point out relevant materials and to locate the relevant passages. For example, treatises with a logocentric focus can be located by retrieval of speech-act verbs of reporting in quotative passages (Taavitsainen 2002), mixed-language texts and functions of code-switching can be detected by searching for Latin lexical items, and recipes that deal with certain ingredients can also be collected on lexical grounds. In addition, the corpus helped us to relate our findings and conclusions to the larger context of different traditions and genres of scientific writing (see the individual chapters for details; for the list of texts included in *MEMT* see the Bibliography).

1.7   Latin and vernacular

In most of medieval Europe, Latin had a primary position as a written language. It was the institutionalised *lingua franca* of the church, government, and learning; in classical literature it was the standard of literary excellence. Despite the advantage that Latin held as the primary vehicle of knowledge during the first millennium, in the blooming culture of Anglo-Saxon England scientific texts were already being written in the vernacular. All in all, 300 Old English items in manuscripts from the ninth to the twelfth centuries are listed in *eVK*; the majority of texts date from the eleventh century. This substantial body of writings, consisting of astrological and computational treatises of the calculation of time, herbals, and medical texts in the remedybook tradition, forms the earliest collection of vernacular medical literature in medieval Europe (Rubin 1974; see also Carroll, p. 175 below). By comparison, the first extant vernacular medical text composed in France dates from the thirteenth century (P. M. Jones 1990: 7, 10). Although the repertoire of Old English medical writings does not contain learned or theoretical medical texts, the influence of classical learning is conspicuous in extant writings. For example, the *Laeceboc* contains passages derived from several Latin works (Cameron 1983a: 153) and consists of fairly close translations of Latin originals (Kitson 1989: 57). The Old English version of *Herbarium Apuleii* is also translated from Latin (Voigts 1979; see also Mäkinen, pp. 171–2 below).

Materials from the intervening period between Old and Middle English are scarce: only three items from the thirteenth century are listed in *eVK*. This hiatus was partly due to the Norman Conquest in 1066 with its well-known radical consequences on the linguistic situation in England. The complex multilingual situation in the centuries following the Conquest can be described in sociolinguistic terms as polyglossia, where several languages coexisted with different, though partly overlapping social functions (see e.g. Clanchy 1993, Chapter 6; Blake 1996: 107–15, 132–8; or Machan 2003). The three main languages in descending order of prestige were Latin, French, and English, but there were also other minority languages, including Celtic languages spoken in some western and northern areas. Latin retained its position as the prestigious variety employed in public domains, including religion, government, law, education, scholarship, and literature. French had a mixed functional range: it was used in public domains, for example administration, law, commerce, education, and literature, but also for ordinary interaction in the French-speaking social strata. In the period after the Conquest until the mid-thirteenth century, English in general remained peripheral to written culture and was mainly used for interaction in more domestic and casual domains (for English writings from this period, see Laing 1993). The patterns of use changed over time, with English gradually gaining ground from the other languages. The written materials of the period in several registers reflect the dynamic state of societal multilingualism and are characterised to a varying degree by a mixture of languages (see Pahta, pp. 74–5 below).

1.8 Pan-European diffusion of learned medicine

Vernacularisation of science and medicine took place elsewhere in late medieval Europe as well. Advances in science continued to be discussed in Latin in the universities and university curricula provided for the transmission of authoritative medical texts, concepts, and techniques that formed the basis of medical knowledge and practice in society at large. Universities were responsible for the training of a small medical élite, but medical practitioners were a much larger and heterogeneous group (see section 1.13 below). By the fourteenth century, diffusion of knowledge from the university world had begun in several fields of scholasticism, including theology and natural philosophy. Several of the important thirteenth-century scientific encyclopaedias were translated into various European vernacular languages in the course of the fourteenth century. Among these were works by scholastic scientists like Albertus Magnus, Vincent of Beauvais, Thomas Cantimprensis, and Bartholomaeus Anglicus (García-Ballester 1994: 4–5; Crossgrove 1998: 82). By the fifteenth century, texts on scientific and technological subjects in vernacular languages were becoming increasingly common all over Europe. Medical texts originating in learned contexts found their way into several vernaculars and gradually spread through society as they demonstrated their usefulness to all. Two examples may suffice here to illustrate the scope and nature of the diffusion. The *Lilium medicinae*, a Latin medical compendium completed in 1305 by Bernard of Gordon, a Montpellier professor of medicine, is known in medieval translations into English, French, Castilian, German, Gaelic, and Hebrew (see Demaitre 1980). In a recent study of a fourteenth-century Middle High German version of the *Lilium*, Luke Demaitre (1998) places this vernacular translation in its social *locus*. He shows that the text stands in both form and content in the intermediate setting between *ars* and *vulgus*, between the scholastic learning of formalised Latin textbooks and the popular, colloquial medical lore of vernacular recipe collections. The translator aimed at making the learned text more accessible to vernacular readers, for example by simplifying theories, and replacing Latin terms with native variants or explaining them in more familiar words. Demaitre's conclusion is that this text, like much of vernacular medieval medicine, was written and read on a level below the classroom but above the street. The second example is provided by the set of three gynaecological and cosmetic treatises written in twelfth-century Salerno and attributed to a woman author named Trota, or Trotula. These texts were widely disseminated in Latin throughout Europe and are known in 23 different vernacular versions in eight languages: one Catalan translation, three Dutch, five English, seven French, three German, one Hebrew, one Irish, and two Italian (Green 1996, 1997). The vernacular versions of the Trotula texts vary in the treatment of the source material. Some versions are literal translations rendering the Latin source text faithfully into the vernacular. Others are free adaptations, sometimes heavily abridged, sometimes fused with material from other sources.

1.9   The widening use of English across registers and genres of writing

The use of English in professional writing can be traced back to the late fourteenth century, when it gradually appeared as the language of legal proceedings, guild records, religious controversy, and instruction. The spread of the vernacular gathered momentum in the fifteenth century with the nationalistic strivings of the Lancastrian monarchs.[5] The broadening range of genres in English is often attributed to the sixteenth century, but the process started as early as the late Middle English period. Utilitarian writings became available to readers in English on a variety of topics, such as cookery, deportment, grammar, horticulture, hunting, and table manners (Getz 1990a: 3). The introduction of new genres into the vernacular was conspicuous in literature, as Chaucer introduced Italian and French traditions into English. Continental influences can be seen in the multitude of genres in the *Canterbury Tales*; even its frame narrative is an adaptation of a foreign model and the beginning of the prologue a formulation of a commonplace in European literature. In addition, several poetic conventions found expression in English for the first time in Chaucer's shorter poetry. The initial stages of more private writing are also found in this period, for example Margery Kempe's religious treatise can be considered the first autobiography. The earliest letters are extant from the very end of the fourteenth century. The overall trend towards more subjective and individual perspectives is perhaps also one of the underlying motivations for rendering medical texts in English for private use.

In the field of science, medicine was in the vanguard of vernacularisation. The earliest substantial body of vernacular medical texts in England after the Conquest is in fact in Anglo-Norman French, not English. The earliest records consist of recipes and charms in early twelfth-century manuscripts (Hunt 1990; see also Carroll, p. 176 below). The majority of extant Anglo-Norman medical treatises date from the thirteenth century, but Anglo-Norman is also found in later glosses and in polyglot texts and manuscripts (Voigts 1984: 325–6). Some of the fourteenth-century primarily Anglo-Norman records display extensive language mixing (see Hunt 2000; Hunt and Benskin 2001; see also Pahta, p. 76 below). Most of the material belongs to the remedybook tradition, but there are examples of other kinds of texts as well, such as the thirteenth-century translations of Roger Frugardi of Parma's *Chirurgia* (Hunt 1990: 143) and the gynaecological and cosmetic works attributed to Trota of Salerno (Green 1997: 92). Astrological treatises also survive in Anglo-Norman (Taavitsainen 1988: 112–15; Hunt 1990).

After a fairly slow start, the fifteenth century witnessed an explosion in vernacular text production: *eVK* lists *c*. 200 fourteenth-century items, whereas nearly 8,000 of the items included date from the fifteenth century. As remedybooks and recipe collections had already existed in Old English, one of the interesting questions of transmission is how much of the medical lore contained in the Anglo-Saxon materials was carried over to the later Middle Ages (see Mäkinen, p. 152, and Carroll, p. 175 below). Academic and surgical treatises were totally new in the vernacular. Most of the texts were translated or adapted from Latin sources, but works bordering on original compositions were also compiled in English.

To begin with, English often occurred in company with Latin and/or Anglo-Norman French in bi- or trilingual manuscripts. The extent of multilingualism in the scientific register was demonstrated in Linda Voigts's survey of scientific and medical codices produced in England in the period 1375–1500 (Voigts 1989b).

She examined 178 'units', either unified manuscripts or booklets in composite manuscripts: 29.2 per cent (52) of these units were found to be monolingual Latin, 22.5 per cent (40) monolingual English, 42.1 per cent (75) bilingual Latin and English, and 6.2 per cent (11) trilingual, containing Latin, English, and French. A change of code in polyglot materials can be found between texts in codices containing monolingual treatises in several languages, but it was also common to mix languages within a single text (see Voigts 1996 and Pahta, below). The gradual spread of English in scientific and medical writing across time is reflected in the fact that in the early materials vernacular texts in general occur in manuscripts where Latin dominates, whereas towards the end of the fifteenth century predominantly English manuscripts become more common (Voigts 1995b). The first phase of vernacularisation seems to have been largely complete by 1475. By that time the range of vernacular material also includes sophisticated university treatises on medicine and astrology in primarily English-language manuscripts (Voigts 1996: 814). A few medical books were among the first to be printed (see the Bibliography), but the new medium did not influence writing conventions at first; the old practices continued at least till the sixteenth century.

1.10   Transmission

Although the theoretical framework of natural science was largely inherited by the Latin Middle Ages from Greek antiquity through the Arabic world, the transmission of texts and concepts across cultural and linguistic borders was not always straightforward. By the time they reached European vernacular readers, many theories had passed through a multilayered process of text production and reproduction that involved successive stages of copying, translating, paraphrasing, commenting, excerpting, assimilating, adapting, and conflating. On the one hand, ancient authors were revered and many of the prestigious works of the medical canon were passed on unchanged. On the other hand, it was also customary to compile new texts by assembling extracts from earlier texts. In this process not only the identification of texts and authors but scientific theories themselves often became blurred. Compilation was sometimes described as a useful process of collecting and spreading knowledge. For example, the prologue to the Middle English version of Guy de Chauliac's surgical treatise explains the practical benefits of a compilation (see Taavitsainen 'Transferring', p. 43).

The special nature of the manuscript as a medium for preserving and transmitting information is also crucial. Manuscript books offered less material support to the text than printed books, as in manuscript transmission each copy of the text is unique and prone to changes (see e.g. Wallis 1995; Pahta 2001; and Jones, p. 26 below). The physical details of presentation vary: handwriting, script, the quality of ink, and the size and layout of pages can differ from one copy to another. Often the scribe also made some conscious or unconscious changes to the actual text. Some changes may only affect the surface of the text, for example the scribe's wordstock and spelling may reflect regional or idiosyncratic variation in language (see Taavitsainen 'House-styles' and Voigts in this volume). Some scribes assumed the role of an active editor and modified the contents by deliberate additions or omissions for a projected target audience, for example in a version of Gilbertus Anglicus's *Compendium medicinae* apparently intended for monastic use, passages dealing with diseases of women and children were omitted (Getz 1991: li–lii). Unconscious changes include spelling mistakes, inadvertent omission of words, phrases or passages, or confusion of letters and words because of visual association. Some problems are clearly of a more linguistic character. Other languages had difficulties in expressing the philosophical complexities of originally Greek medicine, and every new layer of transmission modified the original material and created potential new problems for translators and scribes of the next generation of texts.

1.11   The composition of Middle English medical texts: Derivative vs. original writings

Most Middle English scientific texts are translated from or, in one way or another, derived from Latin or French treatises. The techniques employed in vernacularising learned science and medicine varied. Multiple translations provide especially fruitful material for analysing the range of translation strategies (see e.g. P. M. Jones 1989, and Voigts in this volume). The distinction between translating 'word for word' or 'sense for sense' had existed in the tradition of translation from its earliest phases, and it became part of medieval translation theory and practice (see Copeland 1991). A survey of Middle English learned medical treatises illustrates the continuum that the texts form on the scale from literal to free translation (see Pahta 1998: 62–72). In this continuum one level of variation is formed by the translator's handling of the source text contents and the other by his linguistic strategies. Medical translations at the most literal end of the scale render the contents of the source text faithfully and rely heavily on its syntactic and lexical structure. Some of the 'word-for-word' translations depend so profoundly on the linguistic structures of the Latin source text that at places they are impossible to understand without the original. Examples of such muddled texts are found among the multiple translations of John Arderne's surgical *Practica* and Benvenutus Grassus's ophthalmologic treatise *De probatissima arte oculorum* (see P. M. Jones 1989; Eldredge 1996). The translation of the pseudo-Galenic *De spermate* and some other learned translations in Cambridge, Trinity College MS R.14.52, apparently by the same person, belong to the extreme end: in some cases the translator of these texts seems to have worked not only word by word, but morpheme by morpheme (see Pahta and Carrillo Linares forthcoming). In 'sense-for-sense' translations the translator has faithfully transferred the contents of the source text into more fluent Middle English. Translations at the other end of the scale come close to original compositions. In these texts the translator also acted as an editor and compiler, freely excerpting, rearranging, and paraphrasing the material of the source text and blending it with material from other sources.

This practice is illustrated, for example, by some Middle English gynaecological texts (see Green 1992). Some vernacular translators explicitly described their method in these terms. The best-known examples are perhaps found in the Prologue to the Wycliffite Bible and in John Trevisa's letter accompanying his translation of Higden's *Polychronicon*. Similar ideas are expressed in less-known texts as well, for example in a preface to a urinoscopy in the commentary tradition (see Taavitsainen 'Transferring', p. 52). Occasional remarks concerning translation methods also occur in other medical texts. For example, in his *Liber uricrisiarum* Henry Daniel claims that he has translated the text 'nerhand word for worde'; however, a closer analysis of the text has shown that, contrary to his claim, Daniel in fact apparently edited and revised his source material to a great extent (see Jasin 1983: 483 and 1993).

Original composition was not a goal to be strived after in the medieval period, when imitation was a virtue and copyright and plagiarism unknown concepts. Intertextuality is striking in recipe materials (see Mäkinen in this volume), but it is equally important in the other traditions of medical writing. Original compositions in the vernacular are said to be extant in the surgical field (see e.g. Voigts 1990: 290, and 1995b). In the light of our present knowledge the texts may be compilations and adaptations from various sources. An analysis of textual components may reveal several layers, for example passages from different sources may be amalgamated in texts. This seems to be the case in the surgical treatise *Philomena* (see Taavitsainen 'House-styles', p. 232 below). John Arderne wrote in Latin and the vernacular versions are translations of Latin originals (see P. M. Jones 1989), but the transmission of recipes attributed to him may be even more complicated. The time of writing may be important here. Arderne was probably born in 1307. He practised surgery from 1349 to 1370 in Newark and in London in the 1370s (P. M. Jones 1994: 294). Thus the vernacularisation boom started only towards the end of his career.

1.12   Traditions of medical writing

A tripartite classification of medieval medical materials into academic treatises, surgical texts, and remedybooks was suggested by Linda Voigts in 1982 (see also Voigts 1984). This classification has become generally accepted in subsequent research. Linguistic evidence supports the division. Recent studies have shown distinct linguistic differences between texts belonging to the three different subclasses. The texts differ from each other, for example, in the use of technical terminology (Norri 1992, 1998); in linguistic features indicating involvement and emotionality, such as personal pronouns, imperative forms, and passive and impersonal constructions (Taavitsainen 1994a); in expressions of evidentiality and modality (Taavitsainen and Pahta 1998; Taavitsainen 2001a); in the use of appositional constructions (Pahta and Nevanlinna 1997); in metadiscursive practices (Taavitsainen 1999); and in nominal structures (Pahta and Taavitsainen 1999).

The three-part division also serves as a frame of analysis in several studies in the present volume. There are, however, some problems in the definition of categories and in assigning individual texts to them. Our initial research has led us to label the categories in a somewhat different way. Instead of calling the top class academic, we have chosen the term 'specialised treatises'. This category contains a range of learned texts dealing with bloodletting, ophthalmology, embryology, urinoscopy, gynaecology, the plague and other diseases, as well as encyclopaedic treatises rooted in the academic tradition. The second category, 'surgical treatises', consists of surgical manuals and anatomical descriptions. Some of them are very learned, and as most of them were originally compiled by university masters and used as university textbooks, they belong to academic texts as well. The third category is labelled 'remedybooks and *materia medica*'. Remedybooks comprise recipe collections with prognostications and charms, and other guides for maintaining health, including regimen texts on diet and exercise that can also be learned writings (see e.g. Getz 1991). *Materia medica* include herbals and some other texts, such as lapidaries.

1.13   Literacy, the scope of readership, and discourse communities

The question of readership is central to vernacularisation, and although the focus has shifted more to the discourse communities, the basic facts of literacy provide the essential background for vernacularisation. The definitions of the terms vary in the literature. For our purposes, it seems helpful to make a distinction between a discourse community, readership, and audience of a text. Members of a discourse community have much in common (for a definition and discussion, see Jones, pp. 24–6 below), but they need not have read the text; readership consists of those who have actually read the text; and audience would be the potential readership the work is targeted at.

As matters of health are of universal interest, the potential audience for vernacular medical texts includes all those who could read – a heterogeneous group in terms of social status, education, and profession. Estimations of the scope of literacy in medieval England vary. University education guaranteed the most advanced level of literacy, including professional literacy in Latin. Fairly advanced literacy, including the basics of Latin, was probably widespread among both male and female members of the aristocracy (Orme 1983: 80; see also Biller and Hudson 1994). With the growth of urban society, the rise of a middle class, the grammar school system and new professions, practical literacy was spreading outside the upper classes. According to the most optimistic estimate, in the fifteenth century people of almost all ranks could read, write, and enjoy books (Lester 1987: 216). A more cautious assessment suggests that perhaps 30 per cent of the population in the fifteenth century could read, although in the largest urban centres the figure may have been higher (see Keen 1990: 224). Yet another estimation, taking social, regional, and gender variation into account, proposes that 40 per cent of the London merchants were literate. Figures for some other groups are 25 per cent for the urban male population, 6–12 per cent for men in general, and for women less than half of the figure for men (Graff 1987: 99, 106). It has been stated that the demand for more writing in the vernacular grew with the increasing numbers of readers, and the growing supply of vernacular texts in turn encouraged more people to learn to read (Parkes 1973: 565–6; Clanchy 1993: 201).

Another facet of vernacularisation is connected with the materials and with the politics of open access to knowledge involving issues of gender, class, education, and community (Evans *et al.* 1999: 322): what was thought desirable and appropriate to offer in the vernacular for wider distribution among different social strata. The choices of rendering learned texts like the *Phlebotomy, De spermate,* or Chauliac's works into the vernacular indicate a conscious choice and the desire for more open access to knowledge among professionals who were familiar with these materials in Latin.

Medical practitioners are an obvious target audience of medical texts. In medieval England they formed a heterogeneous group. Latinate university-trained physicians were at the apex of the social and professional hierarchy. They belonged to the pan-European discourse community, but their role in the promotion of vernacular writing remains to be discovered. They were relatively few in numbers and mostly practised in large cities. Many of them rose to important positions as physicians at court, or in the service of lay and ecclesiastical lords or wealthy townsmen (Getz 1992: 394–5; Rawcliffe 1995: 109). Some master-surgeons, whose tasks were more practical, may also have attended university lectures on general medicine, although apprenticeship was the main form of their training. Other practitioners were trained in apprenticeship. The establishment of the guilds brought institutionalisation to a different level of practitioners. This organisation of learning and training in the medical profession must have contributed to the formation of new discourse communities. Barbers or barber-surgeons were allowed to practise surgery and they conducted operations like bloodletting and dentistry. Apothecaries too were involved in the practice; they diagnosed diseases and prescribed medicine, even though their main trade was supplying and selling medicine. Women were involved in medical practice primarily as nurses and midwives, and in the family. Although these topics were treated in learned treatises, the skills of midwifery were acquired by acting in attendance with an experienced midwife and included assisting in childbirth and offering consultation with gynaecological troubles (see Plate 2). In places where other professionals were unavailable, midwives were probably turned to in other kinds of diseases as well, along with layman practitioners, empirics, herbalists, wise women, and cunning men (see also Jones, p. 26 ff.).

The bulk of medical writing contains texts that were aimed at and shared by different discourse communities.[6] The potential readership is likely to have varied according to the nature of texts and manuscript contexts. Some medical and scientific texts required less advanced reading skills and probably reached a wider audience than others; the difference can be detected, for example, in the encyclopaedic texts of the time that follow the same principal order but on different levels of technical and theoretical detail (see Taavitsainen 'Transferring', pp. 43–44, and forthcoming). Another class of writings for different types of audiences consists of medical recipes and remedybooks, for example some learned treatises include sophisticated recipes containing Latin terms and exact measurement indications, but there are also recipe collections that belonged to household literature. Some treatises originating in learned contexts, like Henry Daniel's *Liber uricrisiarum* in MS Wellcome 225, show efforts to accommodate a learned treatise to an expanded audience literate in Middle English (see Plate 3). Some technical treatises, such as the surgeries of Lanfranc and Chauliac or the ophthalmological treatise of Benvenutus Grassus, were probably aimed at medical professionals. As English texts often appear in polyglot manuscripts, the audience must have also comprised Latinate learned or aristocratic readers.

One special constellation among the new audiences is women (see Green 2000a). An example of a text written specifically with a female audience in mind is *The Knowing of Woman's Kind in Childing* (ed. Barratt 2001). This gynaecological treatise survives in five manuscripts and is based on Latin and Old French sources that derive from Greek. In the prologue, the Middle English writer explicitly states that he has translated the text,

> be-cause whomen of oure tonge cvnne bettyre rede & vnderstande þys langage þan eny oþer & euery whoman lettyrde [may] rede hit to oþer vnlettyrd & help hem & conceyle hem in here maledyes with-owtyn schevynge here dysese to man. (ed. Barratt 2001: 42)

A female readership is implicit throughout the text. Physical evidence of two manuscripts suggests that they may have been designed for practising midwives or women interested in midwifery. The translator also addresses possible male readers, asking them to avoid misogynist readings of the text; one of the manuscripts may have belonged to a house of Augustinian canons in Norfolk (Barratt 2001: 4–5).

In general, an earlier assumption that language marked the social distinction between university-trained physicians, who derived their knowledge directly from Latin treatises, and lower classes of practitioners, who relied on vernacular material (Robbins 1970: 394) needs to be complemented by other social paradigms. One of these is related to the idea of the vernacular, i.e. the desire to use the mother tongue in a domain of writing that traditionally excluded lay people and those illiterate in Latin. It is more likely that the readership of vernacular medical works in late medieval England was heterogeneous, including both lay readers and medical professionals of various levels. The process of vernacularisation must necessarily have been initiated by people who knew what was available in Latin. It is known that some members of monastic orders, such as Henry Daniel and Thomas Moulton, were involved in the process, but the discourse communities of learned doctors may have also been active. Until more sociohistorical evidence is forthcoming, this remains, however, speculation.

Notes

1. For illuminating discussions of the topic from various angles, see, for example, Weisheipl (1965), Manzalaoui (1977e), Voigts (1989b), Crombie (1994), and French and Cunningham (1996).
2. An edition of an alchemical treatise is forthcoming by Peter Grund (Uppsala University); see Grund (2002 and forthcoming).
3. See the introduction to *LALME* for studies before 1986; later studies include Taavitsainen (1988), Beadle (1991), and C. Jones (2001).
4. In addition to *MEMT*, the *Corpus of Early English Medical Writing* (*CEEM*) is also under construction. The text selection in the Early Modern corpus ranges from specialised texts and experimental reports in the *Philosophical Transactions* of the Royal Society to health guides intended for a general audience. The selection demonstrates the widening use of English in this period: the material also contains statutory texts dealing with hygiene, religious and moral treatises on diseases, argumentative texts, and educational works giving guidelines for healthy living. Shorter texts are included *in toto*; longer treatises are represented by substantial extracts of varying length.
5. For arguments of a conscious policy, see Fisher (1992) and Blake (1996: 176); see also Taavitsainen (2001b).
6. For a discussion of parallel issues in Early Modern England, see, for example Wear (1992) and Slack (1979).

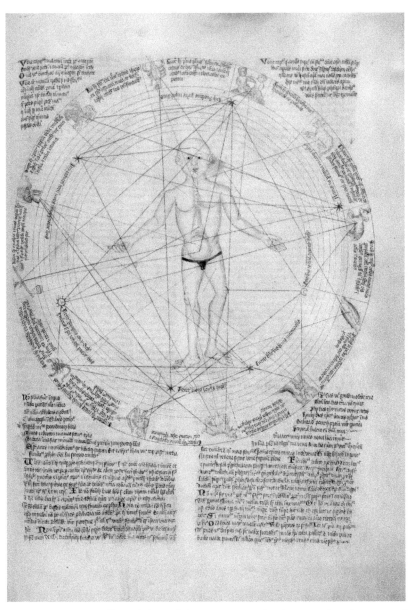

Plate 1 The relations of the macrocosm of universe to the microcosm of man. From a German manuscript, *Apocalypsis S. Johannis* from *c*. 1420. Wellcome MS 49, f. 41r.

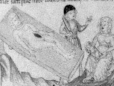

Plate 2 Scenes of medical practice in a learned Latin manuscript, with women and a learned doctor performing a Caesarean section. From a German manuscript, *Apocalypsis S. Johannis* from *c.* 1420. Wellcome MS 49, f. 38v.

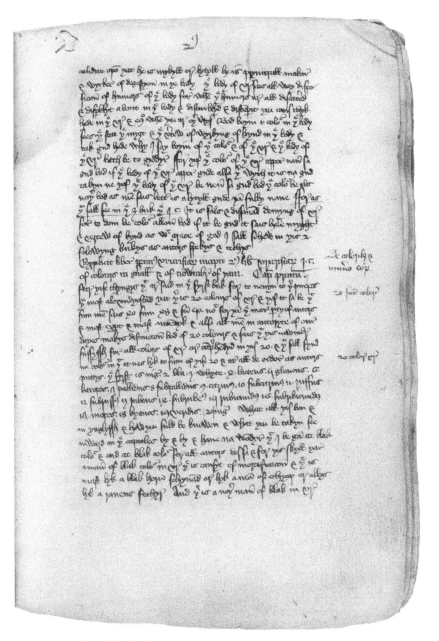

Plate 3 Early fifteenth-century manuscript page from the Middle English translation of Henry Daniel's *Liber uricrisiarum* in Wellcome MS 225, f. 24r.

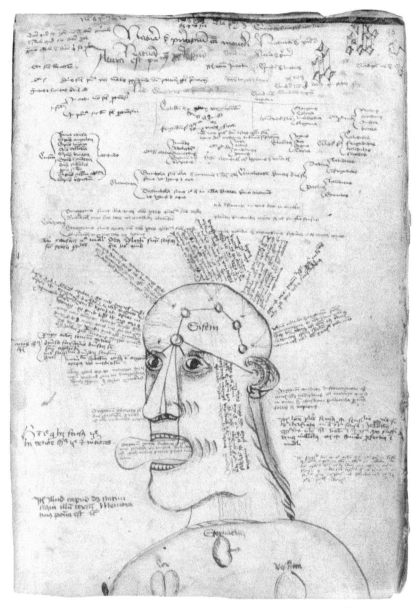

Plate 4 Pen drawing of a human head and torso, with text, illustrating the sense organs. Late fifteenth century, Aristotle, *Analytica priora*. Wellcome MS 55, f. 93r.

2   Discourse communities and medical texts

CLAIRE JONES

2.1   Introduction

In late fourteenth-century England, learned medicine and science from the universities 'leapt the walls and found a readership outside' (P. M. Jones 1999: 433). The nature of this readership has been the subject of many studies. Over the past three decades in particular it has become increasingly apparent that simple dichotomies such as Latin/English, literate/illiterate and especially the anachronistic professional/amateur are simply not adequate to describe the complex patterns of producers, users, and disseminators of medieval medical texts.

In comparison with other genres, medical and scientific writings in English have received relatively little scholarly attention, though this situation is now being remedied. A large proportion of recent research has taken the form of surveys, notably in the work of Linda Voigts (see in particular Voigts 1989b and 1995b), and in more detailed studies of individual books and manuscripts.[1] On the basis of these studies it is now possible to construct theoretical models which will serve as a framework or matrix within which we can place evidence from both surveys and more focused studies and thus build a broader picture of the discourse community for medieval English medical texts: this chapter is intended to serve as a prolegomena to such analysis.

2.2   Discourse community

Modern linguistic theory, with its emphasis on discourse and community, rather than text and audience, is gaining ground within the field of medieval literature. This is notable in the study of medical and scientific writings, too, for example in Linda Voigts's use of contemporary theories of bilingualism (Voigts 1996) and in the essays in this volume. The concept of 'discourse community' is in many ways more useful and accurate than 'audience' or 'readership' when describing the place of texts in medieval society. 'Audience' tends to suggest the passive reception of a text and places the producers at a remove once a text has been disseminated. In a period when many texts were copied by individuals for personal, or at least

23

localised use, this is a misleading picture. 'Readership' is even more anachronistic, given that literacy was still extremely restricted in medieval England, and access to texts did not necessarily depend on an individual's ability to read for him or herself.[2]

The model of discourse community developed and used by discourse analysts is derived from the sociolinguistic concept of 'speech community', but shifts the focus on to the producers and readers of written texts, whilst acknowledging that in many situations spoken discourse can be associated with the texts. Recent research has broadened the concept of 'discourse community' to help explain and define groups of people connected by texts, either as part of their relationships within a particular type of community, or solely by the texts themselves, which may be used for different purposes by different individuals. Such text-only relationships created problems when these theories were first posited. The problems were discussed by Swales (1990), who labelled them 'The Café-Owner Problem'. In brief, Swales argued that three café-owners, A, B, and C, who lived in the same town, read the same trade press, shared clienteles and used the same suppliers but had no contact with each other, could not reasonably be called a discourse community. He argued that to do this would not address 'the logical problem of assigning membership of a community to individuals who neither admit nor recognize that such a community exists' (Swales 1990: 25). This position has been disputed by others, notably Bex, who argues that the problem is 'more apparent than real' (Bex 1996: 64). He observes that in many situations, membership of a group may not be through free choice but through imposition, and therefore 'membership of a community may not always be apparent until faced with an outside threat' (Bex 1996: 64–5). Swales has since modified his original position, and acknowledged that a true discourse community, according to his definition, unaffected by external communicative practices, is likely to be rare (Swales 1993: 695).

A more flexible definition of discourse community is now in general use. Barton offers the following definition:

> A group of people who have texts and practices in common, whether it is a group of academics, or the readers of teenage magazines. In fact, discourse community can refer to several overlapping groups of people: it can refer to the people a text is aimed at; it can be the set of people who read a text; or it can refer to the people who participate in a set of discourse practices both by reading and by writing. . . . More generally, discourse communities are defined by having a set of common interests, values and purposes. (Barton 1994: 57)

We might reasonably add to this definition by arguing that a discourse community can refer to the people who participate in a set of discourse practices not only by reading and writing, but also by listening. We might also add that reading does not simply refer to silent private reading, but also to public readings, or reading aloud within a family or small local circle. All these amendments find numerous examples in contemporary society, and the amended definition is sufficiently flexible to apply to communities with very different types and uses of literacy, such as medieval English society.

Bex also observes that within his own social situation, he has varying allegiances to groups of people, with weak ties to those involved in education in general, but much stronger ties to members of his own university department. This observation is an important tenet of social network analysis, discussed by James Milroy as follows:

> a person may be conscious of, for example, family and friendship relationships, or membership of institutional groups, but he/she is not fully aware at any point of the multiple webs of (mainly informal) relationships that constitute a 'social network'. (J. Milroy 1992: 85)

James and Lesley Milroy's work on social networks, particularly in Belfast, has important implications for our understanding of the role of individuals in language change. They observed that closely knit networks tended to be linguistically conservative, resisting external pressures to change. Such close-knit networks were observed in both high- and low-status groups, which lack social mobility, and are bound by various ties such as kinship, school, church, or common financial interests (L. Milroy 1987: 184–5). Lesley Milroy's book focuses on maintenance of linguistic norms, rather than change; nonetheless she stresses the importance of loosely knit networks and mobile individuals for linguistic innovation, and the diffusion of innovative forms. Following Granovetter (1973), she notes that ' "weak" and uniplex personal ties are important channels through which innovation and influence flow from one close-knit group to another, linking such groups to the wider society' (L. Milroy 1987: 199). Individuals on the margins of closely knit groups serve to facilitate the acceptance of innovative features within the centre of the group:

> Persons central to a close-knit, norm-enforcing group are likely to find innovation a risky business; but adopting an innovation which is already widespread on the fringes of the group is very much less risky. Thus, instead of asking how central members of a group are induced to accept an innovation from marginal members, we can view this as a sensible strategy on their part. (L. Milroy 1987: 203)

The flexibility of both discourse and social network approaches means that they can be adapted to historical contexts, although the means of analysis cannot be so easily transferred. The accidental survival of evidence which was not conserved for the study of linguistic change means that quantitative studies of social networks in history are difficult if not impossible. Nevertheless, qualitative studies using these models have the potential to illuminate means and patterns of linguistic change and textual dissemination.

Studies of present-day discourse communities can work outwards from the members of a discourse community to examine the features of their shared texts.

Evidence for attitudes towards texts and participation in discourses is much more restricted in medieval studies; nevertheless, it does exist, and by combining historical, codicological, textual, and linguistic analyses the reconstruction of medieval discourse communities becomes possible.

2.3   Codicology and literacy artefacts

In the age before print each manuscript was unique, from its size, composition, and handwriting, to the combination and even the wording of texts it contained. Such manuscripts are essentially literacy artefacts and their physical nature can provide us with a great deal more information on their producers, owners, and readers than can the mass printed books of the present day.[3] It is also the case that before the age of mass publication the transmission of texts was more dependent on local sharing of manuscripts and texts than it was even a century later, and so patterns of distribution of texts can also be analysed in terms of the community in which they circulated. The widespread interest in medicine and the increasing use of the written word for the transmission of medical knowledge are well attested by the number of recipes added in free space and on the flyleaves of all kinds of manuscript.

2.4   Medical and social history

We can also use information from medical and social history to build up a picture of the producers and readers of medical books in the period. In many cases we can link these individuals to institutions, towns, villages, or family groups. Talbot and Hammond's list of medical practitioners in medieval England (Talbot and Hammond 1965), together with Getz's *Supplement* (Getz 1990b), contain a wide range of types of practitioner, and biographical information which links them to institutions and communities where this information is available. In some cases there is evidence for families of medical practitioners, such as Katherine, 'la surgeine' of London, who seems to have followed in her family trade (Talbot and Hammond 1965: 200). We can also, through wills, bequests, and surviving manuscripts, link individuals to books and texts. One of the most important surveys of book ownership from the evidence of wills and bequests is Susan Hagen Cavanaugh's unpublished survey, which includes a large number of owners of medical books (Cavanaugh 1980). A project currently in progress at the University of York aims to gather information about the owners and producers of manuscripts in late medieval English towns, using information from surviving manuscripts. This survey includes a range of medical books, and will further assist our understanding of patterns of ownership.[4]

As vernacular medicine was primarily a development used outside the universities, we know much less about the owners and readers of vernacular texts than we do for their Latinate equivalents. Those who trained in the universities could command the highest fees, and often treated prominent families and the royal household. In many cases they could afford to build up substantial libraries of medical works, often in Latin, but also increasingly in English, though their attitudes towards the vernacular texts varied. Linda Voigts's study of a Cambridge-trained physician, Roger Marchall, practising in London, provides a good example (Voigts 1995a). Roger Marchall had a large medical library, and a number of his books survive and can be identified. However, the book lists which Marchall drew up do not mention any vernacular texts, despite the fact that many of his books contain works in English. Academic medicine, like other subjects taught at the universities, used scholastic methods of teaching and learning, and this was reflected in the Latin texts which were used in the universities. However, scholastic features also found their way into the English translations and derivations of these texts. The presence or absence of such features in vernacular texts tells us something of the type of medicine the reader of such a text imagined him- or herself to be practising, and their perceived position in the hierarchy of the medical discourse community (Demaitre 1976; see also Taavitsainen and Pahta 1997 and 1998). A number of other practitioners also received formal training, some of which was at the universities, though this may have been on an unofficial basis.[5] Surgeons received training from guilds, which not only regulated the practice of their members, but also trained apprentices, taking them on for a period of at least five years (Rawcliffe 1995: 126–8). Other practitioners, such as barbers and apothecaries had also formed guilds, and received formal training and recognition of their craft status. Many practitioners from outside the universities viewed their practice as a craft, rather than a learned discipline, and surgical training placed much greater weight on evidence and practice than academic medicine:

> Techynge of bokys, yf at all yt be profytabyll, yet yt ys not allynges so sufficient as ys the othyr maner of anathomie, for the partes of the membyrs may better be sene with eyne in ded than in letters wretyne onn the boke. Never the latter, man ys schorte and slydynge away, ther for yt ys nedfull to have syght of anothomie wretyn in letters (London, British Library, Harley MS 1736, f. 9r–v, quoted in Beck 1974: 109, and Rawcliffe 1995: 128)

A large number of surgical texts written in England survive. John of Arderne, one of the leading surgeons of medieval England, asserted that 'the exercise of bokes worshippeth a leche' (Rawcliffe 1995: 130). As Carole Rawcliffe observes, many practitioners 'sought to improve their knowledge and no doubt their professional status by reading' (1995: 130). Both professional and social status of such practitioners was linked to the type of texts they read, and thus their association with the discourse community depended to an extent on their choice of reading.

The majority of medical care in medieval England was, however, undertaken by people with no formal medical training (see also Pahta and Taavitsainen, p. 16 above). Some made a living, often part-time, from their practice, such as the

Suffolk bailiff, John Crophill, who dispensed medicine and collected rents in the same area, possibly engaging with the same people in two different capacities.[6] Much of the evidence we have for this type of practitioner is anecdotal at present, though an increasing number of studies of individuals and manuscripts enable us to add detail to the wider picture of owners and readers of medical texts. For example, Peter Jones's studies of the manuscript of Thomas Fayreford shed light on the work of a practitioner in south-west England (P. M. Jones 1995 and 1998b; see also Talbert 1942 and Voigts 1995a). Other sources, such as the Paston letters, show how many households, even those of wealthy families, tended to treat their own ills wherever possible, and turned to a doctor as a last resort:

Margaret Paston to John Paston I, probably 1452, 5 November:

> My vncle Phelyppe comaund hym to yow, and he hath be so seke sith that I come to Redham that I wend he shuld never an askapid it, nor not is leke to do but if he have redy help; and therefore he shal into Suffolk this next weke to myn aunt, for there is a gode fesician and he shal loke to hym. (ed. Davis 1971, 1: 244)

2.5   Dialectology as literary geography and historical sociolinguistics

The highly dialectal nature of Middle English provides one means of grouping texts within a given region, and thus enables us to examine local patterns of production and transmission (see Pahta and Taavitsainen, p. 6 above). Such literary geography research may serve to establish links within and between communities (see Beadle 1991). Studies of regionalism in medical manuscripts have been greatly facilitated by the *Linguistic Atlas of Late Mediaeval English* (henceforth *LALME*). Palaeographical and codicological investigations also demonstrate patterns of production which suggest the existence of discourse communities. In this chapter I will be examining three manuscript groups, two derived from textual, dialectological, and provenance research, and the other largely from studies of texts and codicology. The discussion demonstrates how we might find evidence to support the theory that in medieval England, there were medical discourse communities which overlapped with communities using other genres, and with medical discourse communities in other parts of the country.

As discussed above, theories derived from contemporary sociolinguistics and research on discourse in present-day societies also provide a starting point for the analysis of language in historical contexts. For example, the importance of speakers with weak social ties to linguistic change has been recognised in historical dialectology for some time. Close-knit groups could include graduate physicians and university communities in general, craft guilds, such as those for surgeons, barbers and apothecaries, and parishes. Other, more loosely knit groups include medical practitioners and their communities, both local and more wide ranging, for those with large practices, such as Fayreford and Crophill. Family groups, although closely knit in a general sense, are more loosely tied in terms of their use and transmission of medical texts. There is evidence for all these groups, and for interactions between them, to a greater or lesser extent in later medieval England. However, there is evidence that the translation process in medicine was associated not only with those for whom the vernacular was their main medium of communication, but also (and perhaps initially) with members of close-knit groups such as monastic communities and universities (see also Taavitsainen, p. 49 below).

2.6   Professional tensions and the discourse community

The practitioners described above, along with lay readers on the periphery, can be said to have formed a discourse community around medical texts. Of particular interest are the ways in which texts and the social contexts may inter-relate. The transmission of texts from smaller subgroups within a discourse community could lead to a wider dissemination of knowledge. On the other hand, it could also lead to attempts to restrict the professional opportunities of those in receipt of this new knowledge. For example, a petition to the king in 1421 from the senior members of the 'scoles of fisyk' complained that 'many unconnyng and unapproved in the forsayd science practiseth, and specialy in fysyk, so that in this roialme is every man, be he never so lewed, takyng upon hym practyse, y–suffred to use hit, to grete harm and slaughtre of many men'. The solution, they claimed, was to restrict licence to practice to those who had 'long tyme y–used the scoles of fisyk within som universitee . . . That is to sey, but he be bacheler or doctour of fisyk' (*Rotuli Parliamentorum*, 4: 158). Whilst there is no explicit link stating that the proliferation of medical books should also be censured, it is clear from the wording of this petition, which also sought to ban women's medical practice entirely, that these physicians approved of no other forms of medical education than the universities, and were therefore not in favour of the dissemination of medical knowledge beyond their institutions.

Bex observes that 'it seems likely that the degree of identification with partic- ular groups will depend partly on the frequency with which individuals interact with each other in the pursuit of common goals, and partly on the perceived strength of external threats' (1996: 64). The large discourse community I have outlined, including all those who owned or read medical books in medieval England, or within a particular region, for example, may not have been the perceived community of many of its members. Vernacularisation and wider liter- acy in both English and Latin led to a wider dissemination of medical texts, and therefore presented potential problems for the university and guild-trained pro- fessionals who viewed the encroachment of untrained amateurs into the field of medical practice as dangerous and singularly undesirable. Many graduate physi- cians would not have seen themselves as part of the same discourse community as those practitioners and lay people who owned and read medical texts in increasing numbers. They attempted to restrict both the actual membership of the group by petitioning Parliament to legislate against unlicensed medical practice, and also access to texts (perceived membership), arguing that only those who had attended university, and were therefore proficient in Latin, should be allowed to practice. However, the huge increase in numbers of both Latin and English medical texts, which was not mirrored in an equivalent growth in graduate physicians, suggests that the boundaries of the medical discourse community which many professionals perceived and attempted to reinforce, were more apparent than real, were certainly permeable, and that the discourse did extend to all areas of the literate community, and beyond.

Despite the efforts of the graduate physicians, the vernacularisation process continued its rapid growth, and the medical discourse community could not be restricted to the universities. It extended to anyone who could read English, and, by extension, to anyone who had access to vernacular medical texts, whether as a reader or listener. This extension could not have happened without the input of those with access to the original Latin texts. Having observed the essential conservatism of many professional graduate physicians, we must consider the other possible motivations and pressures felt within the institutions. One of the key issues here seems to be religious motivation. Faye Getz has shown that medical translation was often undertaken as a form of charitable work by those within monastic communities. She observes that many medieval translators 'seem to have seen the vernacular medical translation as a kind of medical sermon, with a pastoral, indeed charitable, function in mind' (Getz 1990a: 9). Thomas M[o]ulton, a Dominican Friar, explicitly stated that he made translations out of a Christian duty to assist his fellows. He put it down in English 'so that every man both learned and unlearned may better understand it and act accordingly: be his own physician in time of need against the venom and malice of the pestilence' (Getz 1990a: 12). Although the number of lay students entering the universities was on the increase in the fifteenth century, they were still at heart religious institutions. It seems reasonable to assume that the charitable impulse did not stop at the monastery walls, and that translation as an act of charity may also have taken place within universities. We may consider that those who undertook such charitable acts were more strongly motivated by (and closely linked to) their religious communities than their professional cohorts. We can therefore say that there were loosely knit elements within the close-knit communities, which facilitated the spread of vernacular medical texts to the wider community.

2.7   Literacy practices and the medical discourse community

An analysis of regionally associated texts may enable us to understand more about literacy practices specific to a local discourse community. Literacy practices are the patterns, strategies, and background information which individuals bring to any situation involving the written word. Street defines them as follows: 'Literacy practices I would take as referring not only to the event itself but the conceptions of the reading and writing process that people hold when they are engaged in the event' (Street 1995: 133).[7] For example, practitioners/readers in a particular area may have had a shared cultural knowledge about medicine, and about the *materia medica* available locally, which coloured their approach to the texts they read, and thus their literacy practices. Within this community, however, there were those who were fluent in Latin and had trained in medicine, and who therefore had literacy practices which could not be directly shared by those who had little or no Latin. Many members of a community would not have been able to read or write; however, they would still have had medical literacy practices if they came into contact with medical writings, perhaps through asking another member of the community for assistance. For example, the book of Robert Reynes, a church reeve from the village of Acle, in Norfolk, contains a wide variety of texts, including short bloodletting tracts. It is possible that Reynes served as a local information centre, and gave medical and legal advice to those of his neighbours who did not own relevant texts or were unable to read.[8]

The vernacularisation process was not, of course, restricted to medical and scientific writings, and the wider political and national pressures which encouraged the spread of vernacular writings of all genres across Europe had an impact on scientific works. Recent work examining the use of the vernacular across genres demonstrates the variety of circumstances and motivations which underlay vernacular writing, and these are also applicable to medicine.[9] However, there may have been other pressures more particular to the translation of medicine, such as the charitable impulse discussed above, but also the nature of medical Latin. Little work has been done on the relative difficulty of reading Latin in a variety of different genres, but the survival of translations made for university fellows indicate that translations were not simply for those with a poor command of Latin.[10] An example is the translation of Gilbertus Anglicus made by Thomas Westhaugh, a fellow of Pembroke College, for another Pembroke fellow, John Sperhawke, who was, like Westhaugh, a doctor of canon law. As Sperhawke clearly must have been highly proficient in Latin in order to cope with the complexities of Latin legal texts, we must ask why he needed or wanted a medical book in English. The range of vernacular translations and the various literacy practices of their readers indicate that we cannot simply imagine an audience of a homogenous nature for these texts, but should rather consider them within a flexible discourse community, with shared interest in medicine but varying literacy practices and motivations.

2.8   Evidence for medical discourse communities

2.8.1   The Stockholm Group and Additional 33996 Group

My research on medical books in late medieval East Anglia showed that particular groups of recipes and charms circulated throughout Norfolk and Lincolnshire (C. Jones 2000). One of these groups, which I will call the Stockholm Group, was identified by George Keiser when researching his volume on medical and scientific writings for the *Manual of Writings in Middle English* (Keiser 1998). The texts are contained within a group of medical recipe and herbal manuscripts which circulated in Norfolk and Lincolnshire; it is convenient to name this group after Stockholm, Royal Library MS X.90, one of its most important members, and one of the first to receive serious scholarly attention (Stephens 1844; see also Mäkinen 2002a). Keiser observes that '[f]ull studies of the affiliations among these miscellanies will probably lead to interesting conclusions about the practice of medicine and the transmission of medical writings in the region of their origin' (1998: 3654). Another group, which is distantly linked to the Stockholm Group by one manuscript, contains recipes and charms found in London, British Library, Additional MS 33996 (Keiser 1998, no. 264). The relationship between the two groups is complex and tenuous at present, but bears further examination. The Stockholm verse recipes (Keiser 1998, no. 261), which link the Stockholm Group, are found in San Marino, Huntington Library MS HM 64. This does not contain the group of recipes in MS Additional 33996, but does contain the Charm of St Susan (Keiser 1998, no. 344), which is contained in a third of the Additional Group manuscripts. There is a further link from this charm, to the charm of St William (Keiser 1998, no. 345), which seems to be derived from the St Susan charm, and is found in Stockholm, Royal Library MS X.90.[11] The St Susan charm is found in eight manuscripts; two are localised in *LALME* to East Anglia and Lincolnshire, and another, London, British Library, Harley MS 1600, was considered to be written in an East Anglian dialect, but could not be localised with sufficient precision to be included in the published version of *LALME*.[12] The St William charm is also found in nine manuscripts (including two, Glasgow University Library, MS Hunter 117, and Cambridge, St John's College MS B.15 which were not listed in Keiser 1998). Five of these manuscripts can be localised to Norfolk, and one to Lincolnshire. One has been placed in Nottinghamshire, and two have not been localised.

These interconnected texts and their strong associations with East Anglia and Lincolnshire suggest that certain practical medical texts were circulating within a local community, whose members compiled their medical texts in order to suit their own purposes from material which was readily available. The books are not carbon copies of each other, but many of the texts they contain again survive commonly in manuscripts from East Anglia. The Stockholm Group contains nine manuscripts, four of which have not been localised in *LALME*. One (Cambridge, Trinity College R.7.23) has been described as being written in northern Middle English, with four more placed in Norfolk or Lincolnshire, thus providing clear evidence for the kind of restricted local transmission which we might expect from a local discourse community. Further work on disentangling the relationships and complex textual affinities within these localised manuscripts should provide firm evidence for a network of book ownership, copying, and compilation within one or more overlapping discourse communities.

2.8.2 The Sloane Group

The identification of the Sloane Group by Linda Voigts was based on both textual and codicological evidence (Voigts 1990). In an important and detailed study of the manuscripts, Voigts analysed the relationships between six core and several cousin manuscripts.[13] The main group is made up of London, British Library, Sloane MSS 2320 and 1118 and Additional MS 19674, and of booklets found in MSS Sloane 1313, 2567 and 2948, all of which Voigts dates to the 1450s and early 1460s. These manuscripts share a common core of medical texts and are also linked by common paper sources, *mise-en-page*, scribes, and, in two cases, by references to John Kyrkeby. These main manuscripts are connected to others by similarities in layout, common paper sources, and references to 'R.B./B.R' which Voigts suggests may refer to the Bacon texts in Sloane 2320. Several of the related manuscripts also share the same core of medical texts and some have a similar programme of medical illustration as that found in Sloane 2320.

The main members of the group seem all to have been produced in London or Westminster. Voigts suggested that these manuscripts were produced for speculative sale: 'it appears that there must have been in London or Westminster in the mid-fifteenth century one or more individuals responsible for the production of a specific *kind* of manuscript, uniform in appearance and scientific and medical in subject matter' (1990: 37). On the periphery of this group are cousin manuscripts, which share many of the core texts, but do not have the uniform layout as the core. One of the cousins is Harvard University Medical Library MS Countway 19. This seems likely to have been the 'litil boke of fisik' commissioned by John Paston.[14] It contains texts closely linked to the core texts of Sloane 2320, but does not share the uniform codicological features of the main group. Evidence from this manuscript suggests links within the larger discourse community, and may show how links between non-medical subgroups make connections within the medical community. The manuscript was copied (possibly for Paston) by William Ebesham, a professional scribe who was based in Westminster, but who often undertook work for the Paston family, and sometimes came to Norwich to work for the family there. The Paston men spent a great deal of time in London on business, and it is possible that Paston came across the Sloane Group manuscripts whilst in London, and decided to have a similar copy made for his family.[15]

Such patterns of textual and physical correspondence point to various means of production and circulation. The uniformity of the main Sloane Group manuscripts does not point to a Westminster medical discourse community, as Westminster was a centre of book production, and the book producers and stationers based in the area did business with book buyers from a very wide area. However, there are some links between this group and the East Anglian/Lincolnshire groups discussed earlier which indicate how texts made their way from larger centres, and formed part of the group of texts shared by the Norfolk/Lincolnshire medical discourse community.

2.8.3 Links between the groups

The Pastons were a key family in the Norfolk gentry society at the time, and the women in the family, who seem to have taken on most of the medical practice, spent most or all of their time at the family properties in Norfolk – often at Norwich or Caister. The men of the family did, however, do a great deal of travelling for business, and so had links to both the Norfolk gentry and to London law, business, and trade. We can say that in this case the men were on the periphery of the day-to-day business of medicine in Norfolk, leaving the detail to their wives, mothers, and sisters. The women formed a close-knit medical community within Norfolk, while the men may have been more receptive to innovative ideas in medicine from outside the community. The Sloane Group books, while containing much practical medicine, are still part of the tradition of academic medicine, whereas the origins of, for example, Margaret Paston's plaster for a sore knee are much less clear. It may well have derived originally from a classical remedy, but whether its producers and users in fifteenth-century England were aware of this is highly doubtful. The innovation of literate academic medicine by John Paston may have been more easily accepted by the central members of the medical discourse community partly through the structure of the book, which juxtaposes Latin texts with shorter English translations, thereby catering for a variety of literacy practices within the same family/household, and also allowing the information to be spread through a wider social network.

There is a further link between the Sloane Group and the Norfolk/Lincolnshire manuscripts included in the Additional 33996 Group. London, British Library, Additional MS 19674, which contains a number of the core Sloane Group texts, also contains the Additional 33996 recipes, and other texts, including verses on bloodletting sites (Keiser 1998, no. 288) and diet and bloodletting (Keiser 1998, no. 291), which are also found in East Anglian manuscripts. The latter two texts are found in a wide variety of manuscripts, and further dialectal and provenance studies are required in order to establish what, if any, is the regional or social connection between these manuscripts. The Lincolnshire/Norfolk connection between the manuscripts of the Additional 33996 Group, however, is much stronger. Of the six which have been localised in *LALME*, three are from East Anglia (including Cambridgeshire and Essex), two are from Derbyshire, and one from Hampshire. One manuscript, London, British Library, Harley MS 1600, is considered to be written in an East Anglian dialect. A number of studies which seek to further refine the localisations of *LALME*, and to closely examine the dialect materials of specific regions, may help to place the other manuscripts regionally, and potentially find more links within the discourse communities.

2.9   Conclusions

Until more detailed examinations about manuscript groups such as those discussed in this study have been done, our conclusions must remain speculative.

However, the recent publication of a database of scientific and medical writings in Old and Middle English by Voigts and Kurtz (2000; *eVK*), together with the ongoing work on an electronic version of the Thorndike and Kibre catalogue of incipits of Latin scientific works, and other ongoing projects charting the extant sources will make the identification of textual clusters much easier. More information about the relationship between these clusters and discourse communities can be gained through the *LALME* method and related dialect studies, and ongoing research into production and ownership of manuscripts.[16]

How does this model aid our understanding of the vernacularisation of science and medicine in medieval England? The answer is that it stops us looking at texts in a vacuum. The intra- and inter-linguistic processes which characterise the changing nature of scientific and medical English can only fully be examined through textual work. However, we need to understand not only how the process happened in linguistic terms, but also how and why it happened in social and historical terms. To do this we have to consider all the contexts of the texts; the unique manuscript context, and the sociohistorical contexts in which these texts were being produced and used. Instead of the idea of audience which suggests a homogenous group of people who passively read the texts, do not interact with them or each other, and have apparently the same motivations for reading a given text or genre, the concept of discourse community allows us to link texts and their users in a framework which takes account of people's varying relationships with texts and languages, and which removes the need to force readers into set categories which may be both anachronistic and inaccurate.

Notes

1. For example, P. M. Jones (1995, 1998b); Keiser (1996); Tavormina (forthcoming b).
2. The terminology used here derives from a range of studies, such as Heath's ethnographic studies of the south-eastern United States (Heath 1983). However, for the sake of clarity, I use references to Barton (1994) when discussing terminology, because his work presents various terms woven into a coherent approach. See also the definitions by Pahta and Taavitsainen, p. 15 above. They make a distinction in another way: 'readership' consists of those who read the book whereas 'audience' is a broader concept.
3. I have borrowed the term 'literacy artefacts' from a study into present-day children's literacy by Fiona Ormerod and Roz Ivanic (2000), which bears interesting comparisons with medieval manuscript culture.
4. AHRB project 'Privately-owned English urban manuscripts, 1300'1476: A database', directed by Professor Felicity Riddy, Centre for Medieval Studies, University of York.
5. For a discussion of non-university trained practitioners, see Bullough (1959).
6. Crophill's manuscript survives as London, British Library, Harley MS 1735, and has been edited by Lois Jean Ayoub (1994).
7. For more detailed discussions of literacy practices, see Barton (1994), and Barton and Hamilton (2000).
8. Robert Reynes's commonplace book survives in Oxford, Bodleian Library, Tanner MS 407, and has been edited by Cameron Louis (1980).

9. A recent anthology of extracts and essays provides an excellent introduction to the process of vernacularisation and medieval literary theory in a broad sense (Wogan-Browne *et al.* 1999).

10. A recent study by Peter Jones sets medical Latin in its late medieval English context (P. M. Jones 2000). His study is an excellent starting point, but much more work needs to be done in this field before we can properly begin to understand the complex processes which led to the translation of Latin medical texts at all levels.

11. I am currently preparing a study of the St William charm and its Norfolk associations.

12. I am grateful to Prof. Jeremy Smith for this information.

13. This group is also discussed by Taavitsainen in her chapter on house-styles, p. 217 below.

14. It should be emphasised that this link has not been firmly established, and much discussion of this manuscript has been based on a speculation by Ian Doyle. Much more work on this manuscript is required before any clear links to the Pastons can be established. I am grateful to Dr Doyle for discussing this matter with me.

15. For a discussion of the texts in MS Countway 19, see Harley (1982).

16. In addition to the Urban Manuscripts project (see note 4), large-scale projects in these fields include the Middle English Grammar project (University of Glasgow) and Linne Mooney's research on professional scribes (see also Pahta and Taavitsainen, pp. 5–7 above).

3 Transferring classical discourse conventions into the vernacular

3.1 Introduction

The aim of this chapter is to relate textual variation within medical writing to the dissemination of scientific knowledge in the vernacularisation processes. Besides repertoires of individual features, discourse forms or macrostructures of language use are important for an overall description of variability in texts. Scientific writing in Latin developed conventionalised discourse forms and schematic presentations to organise knowledge. By the late Middle Ages, they had become legitimate modes for disseminating learning. (For a scholastic book illustration, see Plate 4.) These conventions were transferred into vernacular languages in imitation of their Latin models.[1] The focus of the present assessment is on the discourse forms of commentaries, compilations, and question–answer formulae with their origins in Graeco-Latin scientific writing.

In an attempt to identify manifestations of discourse forms in the vernacular, three layers of text reality are taken into account. Text conventions are first assessed in their Latin context. Chronological developments took place already in Latin, which complicates the issues of sources and models. The transfer may have caused further changes, and modifications are likely to be found in the vernacular in their new cultural background. Vernacular reality is assessed at two levels: the manuscript reality and the 'edited truth'. Both can now be searched with modern electronic tools (see below). I shall start my assessment with top-level texts for academic audiences with commentaries and compilations and trace the scale to tracts for a wide readership. I intend to assess the role of *loci communes* in the dissemination of knowledge, for example how some doctrines become stereotypes and find their way into popular literature. The third discourse form in focus in this chapter is the question–answer formula; it also originates from learned writing and found its way into more popular adaptations.

The findings of my study raise further questions as commentaries and compilations seem to overlap at the highest level in the vernacular material. Commentaries proved to be rare and focus on the more utilitarian kind of academic texts. Compilations show a broad range from top-level academic surgical treatises and academic encyclopaedias to assemblies of commonplaces and tracts for practical use. The question–answer formula seems to develop in mainstream medical prose writing fairly late, though some examples can be found in the fifteenth century (see below and note 21). A time-lag with the manifestations of other discourse forms is also possible.

3.2   Vernacularisation of academic discourse – for whom?

One of the issues to be taken into account in the vernacularisation of scientific writing is the intended audience. Latin was the language of education and retained its position until the turn of the seventeenth/eighteenth century. The universities at Oxford and Cambridge used Latin. The scientific discourse community of the Royal Society (founded in 1660) used English, although the *Philosophical Transactions* include articles in Latin as well. According to publication statistics, Latin prevailed in printed scientific books until the middle of the seventeenth century (Webster 1975: 267).[2] Although language, whether Latin or English, cannot be taken as direct evidence of the level of education or social standing of the audience, it has direct relevance to my assessment here. Originally the commentary, the compilation and the question–answer formula were university-based, institutionalised textual forms of learned Latin writing, but in the vernacular, out of the original institutional setting, and some centuries after their heyday, the text forms must have lost some of their original functions and gained new applications. In the dissemination of knowledge to the wider public, when translated into the vernacular and when in other teaching forums, the patterns are likely to have been modified or changed. If these text forms are found in vernacular medical writing, in what form do they occur and how have they been modified? Another pertinent question is how the text forms relate to one another. There are no previous studies about how, when, to what extent and for whom the academic text forms were adopted into English medical writing in the vernacularisation process.

Commentaries and compilations were essential in the dissemination of knowledge, and their range is wide. The university level is represented by Chauliac's texts, as the original audience constituted doctors from Montpellier, Bologna and Paris, three leading faculties of Europe at the time, and the doctors and clerks of the papal court (McVaugh 1997).[3] The distribution of Chauliac's works was wide: 33 manuscripts are extant in Latin; there are translations in most vernacular European languages, including at least three translations into Middle English (anonymous from the second quarter of the fifteenth century). It can be assumed that the audience of the vernacular versions was wider, including learned doctors but also others who could read and had access to books. As compilations were so useful even at the top level, they must have been indispensable in the education of other literate medical practitioners as well.

It is also relevant that the question–answer formula is found earlier in verse than prose in English medical writing. In the Middle Ages, verse provided a more elementary mode of expression than prose, which was more sophisticated and associated with philosophy and higher learning. Rhymes were easy to memorise and had links with oral culture. Earlier studies on the transmission of *The Form of Living* in verse and prose established different audiences for the two modes; prose was for the learned (Blake 1974). This stratification could apply more widely and should be related to the different discourse forms as well.

3.3   Discourse forms: Definitions and theory

Medicine is somewhat different from other scientific writings, and the discourse forms in this discipline have their own characteristics. The position of medicine among the sciences was special as there was a fundamental problem of the relation of theory and practice. The problem occupied learned writers throughout centuries, and various solutions were offered. In his widely disseminated book *Sermones medicinales*, Niccolò Falcucci, an Italian physician (*d.* in 1411 or 1412), offers a solution in which the theoretical part and the practical part are integrated from an epistemological point of view, and yet the status of medicine as a science is guaranteed. Medicine is presented as a special branch of knowledge and the formation of a physician must follow a unified course of study according to a composite pattern. Medical education involves didactic techniques and a form of transmission sufficiently diversified to convey both general theories and specialist doctrines, but it also includes practical apprenticeship. Medicine was both an accepted learned university discipline, with ties to natural philosophy, and an occupation involving technical skills. Epistemological levels of medical education formed a hierarchy: *scientia* was the top level, with general theories not directly orientated to practical applications; next follows *scientia operativa*, defined as 'a kind of *scientia* but not *operatio*'; the third level is *ars scientifica* based not only on the knowledge of theories but on experience and practice, with rules and canons suitable to practical applications, and including presentations of medicine through individual therapeutic acts (Crisciani 2000: 75–6).

All these text levels were transferred into the vernacular. Commentaries are connected with the top level and with theories of natural philosophy, but the twofold nature of medicine being at the same time both text-based and practice-based shows in medical commentaries, as the obligation of the commentator was not only to record the truth and the meaning of the text but also to point out its usefulness (Crisciani 2000: 79). Commentaries are, however, prominently research-based and aim to find the truth of the original texts. If commentaries are connected with *scientia*, compilations could well be linked with the next level, *scientia operativa*, though its definition does not open up easily. *Compilationes* are not practice-orientated either, but more instructional, and the third level, *ars scientifica*, is presented through individual therapeutic acts and is thus directly linked with medical praxis. *Ars scientifica* can perhaps be connected with question–answer formulae. This text form belongs to didactic texts and individual questions are well suited for some particular ailment with answers specifying individual therapeutic acts.

Institutional developments are important as the established settings promoted the creation of discourse forms in a more formalised direction. The origins of several genres of writing and macroforms of discourse can be found in Italy in the twelfth century. In the course of time the numbers of students in monastic and cathedral schools and teaching in urban centres attracted an increasingly numerous and cosmopolitan group of students. The timetable of the academic year and the curriculum took shape. The full institutionalisation in Italy took place between the time of Arnald de Villanova and Falcucci, a period in which there was a general agreement about the delineation of the general features of institutionalised medical teaching. This broad agreement existed throughout Europe at that time (Crisciani 2000: 78).

3.3.1 Commentaries

Commentaries were practised in different ways in different disciplines.[4] They all, including medicine, had a canon of authoritative texts (for the medieval commentary-tradition of 'set texts', see Minnis et al. 1988). Yet prototypical representatives of scholastic commentaries do not include medical texts; the best-known examples are Chalcidius on Plato's *Timaeus*, Macrobius (Antonius Theodosius Macrobius *fl.* AD 395–423) on Cicero's *Dream of Scipio*,[5] and biblical commentaries. Their contents became standardised in the twelfth century, and the visual side was enhanced with refinements of presentation (Parkes 1976: 116). In the vernacular, philosophical texts like Walton's translation of Boethius from the beginning of the fifteenth century continue the classical commentary tradition in the vernacular, and Copenhagen, Royal Library, Thott MS 304 contains manuscript pages with top-quality visual presentation in the vernacular. Boethius's text is carefully written in a textura hand; the commentary runs alongside in the same hand but smaller in size and some diagrams are skilfully inserted. I have not encountered such page layouts in English medical writing.

The sociohistorical context of commentaries in Latin scientific texts places them at the heart of the intellectual mainstream of scholasticism. Textual transmission took the form of systematic and often heavily glossed versions of ancient knowledge. Commentaries reflect the logocentric mode of scholastic science, and consist of expository treatises, comments or explanations. Language was assumed to have the objective status of a natural sign, and the aim of scholastic research was to reconstruct the original meanings of authoritative texts and find the truth by explications of the Bible, Hippocratic-Galenic, Judeo-Arabic, or recent Latin writings. The commentary tradition has several layers from Greek to Latin and Arabic, and the developments continued after the high point of the twelfth century (for the chronological layers, see also below). By definition, commentaries explicate the text and cross-refer to other texts on the same topic (cf. McLean 1980: 4). Thus there is only a small step to a thematic approach, but this connection has not been pointed out before. An important feature that distinguishes commentaries from compilations is that in compilations opinions are attributed to others, while in commentaries the commentator takes the responsibility for conclusions (Minnis 1979: 387). The source of this distinction can be traced to medieval literary theory and most definitions in the literature are based on Bonaventura's explication of the different roles of people involved in medieval book production. In the recent literature this theory has been extended to the vernacularisation processes of the fourteenth and fifteenth centuries (see below). Of the tasks of a scribe, a compiler, a commentator, and an author, those of the commentator and the compiler are relevant here. The compiler writes the materials of others while the commentator adds his own to clarify the sayings of others. As Bonaventura states:

> Someone else writes both the materials of other men, and of his own, but the materials of others as the principal materials, and **his own annexed for the purpose of clarifying them**, and this person is said to be the **commentator**, not the author. (trans. Minnis 1984: 94; highlights in all quotations mine)

In the Middle Ages and at least until the sixteenth century, authorial participation in an intellectually and morally authoritative tradition was appreciated above originality (Wogan-Brown *et al.* 1999: 4). Throughout the period in focus, authorities were texts rather than persons; they were *sententiae* or ideas excerpted from their original context in a work of an author (Parkes 1976: 116). In the vernacularisation process we have one more agent, the translator, whose task was seen as somewhat overlapping with authorship according to medieval opinions. In medieval literary theory, the translator identifies with the expositor and comes very near the commentary tradition (Copeland 1991: 176–7); the translator's role is then comparable to that of a commentator. To illustrate the text form of commentary in the vernacular, I quote below a passage that fulfils the criteria from Thomas Vicary's *Anatomy* from 1541, based on a thirteenth-century surgical text by Henry of Mondeville (Bennett 1969: 108). Following the original, diverse opinions are stated first, and the conflicting statements are reconciled in the conclusions. The author refers to 'the very truth' the discovery of which was the ultimate aim of a commentary. The author clearly takes responsibility for the conclusions and does not attribute them to someone else:

> The Eyes be the instrumentes of sight. And they bee compounde and made of ten things: that is to say, of seuen Tunicles or Cotes, and of three humours. Of the whiche (**sayth Galen**) the Brayne and the head were made for the Eye, that they might be in the hyest place, as a beholder in a towre, as it was rehearsed in the Anatomie of the head. But **diuers men holde diuers opinions** of the Anatomie of the Eyes: for **some men accompt** but three tunikles, and some sixe. **But in conclusion, they**

meane all one thing: For the very truth is, that there be counted and reckoned seuen Tunikles, that is to say, Sclirotica, Secondyna, Retyna, Vnia, Cornua, Arania, and Coniunctiua: and these three humours, that is to say, humor Vitrus, humor Albigynus, and humor Crystallinus. (ed. Furnivall and Furnivall 1930: 35–6)

3.3.2 Compilations[6]

Someone else writes the materials of others, adding, but nothing of his own, and this person is said to be the compiler. (trans. Minnis 1984: 94)

It is generally accepted that before the development of strong vernacular and national intellectual traditions, there was a 'universe of discourse' expressed principally in Latin, but including also texts translated into various vernacular languages. These texts acted as vehicles to transmit conclusions and opinions, they were commonplaces or *loci communes* (McLean 1980: 2). Medical texts had a canon of their own, and the hierarchy of authorities was clear: Galen and Hippocrates were frequently mentioned, especially in learned and specialised treatises; next in frequency were Arab authors, such as Avicenna, Rhases, Haly Abbas and Averroes (Taavitsainen and Pahta 1998: 169).[7] By the side of authentic texts, pseudoauthorial texts were written by near-contemporary authors and transmitted alongside the authentic ones. Thus, for example, Galenic and Hippocratic texts form an extremely complicated body in Latin medical writing. The transmission was further complicated in the vernacular, but the comparison is difficult because the base texts are mostly not known or they have not been edited.

Excerpts from important works were gathered in a convenient and pre-digested way in compilations. The generally accepted definition of *compilationes* points out the contrast to commentaries: compilations list the sayings of others, without taking sides or reconciling conflicting views. No conclusions are drawn in compilations while the author's own conclusions are important in commentaries; if this border is crossed, the compiler assumes the role of a commentator. Compilations were important for the dissemination of knowledge and they gained wide usage in the vernacular. Like commentaries, compilations reflect the logocentric mode of scholastic science, but they are more didactic and instructive than the research-orientated commentaries. The roles of an author and compiler could approximate each other, for example FitzRalph's Ricardus suggests that both be called *auctor* (Minnis 1984: 100). Compilations were reference books with a twofold didactic function. First, they provided easy access to authoritative passages and convenient ways of finding important opinions. Secondly, they made the authorities available to readers not able to work their way through the originals (Minnis 1979: 402–3). Several surgical treatises in the present material disseminate learning in an easily digestible way, providing shortcuts to authoritative knowledge. This is important for the function of learned compilations in the vernacular. The utility and profit of such texts is explicitly stated in the passage of Chauliac's translation:

> The resoun of þis exposicioun or gadryng togedre was noght defaute of bookes, but raþer onhede and profit. Euery man may not haue alle bookes, and if he hadde, it were irkesome or noye to rede hem and goodly to holde all þing in mynde. (ed. Ogden 1971: 2)

By the thirteenth century, medieval techniques of compilation had reached a high level of sophistication, as can be seen in *De proprietatibus rerum* of Bartholomaeus Anglicus originally composed in Latin *c*. 1245 (Minnis 1984: 97; Seymour *et al.* 1992: 11). Other Latin texts to be mentioned in this connection include the *Speculum maius* of Vincent of Beauvais, completed in 1246, and Isidore of Seville's (*d*. 636) *Etymologiae*. Encyclopaedic treatises belong to the learned tradition. They follow an ordered progression and project the medieval worldview so that, for example, the hierarchies of the animal world and the macrocosm-microcosm correspondences are reflected in these compilations. *De proprietatibus rerum* begins with the Creator and the spiritual creation, angels and the soul in Books 1–3; Books 4–7 form the medical section and explore the human nature, the humours that govern the human body, the roles of people in ordered society, and illnesses and diseases. Books 8–9 deal with celestial and temporal contexts, Books 10–18 with the four elements, and Book 19 deals with natural science, for example a herbal is included. Of the contemporary encyclopaedias, *De proprietatibus rerum* is perhaps the most practically orientated and may have helped the friars to cope with outbreaks of pestilence (Seymour *et al.* 1992: 11–14). The ultimate aim of encyclopaedic compilations was perhaps to explain the existing order by linking its various aspects with underlying religious convictions, and combine the knowledge of various fields into a holistic system. In the vernacular, encyclopaedic treatises broadened their scope towards more practical and everyday adaptations of the underlying principles (see below).

At the other end of the scholarly scale, the borderline between compilations, digests[8] and commonplace books is likewise difficult to draw. The distinction lies in the overall structure: compilations have orderly arrangements of materials, while, for example, commonplace books do not. According to the medieval practice, useful texts, which also circulated independently in various forms, were gathered into the same manuscripts. Such collections can be found in commonplace books compiled for one's own personal use. Originally the term meant passages applicable in many different circumstances (Robbins 1952: xxviii–xxx). *Loci communes*, which are components of compilations, provided useful material. The distinguishing feature of a commonplace book is, however, the purpose of the collection. In these books miscellaneous items have been copied for the interest, amusement and instruction of the compiler (Ayoub 1994: 5–6). The materials are not integrated to form coherent longer treatises but parts of different origins are given one after the other in a more haphazard order. As the books were written over several years, they also show how the person's interests, tastes, activities and lifestyles developed over the years (Louis 1980: 101). Perhaps the best-known examples of medieval commonplace books with vernacular texts are the note books of Robert Reynes of Acle (ed. Louis 1980) and that of John Crophill, a rural medical practitioner (ed. Ayoub 1994). A further example from the sixteenth century is found in Stockholm, Royal Library, Huseby MS 78, which has not been edited (see Taavitsainen 1994b).

3.3.3 Aristotelian questions, Salernitan questions, and philosophical dialogues

Debates and disputations were among the teaching methods of universities, in medicine as well as in other fields connected with scholastic philosophy. Questions literature had several layers. By c. 1200 several collections of medical and scientific questions circulated in Latin (Lawn 1979: ix). The written discourse form of questions and answers was based on classical models and originally derived from Aristotelian treatises. It developed into a typical pattern in treating theological, medical, and scientific problems at universities in the thirteenth and fourteenth centuries and the scholastic discourse form developed its own characteristics. The academic formula was elaborate: the question was posed, and the first answer considered the issue with pros and cons, giving an affirmative or a negative answer. Central arguments were accompanied by descriptions, definitions and explanations. A review of authorities on the subject could be included. At the end, the main argument was raised again summing up the previous opinions and viewpoints, and the problem was finally answered. In the course of time, a standard stock was developed which remained valid for centuries (Grant 1974: 199, 610; Cadden 1993: 114; see also Minnis et al. 1988: 212). The roots of questions literature lie in classical antiquity, but medieval commentaries also contributed to its development (Siraisi 2001: 144–8). Salernitan questions in Latin are found in English manuscripts in collections of medical and scientific questions both in verse (ed. Lawn 1963) and in prose, containing the answers as well. The collections also include astrological, theological and philosophical questions, and many are repeated several times. The sources can be traced to Salerno, and in some cases to Montpellier and Paris where both Arabic and Salernitan influences met in the second half of the twelfth century; many of the questions seem to stem from classical collections of Greek problemata as well (Lawn 1979: xiv–xxiii). The characteristics of vernacular texts in the same discourse form can be assumed to have developed from these Latin models but have undergone some modifications and simplification (see Taavitsainen 1999 and 2001b).

Like commentaries, questions had oral counterparts at the highest academic level, and institutionalisation contributed to the establishment of the public dispute as another central form of communicating knowledge orally at the university. Public disputations took place at specific times in the academic year and at specific stages of the curriculum. The academic community with both teachers and students participated in these public disputations. Questions on a set text or problems on any subject formed the basis and, like the written questions and answers, they were expounded with pro and con arguments, responses to contrary arguments, reviews of the competing opinions of authorities on the subject, and a determination or conclusion. The format could vary, but the usual structure was elaborate. Pedagogical dialogues also derive from classical models but they have different underpinnings. The earliest examples of the philosophical dialogue are found in Greek literature and continue throughout history (see Smiley 1995). This discourse form derives from Socrates through Plato, and Aristotle contributed to the formation of a more abstract form (Ong 1958: 152). The tradition continued in the Middle Ages, with Boethius's *De consolatione philosophiae* as its most influential manifestation. Boethius's work portrays a fictional encounter and a 'schoolroom colloquy between a master and a student' (Lerer 1985: 19). This treatise was commented upon by medieval *auctores*, and, for example, the above-mentioned example of the commentary page from the Thott MS of Walton's Boethius provides an example of a philosophical dialogue with a commentary in a vernacular. This shows how the discourse forms described above were all interconnected and, in principle, any written text could be subject to commentary, or a question–answer formula could be imposed upon them.[9]

3.4 From Latin into English: Vernacularisation of the discourse forms

Discourse forms in Latin scientific and medical texts provided the models for vernacular texts. Several parameters are, however, different in the original Latin material and in the vernacular.

The original setting of the three discourse forms in focus here, commentaries, compilations, and question–answer formulae, was institutional. All these forms were academic, with research-based commentaries having most scholarly prestige. In the vernacular the original function was lost in the non-institutional setting. Modifications and a wider audience may be expected in the vernacular, and some may have developed already in Latin. For example, *loci communes* were indispensable to all practising doctors regardless of their rank. It can be assumed that the lower down the scale the more important such vernacular compilations were. Such compilations would become useful even to a lay audience, with the increasing literacy of the upper-middle classes in the aspiring atmosphere of the fifteenth century. The character of *loci communes* needs closer scrutiny as it seems probable that the doctrines tended to become stereotyped when repeated. It may be possible to trace the transmission of some of the doctrines from academic treatises to popular adaptations, for example in astromedical literature, from texts described as commentaries to almanacs with miscellaneous useful materials, and jottings in commonplace books for individual use. The *homo signorum* principle is a case in point: it is found in all layers of medical literature in a fairly constant form

Table 3.1. *Transferring classical conventions into the vernacular: some parameters*

language	time	audience	setting	discourse form
Latin	12th c.–	academic	university	commentaries, compilations, questions
English	1375–	wider	non-institutional	modifications?

and fixed wording, but there are differences in the connotations and meanings ascribed to the doctrine. Another relevant example may be found in explanations of the underlying medical theory of humours, for instance, and in this case there may also be differences in wording (see below). Questions literature also developed a standard set (see below) and the discourse form of questions and answers was particularly suitable for elementary instruction, which was doubtless the basic function of vernacular medical texts. In the following, I shall discuss the different parameters of the vernacularisation process.

3.4.1 Time and stratification of materials

As the above account shows, scientific writing in Latin developed conventionalised discourse forms to present and organise knowledge. The time factor complicated the dissemination of knowledge in Latin writing, and different layers of material can be discerned. Works by classical authorities, Galen and Hippocrates at the top, reached the readership through commentaries and compilations, which evolved in the course of time. The earliest stratum derives from the classical period, for example Galen wrote commentaries of Hippocrates' works (Cadden 1993: 112). The ideas of authorities form the principal material which is then discussed, explained, and commented upon. From the eleventh century onwards the Latin West began to seek out and contemplate a fuller version of ancient wisdom. Italy was in the forefront of the developments in the formation of writing conventions and establishing textual traditions, shaped by new institutions and expanding scientific horizons, and by a new disease environment, with the plague, for instance. The twelfth century has come to be seen as the starting point for a long medical Renaissance, for intellectual traditions that, evolving over four hundred years, eventually began to resolve a broad range of issues defining a new science of medicine (McVaugh and Siraisi 1990: 9), growing out of a range of equally new areas of scholarly investigation (Siraisi 1984). The influence of the new translations from the Arabic in natural philosophy and medicine started in the twelfth century, and the Constantinian translations date from this period. The centre of medical knowledge at that time was Salerno in Italy, and the important literary product of the school of Salerno was the *Articella*, a collection of classical medical texts.[10] It has been described as a compilation of classical medical knowledge with Arab learning (Ottosson 1984: 60), but as it was a university textbook, it soon became an object of commentary. The practice of writing Latin commentaries on some of the texts was taken up by Salernitan masters. Both physicians and natural philosophers became aware of, and started discussing, the differences between Aristotle's and Galen's views of such central issues as the function of the heart and brain, and the roles of parents in conception; these debates went on until the seventeenth century (Siraisi 2001: 144). The textual histories of its components are extremely complicated and may contain several layers with commentaries and compilations intertwined. This development can be seen in various texts of the original composition: the *Isagoge* by Iohannitius was later commented upon by Taddeo Alderotti (*d.* 1295), as the result of his lectures and disputations held at Bologna in 1277. A little later, Dino del Garbo (*d.* 1327) chose the form of commentary for his work on the surgery of Book 4 of the *Canon* by Avicenna, which was itself a commentary on Galen's works; it combined a family tradition of practice with the teachings of learned authorities for medical instruction (Siraisi 1994: 96, 2001: 147). Accordingly, it should contain all epistemological levels of medieval knowledge embedded into one text. This practice of combining and building upon various discourse forms was probably more widespread than has been realised (Lawn 1993: 72). In Latin, the commentary tradition in the form of interpretation and discussion of authoritative texts continued throughout the Renaissance, and humanistic medicine was primarily a movement for better and more translations of ancient medical texts (Bylebyl 1979).[11]

Chronologically, the tradition of commentaries was stratified with several layers of Latin commentators building upon one another. In an appendix to his book *Scholastic Medicine and Philosophy*, Ottosson (1984: 289–99) lists the references in the commentaries on Galen's *Tegni* by Taddeo Alderotti, Torrigiano, and Jacopo da Forlí, supplemented by the authoritative textbooks of the university of Bologna in 1405. His purpose is to demonstrate the wide range of literature employed in the commentaries. The earliest chronological layer contains classical Greek authors, Arab commentators come next, and contemporary commentaries are the most recent layer. References are found to a long list of authorities, given here in alphabetical order: Aegidius Romanus, Albertus Magnus, Algazel, Alkindi, Aristotle, Augustinus, Averroes, Avicebreon, Avicenna, Biblia Sacra, Boethius, Bruno da Longoburgo, Constantinus Africanus, Euclid, Eustathios, Galen, Gentile da Foligno, Haly, Haly Abbas, Hippocrates, Horatius, Hugh of St Victor, Johannes Alexandrinus, Johannitius, Isaac Judaeus, Isidore of Seville, Mesue, Ovidius, Pietro d'Abano, Plato, Pliny, Porphyry, Ptolemy, Rasis, Seneca, Serapion, Taddeo Alderotti, Thomas Aquinas, Themistius, Torrigiano, Valerius Maximus, Vergilius, Zahel. Ottosson's study also confirms that scholastic commentators relied primarily on the original works of Aristotle and Galen. The authors had studied a large number of different works and made an effort to use only the best translations of authentic works (Ottosson 1984: 288). Avicenna's *Canon* seems to have been the outstanding handbook without which no medical problem could be discussed. Yet it is somewhat surprising to note that well-known authorities like Arnald de Villanova, Dino del Garbo, etc. are missing from this list, though it was supplemented by university textbooks until the beginning of the fifteenth century.

As an overall trend in the Middle Ages, the traditions of commentary and compilation approached one another. The literature is of little help as the terminology seems somewhat confused. The genre of compilation was old but acquired sophistication and refinement in the later Middle Ages, especially in the thirteenth and fourteenth centuries (Minnis 1979: 386–7). This merging of discourse forms can be detected both in the texts of late medieval authors like Chauliac and in the present-day literature dealing with these issues; the difficulty of keeping the two terms apart may ultimately go back to the medieval texts themselves. Medieval commentators were influenced by the practice of compilations, and attitudes changed as works of revered *auctores* were noticed to contain compilations as well (Minnis 1979: 413). It is no surprise that commentaries and compilations overlap and merge in vernacular texts, as this development had already taken place in Latin texts of an earlier period.

Combinations of other discourse forms can also be found. *Sidrak and Bokkus* is an encyclopaedic compilation in the question–answer format, which provided a useful pattern commonly found in later instructional treatises in the vernacular. The classical model of the philosophical dialogue referred to above was also one of the underlying trends. Boethius's text may have influenced discourse forms as well as the linguistic repertoire of scientific writing in English through its several translations at various times with schematic interaction and turn-taking patterns. By the late Middle Ages, a standard stock of questions, for example about conception, had developed at the academic level (see Cadden 1993: 106, 116), and popular adaptations and commonplaces started to appear as well. The most widely spread were the *Questions of Aristotle*, ultimately stemming from classical collections of *problemata* ascribed to pseudo-Aristotle (Burton 1998, 1: xxiii). Salernitan questions were also transferred into the vernacular in a somewhat simplified form and survive mainly in references to the school of Salerno in late medieval medical literature in English.[12]

3.4.2 Audience and setting

The readership of early medical texts can be assessed through text external evidence in library catalogues, wills, and inscriptions of ownership (for the methodology, see Pearson 1994). They give us indications of the users of the books. Text internal evidence may also be found as prologues and dedications increase with time, albeit the information is scanty and difficult to access (see Jones in this volume).[13]

Three features are central in the institutionalisation of medicine, and are common to all scholastic science: the first was the importance of the written text, the second the role of authoritative texts in defining the discipline, and the third the demand that the insights acquired by experience should be checked with authoritative texts and transferred by writing into doctrine, thus making them valid and transmissible (Crisciani 2000: 77–8). Institutional developments promoted the creation of discourse forms in a more formalised direction. Oral practices interacted with written discourse forms and contributed to the development of written genres at the universities. The treatment of the material at the university could range from cursory or literal explication to freer discussion. Conventions of scientific argumentation acquired set formats. The oral and the written modes interacted: the *lectio* shaped the literary form of the commentary, and oral disputations helped to form the basis of question–answer formulae in written discourse. The forms could also combine theoretical and practical experience, for example Taddeo Alderotti's commentary was the result of ten years of teaching, but it also incorporated the experience of a long professional practice (Crisciani 2000: 79). Likewise, Guy de Chauliac combined a university career with a long practice. It can be assumed that this practical side of medical writing was particularly important in non-institutional vernacular texts, and practical concerns influenced the choice of texts to be translated and adapted into the vernacular.

The settings of medical knowledge vary from the more formalised teaching at the universities with established and even elaborate forms of discourse to more lightly organised medical settings. At first the households of noble patrons provided environments for medical learning and medical schools could be attached to monasteries or cathedrals. Universities became fully institutionalised in the thirteenth century (Siraisi 1994: 92), and there was a general agreement about medical teaching throughout Europe (Crisciani 2000: 78), including Oxford and Cambridge, which were monolingual in Latin and part of the pan-European educational network which paid no regard to the vernacular. An important step in the institutionalisation of professional medical training at a lower level than the academic took place with the establishment of the guilds of barber-surgeons in the late fifteenth century. Guilds had started to record their official documents in English, and, for example, the barber-surgeons of York gathered all kinds of useful information into their guild book from the year 1486. It is likely that the medical treatises in these books were used in institutional instruction, but otherwise vernacular medical literature was probably non-institutional, for private use only.

3.4.3 Discourse forms

Vernacularisation of medical writing and the transfer of discourse forms took place almost simultaneously along a broad front in several European languages from the latter half of the fourteenth century (see the issue on vernacularisation of *Early Science and Medicine*, ed. Crossgrove *at al.* 1998). The chronological development is presented below.

My research question focuses on the discourse forms in vernacular medical texts. It has been noticed that the transmission of surgical texts in the vernacular

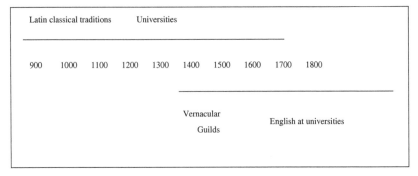

Figure 3.1 Latin and vernacular: chronological development

obeys laws which are different from those applying to Latin, as the translators have acted as editors by selecting and excerpting materials (P. M. Jones 1989: 88). It is possible that the vernacularisation of the discourse forms shows unexpected features. Next I shall illuminate the scope of the transfer of textual conventions and special developments of discourse forms in English texts with a series of case studies.

3.5   Dissemination of discourse forms in the vernacular: Case studies

To find the examples for the case studies I charted the manuscript reality with the *eVK* database and followed the leads by checking the manuscripts to the extent it was possible. The method of detecting discourse forms in the electronic *Corpus of Middle English Medical Texts* (*MEMT*) was based on lexical searches. As there are no previous studies on the dissemination of scientific discourse forms in English, the first task was to chart whether there are texts that show characteristics of these forms, and how common they are according to the criteria in the above definitions.

Both commentaries and compilations are connected with the logocentric mode of knowing. The search for passages composed with the quotative techniques focused on speech-act verbs of reporting, of which some have already proved useful in assessing more learned texts and some for locating dialogic passages and question–answer formulae (see Taavitsainen 1999 and 2001b). In addition, the more personal mode of writing indicated by personal pronouns reveals the author's role in scientific argumentation and in shaping the discourse with metatext (Taavitsainen 2000a). The following verbs with different spellings were assessed using computer-generated word lists of specialised treatises and surgical texts in our electronic database:

> *accord, account / accompt, acknowledge, admit, affirm / confirm, answer, approve, argue, ask, bid, charge, command, commend, conclude, counsel, declare, discourse, discuss, forbid, inquire / enquire, mention, note, number, praise, pray, quote, rehearse, say, speak, swear, teach, tell, treat*, and *write*.

The contexts of these verbs were checked, paying attention to who says what, how the sayings accumulate and relate to one another and reveal features of discourse forms according to the criteria discussed above. In the following, I shall rely on qualitative assessment to illustrate the scope of vernacularised texts with different discourse forms.

3.5.1 Commentaries[14]

Searches in the *eVK* database covering all fields of medieval science indicate that commentaries are few in the vernacular. For example, none of the famous commentaries by Taddeo Alderotti or Jacopo da Forlí mentioned above seem to have been translated into English. Commentaries are typically connected with top-level knowledge and theories of natural philosophy. As English was not used at the highest institutional level, the assumption is that the practical side would be enhanced in vernacular texts. The list in Table 3.2 was retrieved by searches in the Title Index of the *eVK*. The topics of the texts given as commentaries indicate that three texts focus on urinoscopy, three on astrology, three on alchemy, and the last item is a psychological treatise from the sixteenth century.

Table 3.2. *Texts given as commentaries in* eVK

Urinoscopy:
Walter Agilon, *Commentarium Urinarum* (*Compendium Urinarum*)
John Arderon, *Opusculum de Iudiciis Urinarum* (commentary on Aegidius)
A Judicial (commentary on Aegidius)

Astrology:
Commentum super Versibus Egidii (interspersed notes)
Bartholomaeus Mariensuesz, *Commentary on the Ephemerides* (ed. Laird 1966)
Alcabitius, William of England (attr.), *Introductorium ad Scientiam Astrolologiae Iudicialis*; commentary by John of Saxony (ed. North 1976)

Alchemy:
Blamekyn (attr.), Commentary on George Ripley's Compound of Alchemy (16th c.)
Hortulanus (attr.), Commentary upon the Smaragden Table of Hermes (16th c.)
Arnaldus de Villanova, Exposition of Magister Arnald of Villanova upon the
    Commentaries of Hortulanus (16th c.)

Psychology:
Aristotle, *Parva Naturalia* or Commentary (16th c.)

A closer scrutiny revealed that only the uroscopies in the above list are strictly medical. The astrological commentaries also contain some material relevant to the present concerns, as, for example, the *homo signorum* doctrine and astrological advice for the right timing of medical treatment was included in the above commentaries. The time-lag seems to be real: four of the above texts date from the sixteenth century. Another way of searching the *eVK* database gave somewhat different results. The search for the lexeme 'comment' in the index of incipits gave several hits. Most of the hits were to different manuscript copies of Guy de Chauliac's *Chirurgia magna*, to Geber's *Testament*, which is an alchemical text, and to a uroscopy.[15] The titles and incipits give valuable evidence of the top discourse form in the vernacular, but recent textual studies have led to new discoveries which prove that more commentaries were translated into English.

3.5.1.1 Uroscopies. Uroscopies were obviously part of the commentary tradition and well-represented in vernacular texts. One of the seven manuscripts containing copies of Walter Agilon's *Commentarium urinarum* is Cambridge University Library MS Ii.6.17, ff. 5–29. Its prologue (ff. 2–5, division according to *eVK*) confirms the commentary nature of this treatise; it was perceived as a commentary by its translator, and the translation techniques are also explicated.[16] The translator seems to assume the role of a commentator in his exposition of 'hard' words:

> This boke that we haue now in hande to turne in to englissh is of the craft of vrines but whoo it is that werketh it we knowe not sauf only god. Nathelesse we suppose and vs thenketh therby **it is a coment vpon a text** of vrines that a worschepful doctor aboue rehersed seith this verified in latine . . . [illegible]. And in as moch as we may by the grace of god we wil folowe trouth through oute al this translac*i*on. Auctours seine ther ben 20 colours in vrines. . . .
>
> Here note that euer through oute al this translac*i*on we vse to write ij thinges that oon is the plaine entent of **this co*m*ment** sum time the le*tt*re in englisshe aftre the lettre in latine and sum time when the lettre is ferre fro simple menis wittes then we folowe as nighe as we may the witte of the lettre. Alsoo **we vse in this translac*i*on oure exposic*i*on of harde wordes** wherfor this thou shalt knowe that oon from that oth*r*e by the paraffes imerked that begynnyth thus here note that is *our* exposic*i*on and ther*e*with he hath a tra on this wise merked [*] ayenst him in the mergyn and euery paraff that beginnyth not w*it*h this worde here note that is the plaine entent of **this coment** and blithely it beginnyth w*it*h this worde alsoo . . . (Cambridge University Library, MS Ii.6.17, ff. 2–3)

The commentary nature of the text itself is not explicit, and though the prologue promises indications in the margin, there are no special marks, though occasional eye-catching notations, *Nota (hic)*, *Alba*, *De sanguineo*, etc. occur. The exposition of the hard words shows a concern for language, the consciousness of the need for explicitness and an effort to give precise definitions in scientific writing. The passage is marked off from the main text with impersonal metatext at the beginning and at the end, but the narrator assumes a more personal role with the authoritative first-person plural pronoun. The exposition of the hard words must have been added to the original in the translation process, thus confirming the view that the vernacular version is an adaptation rather than a faithful translation:

Nowe this said we wil expoune the harde wordes that ben said befor*e* as of adustion is brennyng of kinde for to moch hete. Digestion is diffieng and lousing of noieous mater that is aboute to make a sekenesse to man. Diuisiff is co*n*uenable departing by diuerse limmes of noious matier that is diffied. . . . These harde wordes now thus expouned turne we ayein to the 6 werkes of kinde . . . (MS Ii.6.17, ff. 3v–4)

The text has a rubric in Latin containing a statement of the audience and the time of writing 'Tractat*us* Mag*ist*ri Bartholomei ordinis Sa*ncti* Francisci *et* composuit brevit*er* in lingua materna magis plane ad intelligenti*am* laicor*um* . . . ad requisi*tio*nem Regis Ric*ardi* secundi et Anne Regine' (f. 2). The lay audience here seems to contrast to the clerical readership, and the treatise seems to be for medical doctors. They are mentioned in several places in the text, but no exact knowledge of the target group can be inferred from these references as they remain on a general level, for example 'but a leche be he phisicion or surgion but he kepe this ordre in his pacient . . .' (f. 3v), 'Note here . . . and therfor herto nedeth a phisicion to take good hede . . .' (f. 8v), 'uncunnyng leches and negligent ben cause of mannys deth' (f. 9v), and 'here thou may clerely knowe that leches oftime fallen . . .' (f. 11v).

The readers of the text encounter vivid imagery. Battle imagery is found in the introductory part of the tract, and the same theme continues throughout large parts of the text:

That when a man is seke there is withinne him a bataile betwene his kinde and his euel that is to seie sekenesse and his kinde striueth. Kinde striueth to the liff and his euel striueth to the deth and soo eithr*e* of thaim ayeinst othr*e* . . . (MS Ii.6.17, f. 3)

The humours are divided into 'friends' and 'enemies' (cf. the passage of *De proprietatibus rerum* given below). The same ascription is often attributed to planets as they are divided into the same two categories (see *eVK* incipits). The battle imagery is varied to imply captivity at this point, but goes on later, for example 'to deth if the sekenesse ouercome kinde in batail' (f. 8v).[17]

Note that ther be 4 humeros in man and 2 of thaim be frendes and 2 enemyes his 2 frendes be blode and fleume his 2 enemies ben colre and malencolie and for they be enemies kinde hath prisoned thaim wher colre in galle and malencolie in the milte. And if any of thaim breke prisone . . . they engendereth dedely sekenesse. And for blode and fleume ben frendes kinde hath yeue thaim leue to goo at large / but thair principal dwelling is in the blode and in the liuer and herte and fleume in the longes. Blode for he is hool frende goeth in al the veines of the body wher*e* that him list. And for fleume is but half frende he hath but certain places lymyted to him . . . (MS Ii.6.17, ff. 5v–6)

The text continues by providing analogues of the physiological processes, for example immediately after the above passage:

Note here howe these iiij humeros be engendered in man and that it may be bettre iknowe **haue here ensample when mete is sette ouer the fier the riseth a stome** thereupon and then it is alwaie istomed til it be ful sode and when it is ful sode the fier is withdrawe and in keling ther*e* riseth a creime . . . able to mannys mete. **On the same wise digestion wercheth** . . . (MS Ii.6.17, f. 6)

This device can go back to classical models, to the use of analogy in Greek medical treatises, for example in Hippocrates' texts; the method is connected with the induction of general laws from individual cases. Analogues often involve homely comparisons, for example the seed in the womb and burning substances, baking bread, growing plants (see Lonie 1981: 77–86). Similar devices are used in present-day scientific writing, and imagery drawn from everyday experience serves to render the subject matter more readily accessible, for example in elementary textbooks, but here the question concerns the adoption of the classical model. The intention of making the text accessible is explicitly stated in the prologue, and the translator has not only explicated difficult words but extended his explications to the physiological processes.

Another text in the same field worth mentioning in this connection is Henry Daniel's *Liber uricrisiarum*, extant in 22 manuscript copies. It is not given in the above lists as a commentary, but a closer scrutiny of the text reveals that the role of the 'I' in the text, the narrator, can at places be compared to that of a commentator.[18] However, it is not so clear who this 'I' is, as there may be several embedded text layers (cf. below, *Benvenutus Grassus*). The narrator guides the reader carefully through the text, giving his explanations with personal pleas of attention in the second-person singular. At the end of the passage the narrator employs 'we'; it could be authorial, as it does not seem to include the reader in its reference (see Wales 1996).

Quid sit vrina et vnde qualiter fit. 2^m capitulum

As seyth Gilis in his text an all auctores and commentoures, this is discripciown of vryn. Descripcioun of a thing is þe telling whate a thing is. **[Vryn is] a late and a suptyle meltyng and clenesyng of bloode and of humuris; et take hede þat I sey** 'late' for this skyll: For sumtyme þe watir passith oute of the body sone after that it is dronken . . . **Also, I sey** 'suptill,' for the more that he is decoct and digested in the body, þe more suptill is he in himsilfe and þe better profowndid in colour, as þu maiste sene in þe 2 boke. Suptil is as mykell to seyn as 'thenne, clere, and bryght.'

Item, id est also, I sey 'a meltyng, a clensing,' of þe blode and of þe humuris for þis skyll: For right **as þou sest** . . . right so the vryn is pressed . . . **Vnderstond that** massa sanguinis is not els but a collectiown, id est, a gedering togidre, of the 4 humuris . . . **as þou maiste sene** in the nexte capitle folowend. And to this forsaid descripcioun of vryn that **Gilis gevyth** acordith well þe **diffiniciown þat Ysaac and Theophele gyven.** Diffinicioun and descripciown arn all one to sayne. . . .

> Item, anoþer similitude, id est, anothir example, . . . **puttyn auctores** also, for thei callin vrin a cribracioun, id est, a sifting, . . . For right as þou sefte . . . right o the same wyse in þe secunde digestion, . . . , that we callen in Latyne epar, the lyuere in English. Of this maner of siftyng and of werkyng, se in the folowende capitle. (ed. Hanna 1994: 195–7)

The authorities are discussed throughout the treatise, but the main line remains clear: there is an authorial voice that gives the references and controls the situation and the reader's reception of the text:

> And þarefore **yu moost tak hede** at godness of þe seignes & wykkydnes, & noght anely at þe nowmbre of þame. For **Galyen sayes opon Ypocras' Empidiis** þat yef þe seik mak blak uryn in þe begynnynge . . . Alsa Galyen says þat ʒif fyrst in þe begynnynge of þe seiknes com a blak uryn, . . . And undrystand blak colour in þise 7 rewlys, ryght **as I said** in þe rewle next before þis 2 rewles. . . . **Theophile in hys Bok of Uryns** sais þat ʒif þe uryn in a fe[ver] causonides have an ypostasis blak. (ed. Jasin 1983: 145–6)

3.5.1.2 Chauliac's surgeries. Some surgical texts also belong to the academic level. Chauliac's learned anatomical and surgical text has been characterised in various ways in the literature. His *Cyrurgie* (original from 1363), for example, has been described as a compilation that urges its value as a compendium (Curtius 1990: 83–5) and as an assembly of authoritative statements with indications of sources (Demaitre 1976: 88). However, when Chauliac's position and learned background combined with his long career as a successful practising surgeon are taken into account, the logical expectation is that the writings also incorporate his own conclusions; the hits in the *eVK* database also confirm this. The following text extract illustrates Chauliac's technique: first he presents Galen's views of the structure of the skull, then mentions the views of William of Saliceto, Lanfrank, and Henri de Mondeville, and goes on to refute them. Finally, he presents his own argument in favour of Galen's view:

> So þat þer ben vij bones of þe braine panne, and so þei be noumberde in dede mennes heuedes, þe whiche ben soþen & diuidid wiþ boilinge water. . . . Also **galien noumberþ** hem in þe same maner **in þe 20. chapiter of þe elleuenþe boke de vtilitate particulari**, wher-fore it semeþ wele þat **Willelmus de Saliceto and lamfrank and henricus de hermonda-villa** also sawe euel her anothomie, for þei seien þat os passulare is vnder þe bone þat is cleped lauda . . . And þei seien also þat þe bones þat ben cleped petrosa ben added vppon þe bones þat ben cleped parietalia & þat þei touche not þe brayne, neiþer þat [þei] ben enye of þe principal bones; **but þe contrarie þer-off is soþe. And þerfore it foloweþ þat** þer ben vij. principal bones þe whiche contenen þe braine; but, neþelesse, þer ben summe oþer litil bones þat ben not principal be cause of helpinge, as þe bone of þe creste þat diuideþ oþer departeþ þe

colatories of þe nose wiþ-inne þe coronale, & bones þat ben cleped ossa paris. þe whiche ben of þe visage & nouȝt of þe braine panne. (ed. Wallner 1995: 20–1)

Chauliac's approach to individual topics is often that of a commentator, and in many cases he begins by giving a final judgement. Thus his work could perhaps be characterised as a collection of thematic commentaries, a view further corroborated by Chauliac's own vision of what he was doing (see above).

3.5.1.3 Hippocrates' Prognostica *in Middle English translation.* The impression of vernacular commentaries being biased in favour of practical applications is further enhanced by a recent discovery by Teresa Tavormina. She detected a fifteenth-century English translation of a commentary of Hippocrates' *Prognostica*, one of the *Articella* texts, in Cambridge, Trinity College MS R.14.52, ff. 62–104. The commentary nature of the text was revealed only by a meticulous analysis of the sources. The word 'comment' does not occur in the title, incipit, or rubric of the text, and its true nature has not been identified earlier. Other such cases may well be detected.

Hippocrates' *Prognostica* deals with the signs of death to be recognised in the patient. The commentary technique is illustrated by the following extract which begins with a passage from the original Hippocratic text listing visible signs of approaching death on the patient's face. It is followed by a list of comments by several later scholars. All three layers of commentary tradition can be detected: Greek, Arab and medieval Latin. The passage ends with a first-person singular commentary in which the author, the last commentator, expresses his own opinion and takes responsibility for the conclusions.

> And the maner of it is as that his nose be sharp or his nosethrilles sharp holow eyed . . . **The Cardynal saith** th'auctor descendens to the parties of the face, that if his nosethrilles bien sharp and holowe eyen &c., al thiese bien dedly. . . . **after Bartilmew.** . . . **Galien saith** vpon this in prouerbis that al thiese significaciouns . . . **And Galien saith** furthermore in the same place that in the nose is . . . **And Ipocras of sum markith** nat the nose bi the sharpnes . . . **After Haly therfor** this maner seemyth the extremytes of the sharp nose fforsoth the depnesse of eyen . . . **This Galien and Bernard of Gordien iiij particules in their prouerbis:** of signes appieryng in the face and of eyen, sum bien whiche appieren in the first daies; bien thiese: holowe eyen . . . **I sey than that thiese bitokenen nat deth,** forwhi yit standith vertu and strength in the herte and in the principal membris. If forsoth suche thynges comen for the sikenes, thei don nat only in the vtter parties but rather first and principaly in the mynes, with as fervent heete in the herte as in the forhede. (ed. Tavormina forthcoming)

Yet the commentary style is not consistent throughout the text. For example, opinions by Galen and Cardinal are listed in a lengthy passage without conclusions or overt expression of the author's own opinion. This passage is in accordance with compilations rather than commentaries, and shows how intimately these two discourse forms are connected:

> That if in to the xl day so it abide the fever nat failyng in to filthed it turneth and al the apostem aboute the wombe to this maner shal be demed. That if &c.: **Galien saith** vpon this place in the precendentis it is spoken **Ipocras** in hote apostemes that helth gadrith in hem whan fever restith nat nor exspirith aposteme and resoluith bi xx daies. In this sermon he settith the terme of helth in cold apostems in the xl day. And **after the Cardynal** if this maner aposteme be nat endid and determyned bifore the xl day, thei turn in to filthed; and in suche thynges if vertu be founde strong in the xl day it is goode to pronostik. If it be fieble to pronostik is tourned from aposteme in to stinche and in to deth. And **the Cardynal seith that Galien** puttith the craft general to know the termynacioun of al apostemes, forwhi **after Galien** the matiers other thei bien hote, colde, or myxt. If hote, so thei han to be determyned in the xx day; if cold, in the lx day; if myxt, other the filthed tornyth to hete or to cold and after that is to be pronostikt of determynacioun bitwene-while. (ed. Tavormina forthcoming)

3.5.1.4 Texts in the natural-philosophical tradition in Middle English. In the Latin academic tradition, texts with a focus on natural-philosophical theory and the topic of human generation, are frequently subject to commentary (Cadden 1993: 69). A Middle English translation of the pseudo-Galenic *De spermate* in the same Cambridge, Trinity College MS R.14.52 is a representative of this genre in the vernacular (ed. Pahta 1998). It is, however, more typically a compilation as the following example discussing the nature of the soul shows. Several authorities are cited and their opinions are explained, but no conclusions are drawn.

> **Porphirius sum considerith** nat the soule but considerith the lifly spirite racional. And therfor **Porphirius hath compowned and made Ysagogas as bi theym shal be shewed** that corporat spirite to be to thuse of the soule, nat the same soule. But **Socrates, Plato, Aristotil, Theodorus, Platoniciens, Andronices, Perypaticis, Pophilijs, and many mo other of oon wil affermen** that . . . Ginnomios the philosopher saith no wounder to be the soule, whiche is the substaunce in body, may be separat and departed from the body with fuyre . . . **Aristotil saith in Phisic** to be v parties of the soule . . . The soule, whiche whan he is greved of nature of the bodie, whan nature of his body goeth to the iiij elementis . . . yieldith þe soule cliere in hevene. But **Porphirius, nat consentyng to Aristotil,** saith that non of thiese partes departith from the substaunce of soule . . . **Porphirius shewith** this maner . . . (ed. Pahta 1998: 217–25)

Even if some conclusions are occasionally drawn, it remains unclear who is responsible for the conclusions, the author himself or Hippocrates, whom the author quotes.

> **Witnes Ipocras seyeng,** 'I sawe a womman preignaunt with chield leten bloode bi the arme and so the thrid day sent out abortief.' **The causes therfor considred whi it fille, it appierith** the nature of the womman to withold bloode to the reformacioun of hir chield. **No wounder that** a man hath nat menstruat so as womman, for whi a man hath poores bi whiche his bloode issueth, whiche torneth into pilis, as it appierith in armes and in feete and in other parties, bi mowth and nose sendith out a strengger spirit than a womman, bi whiche is dryed the humour of that bloode whiche is sent out bi swet. (ed. Pahta 1998: 169–71)

It is impossible to know the source manuscript of the translation, but it is certain that the role of the translator in this case cannot be compared to that of a commentator (Pahta 1998, Pahta and Carrillo Linares forthcoming).

3.5.1.5 Benvenutus Grassus's ophthalmological treatise.   The ophthalmological treatise associated with Benvenutus Grassus (ed. Eldredge 1996) also comes close to the thematic commentary. The beginning of the text states in the third-person singular that Benvenutus adds his opinion to those of ancient authors of philosophy and physic, particularly Johannitius.

> A grete phylosopher and a profunde phycycyane clepid **Benuonucius Grapheus, after the sentence of þe [of] olde auctors of phelozophie and of phisyk** whiche he had radde, **and after hys propre experyence** the wych he had by long contynuance of his owne practik yn dyuerse parties of the world, boyth yn hote regyons and colde, by influence **and help of goddys grace, compilyd and made a** boke of the sekenes of eyon and of her curys. . . . Consequently **he shewyth** how an ey is made. Ffirst **he rehersyth** the opynyon of a gret leche clepid Johannicius and **after he puttyth hys owne opinyon. Johannicius in his Ysagogys seyth** that an ey hath vij tunycles, or vij cootis, iiij colors, and iij humors. . . . Thus sayth Johannicius. **But Benuonucius varieth** from hym in cotys and yn colours, ffor as **he seyth** an ey hath but ij tonycles or cotys. (ed. Eldredge 1996: 49–50)

The text has a special feature not encountered so conspicuously in other texts. The vernacular treatise seems to be written by someone else, not Benvenutus himself (cf. Henry Daniel's text above), and it may contain several layers. As can be seen in the above passage, Benvenutus is mentioned in the third-person singular, and the text gives the impression of a paraphrase or report of his work. If this layer is an addition in the vernacular, it could perhaps reflect the translator's more prominent contribution in text production as he seems to be the narrator in this text, taking an outsider's role. He comments upon the text, asserting something in his own right, and the text is an adaptation or a paraphrase in the vernacular rather than a direct translation. Eldredge (1996: 37–8) pays attention to this peculiarity and identifies three phases of distancing: in the first the authority of the original author is asserted in the third person in phrases like 'After hys doctrine'; in the second impersonal constructions are used, and the passive voice prevails 'Thyes iiij speces ben curable'; and in the third direct instructions are given to the reader in the imperative mood. At places the translator puts himself in the author's place and gives statements in the first-person singular. An example below shows how the commentator's own views and conclusions are incorporated into the text:

> And as for the humors **thys auctor and [Johannicius] accorde yn.** Ther ben thre humours of the whiche the first is said albugineus . . . Therfor **y saye** that the complexioun of the first albuginosi humour is colde and moyste. (ed. Eldredge 1996: 52)

Yet in some interpersonal passages the 'I' seems to be Benvenutus, especially in efficacy phrases like 'as I haue prouyd by experience'. The alternative is that the translator places himself on an equal standing with the original author as a practising physician and assumes an authorial stance (cf. quotations above), and it is perhaps impossible to discern who is who in the layers of writing.

3.5.2 Compilations

A typical form of compilation from various sources can be found in treatises which purport to explain the order of the universe, beginning with the Creation, from God and angels proceeding in a hierarchical order to the macrocosm of the universe and the microcosm of man, animals, herbs and other manifestations of nature (see above). In the vernacular, the scope of encyclopaedic treatises seems to have been wide as it encompasses both texts that mediate knowledge to the learned and to a more popular audience. Middle English astrological literature provides several examples of encyclopaedic compilations of both kinds (see Taavitsainen 1988: 34).

3.5.2.1 Encyclopaedias on the learned level.

On the Properties of Things is John Trevisa's vernacular translation from 1398/9 of Bartholomaeus's learned encyclopaedic work De proprietatibus rerum, which contains medical sections (see above). The chapters with knowledge of this field bring together views expressed by a large number of medical authorities, but they do not contain explicit comments or opinions by the author himself. Trevisa's translation seems to be faithful to the original. In the book on human anatomy, Bartholomaeus adopts a consistent organisation: the description of each organ begins with an explanation of its name, exact configuration and activity, followed by a diversity of facts and comparisons; usually the chapters end by describing ailments and their symptoms (Seymour et al. 1992: 59). The example below illustrates the form of this work as a thematic compilation where opinions of early authors on the properties of the nose are given in a straightforward listing.

> De proprietatibus nasy. Capitulum 13m.
>
> Isidir seiþ þat þe nose is þe instrument of smellinge, and haþ þe name of þe noseþrilles . . . Constantinus seiþ þat þe nose haþ tweye hooles þat ben departid atwynne by a maner grustelbone . . . instrumentis of smellinge ben tweye holowȝ fleischly gobettis þat hongiþ from þe nosetrilles . . . So seiþ Constantyn . . .
>
> Constantinus seiþ þat þe nose is nedeful to drawe in aier temperatlyche, to clense and purge þe brayn . . . And þerfore libro 12° Aristotel seiþ þe witt of smellynge is departid as þe witt of hierynge . . . As Constantinus seiþ, þe nosethrilles ben isette . . . And also super Cantica Galyen seiþ þat þe nose hyȝteþ most þe face . . . Þe disposiciouns of þe membres of þe body tokeneþ and bodeþ þe affecciouns and wil of þe soule, as þe philosofir seiþ in principio physiognomie. For þe chaunginges of þe soule ben ofte ilikned and iknowe by þe changinges of þe body . . . as þe philosophir seiþ in libro suo, in principio. Super pronostica Galien seiþ þe nose is ilette of his doynge and worchinge . . . as Galien seiþ . . . Libro 9° capitulo 15° Constantinus seiþ þe nose is somtyme ilette by euel disposicioun of þe brayne . . . And in amphorismorum particula vi°. it is iseide: mulieri deficientibus menstruis it is good to blede atte nose. (ed. Seymour et al. 1975: 192–4)

The sources are nearly consistent in each passage (Seymour et al. 1992: 59–60). The academic quality of the work can be seen in the frequency of definitions, showing that accuracy was a concern of the author. Other passages are constructed according to the same pattern, as the following passage about humours and elements shows. The title is in Latin and the text begins with a relational definition in which two noun phrases are conjoined with 'is' and the equation is then elaborated. The definition is followed by quotations from authorities, and an important definition of health is embedded.

> De humoribus et eorum generacione effectu operacione. Capitulum 6ᵐ.
>
> An humour is a substaunce fletinge in dede, and is ibred and comeþ of gederinge of þe element qualitees, and apt to norische and fede þe membres and to counforte þe worchingis þerof kyndeliche, . . . Constantinus seiþ þat þe humoures beþ iclepid þe children of þe elementis, for eueriche of þe humours comeþ of qualite of elementis. And þere beþ foure humours: blood, flewme, colera, and melencolia. And beþ iclepid symple . . . Þise foure humours, if þey beþ in euene proporcioun in quantite and qualite, he fediþ alle bodyes þat haþ blood and makeþ hem parfite and kepiþ in þe beinge and state of helþe; as aȝenward, if þey beþ vneuen in proporcioun and infecte, þanne þey brediþ eueles. . . . Constantyne seiþ þat among þe foure humours blood is þe moste ipreised and most frend of

kynde for euene and parfite seþinge; þerof temperat hete makeþ blood of clene aier[y] mater to þe norischinge of þe body. **Constantine** [s]eiþ þat þe blood is kindeliche bloode and som vnkindeliche. . . . . **Aristoteles in libro de animalibus 3° capitulo** [setteþ] oþir propirtees of blood . . . (ed. Seymour *et al*. 1975: 147–50)

The sources are Aristotle's zoology; translations and commentary of Constantinus, viz. *Viaticum, Pantegni*, and *De melancholia*; Galen's commentary in Gerard's translation; Hippocrates' *Aphorisms*; and other authors like Avicenna and Isidore (Seymour *et al*. 1992: 54). The topic of this passage is also treated in the uroscopy text in Cambridge University Library MS Ii.6.17 (see above), but the passage in *De proprietatibus rerum* seems to differ from it in several respects: it contains direct quotations from authorities and refers to them with specific references; it employs Latin much more extensively, and the whole discourse is more specific. This encyclopaedia is a seminal achievement of the mid-thirteenth century, and some chronological developments have been detected in its transmission. In a recent study (Holbrook 1998), the structure and the expository style of Bartholomaeus's work were related to the practices of memorial reading and textbook use of the work. In Wynkyn de Worde's first printed edition from *c*. 1495, adaptations could be found, perhaps according to its intended audience. The overall design of the book with its layout supports the idea of system as in the original composition. The pictures function as visual texts, carrying scientific ideas (cf. religious illustrations for the public); their function is to introduce readers to the circle of learning, making the contents of the learned text accessible to a wider readership. The use of Latin in the rubrics relates to the vernacularisation process and forms part of the scheme (cf. Pahta in this volume).

3.5.2.2 An astrological encyclopaedia. The lower end of the scale of compilations in prose is represented by the anonymous *Wise Book of Astronomy and Astrology*. The encyclopaedic form of discourse imitates the more learned type. The treatise begins with cosmology and the order of the angels, as in Bartholomaeus's treatise. The organisation of the text is not, however, as consistent. The beginning of the text is similar in various manuscripts and forms a coherent whole, but after the common core, the texts differ and the compilation process seems open-ended. There is no clear division into chapters and it is difficult to determine where the book ends in some cases.[19] The items consist of various prognosticatory tracts and may have been copied from various sources. Thus the manuscripts show different biases perhaps according to the individual interests of the compiler (cf. commonplace books), or perhaps in adaptation to the intended audiences and their interests. Some are more matter-of-fact, while some include more superstitious and magical materials. A survey of the manuscripts of the *Wise Book* in the *Handlists* of the *Index of Middle English Prose* shows that the incipits do not differ much, but the explicit was different in each and the cut-off point varies. Further studies of this text are needed, and they may reveal interesting aspects of the transmission of practical adaptations of informative texts.

3.5.2.3 The Guild-Book of the Barber-Surgeons of York. The medieval scheme of encyclopaedic knowledge included the correspondences of the microcosm of man and the macrocosm of the universe, with projections to the natural world, for example the seasons, and the system covered everything (see Burrow 1986, cf. *Sidrak and Bokkus* below). The Guild-Book of the Barber-Surgeons of York contains tables of correspondences, treatises of astrological medicine, and explanations of the basic conceptions.[20] Texts with explicit knowledge of the readership are valuable as they provide anchorage points for the scale from learned to more popular. The Guild-Book of the Barber-Surgeons of York, London, British Library, Egerton MS 2572, may well illuminate what kind of knowledge was considered necessary and appropriate for professional practitioners with a guild background. It contains a calendar and fine illustrations of *homo venarum* (f. 50) and *homo signorum* (f. 50v), a volvelle with the patron saints, and illustrations of the complexions with Christ's head in the middle. There are also tables and charts of astrological influences (ff. 52–54). A treatise with a reference to Salerno as the place of origin is given under the title 'Here yt tellethe of Mannys kynde of the Elementis that acordis to mane' (f. 54v). It begins with explanations of the theoretical basis of medicine, but it soon turns to practical applications. Praise of the usefulness of the knowledge is prominent, but the text itself is a matter-of-fact account of the basic concepts with some simple advice:

> There er 4 Elementes of the Worlde that ys to wytte Aer & Eyr Ignis & ffyer Terra & Erthe Aqua & Wattir
>
> Also there is 4 Humours in a Mane that ys Sanguis & Blode ffel rubi*um* & Rede colowre ffel Nigr*um* & Blake colowre malicoly ffluma & fflume
>
> Also there beyne 4 tymes of the ʒere that ys to weyte Ver*e* Estas Autumpnus and Iemps and thoo tymes lastes os ytt telles eftirwarde and tho 4 tymes <acordes vnto the 4 Elementis of the Worlde & to the > 4 humours in a man and howe a man sholde gouerne hym selfe be all thyes tymes to leue in heyll that he ne gendre no corupcione within hym ne no pestelence . . .
>
> Here ys the fyst tyme of the ʒere and fyrst humoure of man and fyrst Element
>
> Ver ys the ffyrst tyme of the ʒere and in hym abundithe sanguis blode that ys the ffyrst humoure in a man and yt acordis wyth ayre that ys the ffyrst Element of the Worlde an yt ys most and hote as Ver ys. **In this tyme ys gude solyble drynke to purge** mane frome wykyde / humouris **And ys gude to blede** skylfully i*n* tyme for blode ys þane habundant in man And **a** ma*n* **sholde not eytte** that tyme mekyll . . . (London, British Library, Egerton 2572, ff. 54v–55r)

More advice on food and drink follows. Canicular Days are given next, with concise *homo signorum* explanations and advice (f. 57), 'And therefore eu*ery* leche shall be were and not carffe no member yf the mone be in the signe of the signe of the member'. Other astrological information forms a considerable part of the contents: a practical adaptation of lunar astrology is included as well as nativities according to the planets. The contents are partly similar to the prognostications that are often found in the manuscripts with the *Wise Book*.

3.6   The question–answer discourse form

The question–answer formula appears first in verse in early English scientific writing, in a rhymed encyclopaedia *Sidrak and Bokkus*, which has medical components. The edition of *Sidrak and Bokkus* is only recent (Burton 1998–99), and this treatise has not been widely discussed in the literature. To check if any other texts in the same format can be found in unedited material I consulted the *eVK* database, the *IMEP* handlists, and Keiser's *Manual of Writings in Middle English* (1998). A search of the word 'question' in the index of incipits in *eVK* gave several hits, but only a few indicated an interactive text form with questions and answers.[21] These treatises are either alchemical or astrological, so that some overlap with medical texts can be expected. Some of the incipits point to expert-novice dialogues, but the text itself may unfold without the interactive pattern. The contrary may also be true: a treatise called *Thesaurus pauperum* is a dialogue with useful information on the basic concepts of health as humoral balance, etc., ending with a collection of recipes.[22] Titles with the word 'question' in the same database belong to sixteenth-century alchemical or astrological texts. A search in the *Corpus of Middle English Medical Texts* (*MEMT*) proved that questions are encountered sporadically in edited materials.[23] The discourse form appears in early printed books in the sixteenth century (see below). In the following, the scope of treatises in this text form is outlined through case studies.

3.6.1 Sidrak and Bokkus: *'La fontaine de toutes science'*[24]

Sidrak and Bokkus is an encyclopaedic treatise in the question–answer format, cast as a dialogue between Sidrak, a Christian philosopher and prophet, and the heathen King Bokkus. The frame story leads the reader to expect a saint's life or medieval romance in the world of fiction, but the contents prove to be a digest of medieval knowledge of theology, dogma, morals and scientific matters, amalgamated from several sources. The date of the original composition in French is probably as early as 1246, and there are several dozen manuscripts extant from the medieval period in French, English (seven), and other European vernaculars. There are also early printed books from the sixteenth century (Burton 1998, 1: xxi–xxv).

The readership of the text must have been fairly wide. The prologue to the Reader of the printed version from 1530 assures the utility of the book for 'al men', even the illiterate are addressed with a direct admonition to listen carefully:

Than is this boke necessary to **al men.** For it exhortyth to wysdome, good maners, ensamples hystoryis, wherefore it may well be called a boke of philosopfye, that is to say a stody of wysdome. Than **I consayle euery man to rede** this boke, **or that cannot rede to geue dylygent eere** to the reder for they shal fynde therin great frute bothe to the soule and body. (Cambridge University Library, Peterborough. Sp. 27, p. ii, not numbered)

The treatise seems to have been a valued source of information, for example the above-quoted copy of the early printed book in Cambridge University Library shows signs of serious study.[25] There are marginal notes, underlinings, and attention marks in passages on moral matters, behaviour, or dealing with skin colour and climate, and the passage of the seven deadly sins enumerates them carefully in the margin (f. gj^v). The few medical sections with study markings deal with childbirth or natural philosophical matters, for example, the following answer to the question about the abode of the soul is marked as important:

Blode is vessel for the sowle truly
And of the blode is the body
And where as blode raynyth nothing
There hath the sowle no dwelling
As in teth and heer also.
(Peterborough. Sp.27, h.iij)

It is also indicative of a wide audience that copies of the French *Sidrak and Bokkus* were owned by important figures in the English political scene in the fourteenth and fifteenth centuries, including Simon Burley, tutor to Richard II (Burton 1998, 1: xxxiii). Thus there is external evidence of its use by the learned élite of the time, but whether it reached the illiterate audience remains open.

Unlike the learned prose encyclopaedias discussed above, the structure of *Sidrak and Bokkus* is not coherent. The scientific questions are dispersed in the text, and they do not form a whole. Some of the topics discussed in *Sidrak and Bokkus* are also treated in the learned encyclopaedias, for example in *De proprietatibus rerum*. Burton (1998, 1: xxxi) illustrates the difference between these two works by commenting on the sections on intestinal worms (*Sidrak and Bokkus* question 251, *De proprietatibus rerum* VII.49). *Sidrak* tells that worms are bred and live off 'the mukke of the grettest metes / That a man other woman etes' (B7541–2), whereas the learned encyclopaedia discerns several different types of worm according to the part of the intestine and the type of humour from which they are bred, their effect on the body, and methods of getting rid of them. The levels of specificity are very different. The literary form is simple verse in rhyming couplets with a common stock of rhyme words.[26] The dialogue form has been characterised as a 'cathecism' without conflict (Burton 1998, 1: xxvii). The pupil accepts the teacher's answers without argument or further queries, and the text proceeds to the next question, which total 362 in all. The following passage introduces the basic concepts of the humours (cf. above):

Ca. xxxviij Telle me now, if þat þou can, / Þe perilousest þinges þat ben
    in man.
Foure colours a man haþ him ynne / Þat of foure complexiouns bigynne:
Þe firste is blood, þat may not misse; / The seconde blak colour is, ywisse;
Þe þridde is flewme, white on to se; / And ȝelow colour þe fourþe is he;
And if a man of þise wantid oon, / His body were deed anoon.

(ed. Burton 1998, 1: 497)

The representation is straightforward and simple.[27] The last line refers to the
conception of health as balance (cf. the quotation from Bartholomaeus), but it
has been reduced to a blunt statement of the cause of death. The didactic tone
of the treatise becomes very clear in instructive passages, for example the above
extract continues with links to the seasons (cf. the Guild-book):

And eueriche bihoueþ to be / At his sesoun in his pouste;
And if any maister hem alle / Out of time þat it shulde him falle,
To þe sikenesse þe body falleþ: / Perilous þerfore men him calleþ.
And eueriche haþ his powere / In diuerse quarters of þe ȝere:
Capricorne, Aquarie, and Pisses – / Þre þinges þe firste quarter ches;
And of flewmes haue þei mighte / And wete and colde is her righte:
In Decembre þei begynne / And in þe midle of Mars þei blynne –
Þat is þe coldeste time of alle / For þat is þat we winter calle . . .

(ed. Burton 1998, 1: 499)

The application of the theory of humours is very basic, and illustrates dissemination of knowledge in an easily memorisable form. The aim here is obviously to
explain the existing order according to the correspondences. The lines dealing
with autumn end with a promise of a reward by taking heed of the contents of the
book; this is a common formula in practical medical lore and resembles efficacy
phrases in recipes.

And whoso þise foure times couþe him ȝeme / And serue his kinde in
    him to queme,
From perelles he miȝte kepe him longe, / And in hele holde his lymes
    stronge.

(ed. Burton 1998, 1: 501)

3.6.2 Guido's Questions

A fully-developed question–answer formula in a purely medical treatise is found
in a text from 1542 (*STC* 12468), in *Questyonary of cyrurygens*, reissued in 1579
as *Guido's Questions* (*STC* 12469). The name refers to Guy de Chauliac, and a
comparison with his anatomy book confirms the source. Both follow the common pattern of starting with definitions about surgery, the qualities of a good
surgeon, and reasons for studying anatomy, and then proceed to deal with the
different parts of the body and their functions. The answers vary in scope: some

are treated in a cursory manner, though the original has lengthy explications, some others are more faithful renderings of Chauliac's text. The text components are not, however, in the same order, which makes it more difficult to detect the resemblances. The following passages illuminate the technique of adapting and transforming the basic text into the question form. The first is the definition of the term 'anatomy'. In Chauliac's text the passage is brief:

> And þis word **anothomia** is seide of þis worde ano, þat is it to seyen, riȝt oþer euen, and of þis worde thomas, þat is to seien, departinge, as a riȝte diuisioun oþer a riȝte departinge. (ed. Wallner 1995: 4)

In *Guido's Questions* a straightforward pattern is imposed upon it:

> Question. What is Anatomie, and whereoff is it deriuate.
>
> Aunswere. Anatomie is the right determination and diuision of euery particuler member of the bodye of mankinde. And is deriuate of Ana, that is to saye, (right) that is to say (diuision.) Thus Anatomie, is called right diuision of members, done for certeine knowledges.
>
> (*Guido's Questions* 1579, f. 5v)

Other question–answer sequences are constructed in the same manner, for example the following:

> **Anothomie is founden in two maners:** þe tone is bi **doctryne of bokes,** þe whiche manere, alle ȝif þat it be profitabel, ȝit it is not sufficient for to tellen openlye þo þinges þat be knowen to mennes wittes allonelye, as **Galien** seiþ in þe eiȝtene chapiter of þe firste boke de vtilitate particulari. And þerfore **Aueroys** seide in þe first boke off Colliget: We make not schort to speke of þe anothomye but be cause þat oure ymaginacioun is schorte in sucche þingis and litil in comparisoun of þo þingis þat ben in þe anothomie. **þe toþer maner** of ffyndinge of þe anothomye is þurȝ **experience** of dede bodies[;] we haue experience off oure anothomye in bodies . . . as **Mundyne of boloyne** treteþ, þe whiche Mundyne wrote a boke of þe anothomye, . . . (ed. Wallner 1995: 5)

> Question. In how many & which manners ought the science of Anatomie to be taught.
>
> Aunswere. **In two manners,** that is to say, by way of **doctrine as by bookes** written thereoff. In seeing & reading that which hath bene written by **auncient Doctors,** and **by experience,** in deuising and Anatomising the deade corpses. As did **Mundy and Boloine,** and as lykewise did master Bertuce.
>
> (*Guido's Questions* 1579, f. 5v)

The above examples demonstrate the technique of recasting a medieval text into a new format. The reason for doing it may be the suitability of the question–answer formula for didactic purposes and textbook use.

3.7   Conclusions

The research questions outlined at the beginning deal with the extent and character of the discourse forms of commentaries, compilations, and question–answer formulae in the vernacular. Originally all these text forms were institutional and academic, and there was a hierarchy with research-based commentaries at the top. In the vernacular, the texts lost their original function in the non-institutional setting. It is likely that they were targeted at a wider audience. Compilations in particular were valued as useful and economic, saving the trouble of extensive study. They were useful to medical professionals and to lay people. In this study, I tried to follow up the transmission of some basic doctrines and assess how some underlying principles are explained in these texts. Differences are obvious especially on the level of specificity. Translations of learned texts are detailed and accurate, while elementary instruction in verse omits details and gives generalised rules.

The top-level discourse form, the commentary, is not very common when defined according to modern criteria. There is evidence that classical Greek authors were translated into the vernacular, for example commentaries on Hippocratic texts exist, but no editions are available yet and few texts have been studied in detail. According to prior expectations, vernacular commentaries have a practical orientation. A closer scrutiny revealed unexpected features: a text may be explicitly called a commentary but prove to be an explanation of basic concepts and physiological processes, without any discussion of learned opinions or authorial conclusions. My study indicates that the word 'comment' in the title or prologue shows how the treatise was perceived in its own time, but the discourse features of the ensuing text may deviate from the expected norms. According to the definition in the literature, the vernacular version of Walter Agilon's commentary is not a typical commentary in its structure and organisation. It does not build upon quotations of authors in an attempt to conciliate the views, but the focus is instead on making the contents of the uroscopy available for an audience studying the text in the vernacular and guiding the reception, making the contents as easily accessible as possible. Thus a great deal of attention is paid to the explication of terms and presenting the processes by analogues. In comparison, Henry Daniel's text builds upon passages quoted from various authorities, comparing them but keeping the discourse under control by frequent metatext and by presenting the commentator's own opinions. The role of the translator seems to vary in texts, and several layers can be discerned in some texts. It is possible that the translator was instrumental, for example, in distancing the text into the third-person commentary, but the present examples are ambiguous and more studies are needed to make more definite statements. The reverse is also true: the text may show typical commentary features without being explicitly entitled or described as such. It is evident that the criterion of taking responsibility for one's opinions, drawing conclusions and conciliating conflicting views, does not hold. Commentaries often contain quotations without taking sides, and they can be characterised as thematic compilations, i.e. they bring together opinions of various authorities on a particular topic, but no conclusions are made nor is conciliation attempted. It seems that commentaries and compilations overlap to a great extent in the fifteenth century. Chauliac's learned texts combine both forms, and the hierarchy of text forms applies to the earlier medieval period only.

Encyclopaedias are compilations of knowledge. The texts in this category range widely from learned compilations to elementary instruction in easily memorisable form. Yet it seems hazardous to draw any conclusions about the level of learning of the audiences, as according to the surviving evidence the readership of texts that seem popular included people of the highest ranks of society and professionals in the field of medicine (see *Sidrak and Bokkus* above; Taavitsainen 1988, Slack 1979). The question–answer formula was particularly suitable for elementary instruction, but some differentiating features between the levels of writing can perhaps be discerned. The discourse form is found sporadically in medical prose writing in the fifteenth century and in a consistent form only in the sixteenth century, while some other branches of science may have adopted it earlier. At one end of the scale such texts seem to have gained an entertaining function alongside of instruction, which is their primary function. The utility and profit of the texts is constantly emphasised.

Latin discourse forms have not been studied in detail yet, but on the basis of the above examples, it seems that the core forms were adopted from classical texts. It is impossible to say at which stage the discourse forms start to overlap and merge. The converging development of commentaries and compilations, for example, is likely to have taken place in Latin writing. Compilations prove to be a broad category in the vernacular. At one end thematic compilations become fused with commentaries, while the compilation process seems to be at work at the other end, and verges on the type of activity found in commonplace books. In general, vernacular medical texts were useful texts of instruction and practical knowledge, with some theory in a basic and easily memorisable form. This study shows that the epistemological levels of medical education are not found in the vernacular writing as such, but even at the top level practical applications dominate and basic instruction is included. There is a great deal of variation between individual texts. The discourse forms are perhaps more mixed than expected. The scale seems to be wide: there are texts with theoretical considerations transferred from the Latin exemplars without changes, but the same doctrines have become reduced in some adaptations. Great differences are found in the degree of specificity, for example. It may be possible to trace the transmission of scientific ideas to various audiences with a detailed comparison of the content and styles of writing (see Taavitsainen forthcoming). More definitive conclusions would require a larger textual basis, and more studies on the Latin background.

Notes

1. Original compositions are said to have been written in English, especially in the field of surgery, the spearhead of medical advancement in many respects (Voigts 1984; 1989b: 390). Most treatises even in this field were translations and compilations (see note 3).

2. Several scientists wrote in both languages. John Caius wrote his other works in Latin, but his book on the sweating sickness was written in English in 1552. In the following century Francis Bacon's *The Advancement of Learning* (1605) is in English, but *Novum Organum* (1620) in Latin. Harvey wrote his treatise on the circulation of blood (1628) in Latin. Newton's *Optics* (1704) is in English. All lectures, disputations, and orations were in Latin at the universities in the medieval and Early Modern periods. The rule of speaking Latin prevailed in Queen's College, Cambridge, as late as 1677 (Burke and Porter 1987: 7).

3. Surgical treatises by Lanfranc of Milan, Roger of Salerno, William Saliceto and Henri de Mondeville, also translated into English, originated in university teaching texts; John Arderne was a practising surgeon without a university background, but he, too, wrote in Latin (P. M. Jones 1989: 61, 64).

4. The *Middle English Dictionary* (*MED*) gives the following definition of the word *comment* (n.):
(a) An expository treatise; (b) a comment or explanation, pl. a body of comments, a commentary or exposition. The examples of (a) come from Lanfrank (Ashmole 1396), Chauliac (Paris ang. 25), and the *Babee's Book*; of (b) the quotations are from Trevisa's translations. Other relevant words in *MED* include *com(m)entacioun* (n.) An exposition (of a field of knowledge); *commentaries* (n. (pl.)) A body of comments, a commentary; *commentaten* (v.) To write an exposition or commentary, expound (a text); *com(m)enten* (v.) (a) To expound or explain (sth.); *commenting* (ger.) Exposition (of a field of knowledge); and *glose* (n.) (a) A gloss or explanatory comment on a text or word; a series or collection of glosses. This word also occurs with pejorative connotations.

5. Chaucer's frequent references show that the knowledge was widely spread throughout Europe and the target audience of, for example, the *Parliament of Birds* must have understood them. See the *Riverside Chaucer* (ed. Benson).

6. *MED* defines *compilacioun* (n.) as (a) composing; (b) composition or compilation. The examples come from Lydgate and religious verse. *Compiling* (ger.) is defined as (a) compiling a report; (b) a compilation (as of papal degrees). No examples come from scientific texts.

7. According to our study, Greek physicians are predominant in learned theoretical writings, while surgeries also mention near-contemporary authors. Recipes quote a wider range of authorities but, in general, the references are less frequent and less precise.

8. The *MED* entry of *digest* (n.) gives it as a collection of laws; esp. the compilation of Roman laws made by order of the Emperor Justinian. The *Oxford English Dictionary* (*OED*) gives an example from Bacon's *The Advancement of Learning* II xv § I.58 where the word is used in the modern sense: 'The Disposition . . of that Knowledge . . consisteth in a good Digest of Common Places'.

9. Even remedybook materials such as recipes could be commented upon; there is only a small step from marginal notes testifying to the efficacy and the uselessness of various recipes to more comprehensive explications and comparisons between various cures, with the author's own conclusions and recommendations.

10. The *Articella* and the Constantinian translations differed significantly, as the former derived from Greek texts and was in accordance with the practical orientation of early Salernitan medicine. The Constantinian translations derived from Arabic texts and incorporated theory and natural philosophy as well. Both were manifestations of a trend towards learned, written medicine (Cadden 1993: 68).

11. The list of textbooks used in the Faculty of Medicine at Paris in the late twelfth century illustrates the repertoire: *Isagoge* of Johannitius, *Aphorismi* and *Pronostica* of Hippocrates, *Tegny* i.e. *Ars parva*, *Viaticum* of Constantinus Africanus, *De urines* and *De pulsibus* of Theophilos Protospatharios, *Materia medica* of Dioscorides and its abbreviation *De simplici medicina*, *Macer floridus* and *De arte medica*. These works also constitute the major medical sources of *De proprietatibus rerum* (Seymour *et al.* 1992: 23–4).

12. Such references are found mostly in recipes stating the source of knowledge. Some authorities are mentioned by name, for example 'Cophon þe leche of Salerne' and 'maystyr Peers of Salerne'. The formulation may also be more general, for example, to 'the fyrst lechys of Salerne', 'the grete lechys of Salerne' (Benvenutus Grassus, ed. Eldredge), or just to 'the scoll of Salerne' ('Morstede', ed. Beck).

13. Some manuscripts give detailed information about their provenance, for example Cambridge, Gonville and Caius College MS 176/97 was commissioned by a London barber-surgeon Thomas Plawdon, and Cambridge, Trinity College MS 0.9.37 was owned by Richard Dod, another London barber-surgeon (P. M. Jones 1989: 61–2). Studies of the library catalogues give valuable information about the readership of texts. There are detailed studies, for example, about Roger Marshall (Voigts 1995a), and John Argentine (Rhodes 1956).

14. Parts of this section, especially 3.5.1.3 and 3.5.1.4, are based on joint work with Dr Päivi Pahta for a paper 'Transferring classical discourse forms into vernacular: Commentaries in early English medical writing', read at the Kalamazoo Medieval Studies Conference in May 2001. I am grateful to her, and to Prof. Teresa Tavormina for the background information on the Hippocrates' text and for allowing me to quote from her forthcoming edition.

15. The hits were to the following manuscripts and texts: Guy de Chauliac, *Chirurgia magna* (*Capitulum singulare*): London, British Library, Sloane MS 1, ff. 1–7 (incomplete); Tokyo, Takamiya 59, ff. 2–3 (incomplete), Wallner version 1; Tokyo, Takamiya 59 *olim* Manchester Chetham's 27902; New York Academy of Medicine 12, [ff. 1–5], Wallner version 1; ed. Wallner (1964–89). Cambridge University Library Dd.3.52, ff. 3–8v (incomplete); Cambridge University Library Dd.3.52 *Capitulum singulare*, Wallner version 3; Cambridge, Gonville and Caius College 336/725, ff. 1v–10; ed. Wallner (1970), Gonville and Caius 336/725, ff. 1–16, Wallner version 3.

 Geber, *Testament*: London, British Library, Sloane MS 320, ff. 116v–17v (16thc.). University of Pennsylvania, Smith MS 4, ff. 44v–47 (17thc.). British Library, Sloane MS 2532, ff. 74–76v (16thc.). Cambridge, Gonville and Caius College MS 176/97, p. 65. London, Wellcome Library MS 7117, f. 122 (16thc.).

16. Similarly, the translation techniques of the Wycliffite Bible are stated explicitly in the Prologue, chapter 15. The prologues of Trevisa's scientific texts also deal with the ideology of vernacularisation and translation methods (see Pahta and Taavitsainen in this volume).

17. I have not come across similar extensive imagery in other purely medical texts of this period. Alchemical imagery of the late medieval period makes use of the battle and furnace allegories.

18. Most of the first-person singular forms occur in the metatext, and it seems to be one of the leads to follow when assessing the role of the author.

19. The endings of the treatise are different in the different versions recorded in the handlists of the *Index of Middle English Prose* (*IMEP*), and there is some confusion which parts belong to the scope of the *Wise Book*. For example, Oxford, Bodleian Library, Ashmole MS 189 continues with a miscellany of similar prognostications with various starting points. In Bodleian Library, Ashmole MS 1477 the preceding item seems to be part of the text. Some versions are obviously defective, for example Bodleian Library, Ashmole MS 1405 breaks off after the section on the four elements. Most versions finish with nativities according to the signs of the zodiac for men and women separately; cf. *The Mervelous Connyng*, ed. as an appendix in Taavitsainen 1994c, for example Bodleian Library, Ashmole MS 1443, Cambridge, Trinity College MS O.10.21, and Cambridge, Trinity College MS R.14.51. Some versions add other prognosticatory texts after it, for example Cambridge, Magdalen College MS Pepys 878 (pp. 1–36) continues with perilous days and a short prognostication according to the 30 days of the moon with lists of unfortunate days, bloodletting advice and preventive herbal medicine. The following text is a urinoscopy. In Cambridge, Gonville and Caius College MS 457/395 the text is indicated as a variant version with the Book of Ypocras incorporated in it (Rand Schmidt 2001: 94).

20. To my knowledge, no editions of the texts of this book are available, except the zodiacal lunary text (Taavitsainen 1994c).

21. Most references were to astrological questions of nativity, planetary questions, or prognostications of life and death. The following entries may indicate an interactive text form:
Magistro de Discipulo, Opus de: London, British Library, Sloane MS 3580B, ff. 131–34v (incomplete) (16thc.). British Library, Harley MS 2407, f. 68v. 'Master saith disciple . . .'; Oxford, Corpus Christi College MS 226, ff. 31–33v; SAa 384; 'Now here follow certain necessary questions of a disciple . . .'. Oxford, Bodleian Library, Ashmole MS 759, ff. 47v–52; 'Seneca in the book of natural questions saith . . .'; Cambridge, Gonville and Caius College MS 451/392, pp. 20–2; *Interrogationes Discipuli ad Magistrum*: London, British Library, Sloane MS 3747, ff. 66–71v; 'Master saith disciple I pray'; 'Master I pray you of . . .' British Library, Harley MS 6453, ff. 25–29 (16thc.).

22. It is extant in two manuscripts, London, British Library, Sloane MS 3489 and Oxford, Bodleian Library, Ashmole MS 1481, and there may be others that contain parts of it (see *eVK*). The text has been edited by Peter A. Cant, University of London, 1973, but the edition is not easily available.

23. The *Canutus Plague Treatise* (see Taavitsainen 1999) is the nearest to the classical model:

> But ij questions ys meued in this case: what ys the cause that on dye & the tother not, and in summe tovne ther deyd men and in another not? The secunde question beth wheter this morbes pestilencial be contagius? Atte furste Y do say that this may fortune of ij maner of causes, i. of the parte that cumme of, & of the parte of the pacient. . . . And to the ij question, that suche morbes pestilencial be contagius: for cause that the bodyes þat be infected, the humors cumme out of there bodyes & enffect them that be clene of complessyon. Wherffore yt ys goode to voyde . . . (ed. Pickett 1994: 272–3).

24. This subtitle is found in the French versions (Burton 1998, 1: xxx).

25. The following signatures are found in it: *Elizabethe* on the title page and, for example, f. iij, and the names of *Thomas Hinton, Ane Hinton, Thomas Enttene, John Blount* towards the end of the book.

26. The diction of this poem resembles that of, for example, *The Prick of Conscience*, the most popular Middle English text if judged by the number of extant copies. It gives elementary religious instruction.

27. For the Hippocratic background, see Lonie (1981: 54–5); the theory is explicated in *De natura hominis* and it is stated that if one of the humours were lacking, man could not survive.

4 Code-switching in medieval medical writing

PÄIVI PAHTA

4.1 Introduction

The vernacularisation of medical texts in medieval England took place in a context where language contact was present in more than one form. The social context was multilingual, as several languages were in use in the country with partly overlapping social functions that at the time were undergoing dynamic change. The disciplinary context was also dominated by language contact: Latin was the main vehicle for learned discourse, both written and spoken, and continued to hold a central position in the domain long after the emergence of vernacular scientific texts. Medical texts were mostly translated from other languages, which by definition provided an immediate channel for contact phenomena in text production. Furthermore, since Latin was the primary language of the whole literary culture of the period, vernacular writing conventions, including a range of features from discourse forms and textual patterns to the physical layout of manuscript pages, were also influenced by contact.

This chapter considers one of the crucial expressions of language contact in the early phases of English scientific and medical writing, namely the coexistence of learned and vernacular languages. Earlier studies have shown that multilingualism is endemic in these writings, explicitly reflecting the context in which they were produced. A mixture of languages is found both in manuscripts where monolingual treatises in different languages alternate and in individual texts containing passages of varying length in more than one language. The focus in this study is on code-switching between English and Latin in texts where the base language is English, but other kinds of mixed-language materials also exist in abundance (see Voigts 1996).

The primary material of my study consists of texts in the *Corpus of Middle English Medical Texts* (*MEMT*) from *c.* 1375 to *c.* 1500 (see Pahta and Taavitsainen, p. 7 above). Evidence from manuscript contexts and some early sixteenth-century texts is also considered. The texts represent different underlying traditions of medical writing, ranging from recipes and accounts of *materia medica* to learned surgical texts and specialised treatises on a variety of topics. In this study, based on a large amount of data, my aim is to provide an overview of where and why vernacular writers switched to Latin. My main focus is on the range of discourse functions in which Latin can be found, but I shall also discuss switching in relation to the underlying traditions of medical writing. The study shows that some generalisations about the typical functions of code-switching in medieval vernacular medical texts are possible. At the same time it becomes obvious that a full understanding of the phenomenon can only be gained through detailed microlevel analyses of individual texts as communicative exchanges reflecting the bilingual competence and performance of the writer and his projected audience.

My analysis draws on sociolinguistic, pragmatic and discourse-analytic approaches to the study of bilingualism and code-switching in present-day societies. Corpus-linguistic methods were employed in the analysis of the data: the switches in the corpus texts were located with the help of computer-generated word lists and retrieval of Latin lexical items or strings using the *Corpus Presenter* software (see Hickey 2000 and 2003). Before data analysis, I shall set the scene by a brief outline of multilingualism in medieval England, the various types of mixed-language materials known from the period, and some theoretical and methodological issues involved in code-switching in general and in medieval medical texts in particular.

4.2   Multilingualism in medieval England

It is evident that in the complex multilingual situation in medieval England there were social groups and individuals who were fluent in more than one language (see Pahta and Taavitsainen, p. 9 above). The majority of the population was undoubtedly monolingual and only spoke English, but for the higher and educated parts of the society, monolingualism must have been rare. It has been pointed out that 'generations of educated Englishmen passed daily from English into French and back again in the course of their work' (Rothwell 1991: 179); this was equally true between English and Latin, and, on a smaller scale, between French and Latin as well.[1] Bi- or trilingual manuscripts containing texts in English, French and/or Latin survive in abundance, providing evidence of polyglot discourse communities comprising writers and users of these documents. English scholars in all fields of science wrote their treatises in Latin, and literary texts of the period show that many authors were proficient in two or more languages.[2] Extensive multilingualism is also suggested by a detailed study of the depositions of 203 witnesses giving their testimony for the canonisation of Thomas Cantilupe in Hereford in 1307. The study shows that many of these people, speakers of Welsh, English or French, and representing different social classes, switched on this formal occasion to a language that was more prestigious than their native language – a phenomenon typical of diglossia (Richter 2000: 58; see Richter 1979: *passim*).

Studies of present-day bilingual communities have shown that code-switching, 'the use of more than one language in the course of a single communicative episode' (Heller 1988: 1), is a widespread discourse strategy and an integral part of communication. Code-switching is also widely attested in written materials surviving from medieval England. In the light of present knowledge, switching is common in business accounts, legal texts, medical texts, sermons, drama and a specific type of mixed-language poetry known as macaronic verse, but it also occurs in longer verse pieces and various other prose texts, including other religious and scientific treatises, letters, and diaries (Schendl 2000a: 79–80 and 2000b: 68). New information about materials containing Latin and/or French beside Middle English is being supplied by the *Index of Middle English Prose* (*IMEP*) handlists, indexing also mixed-language prose in three different categories of 'macaronic texts'. Information on structural features and communicative functions of code-switching in medieval England has also become available in recent studies, but our knowledge about the patterns of use is still fragmentary.[3]

4.3   Multilingualism in medieval scientific and medical writing

Earlier research has shown that multilingualism has an important role in scientific and medical writings produced in medieval England (for discussion, see Pahta and Taavitsainen, p. 11 above). The tendency to combine materials in different languages appears to be more prominent in medicine than in other disciplines, although language mixing is also attested, for example, in astronomical-astrological and alchemical writings of the period (Voigts 1989a, 1989b).[4] The proportions of languages and patterns of switching in mixed-language materials vary. Primarily Latin materials contain parts in English or French,[5] French materials include Latin and/or English passages, and English materials incorporate Latin and/or French.

Numerous examples of scientific and medical mixed-language manuscripts are cited in earlier literature; some of them are repeated here to illustrate the range. Patterns in the use of the different languages in texts belonging to different traditions of writing in polyglot manuscripts have not been worked out systematically, but it is clear that a simple diglossic division of Latin being used in learned materials and English or French only in more popular ones does not hold. For example, the fifteenth-century Cambridge, Gonville and Caius College MS 176/97 contains academic medical treatises in Middle English and 'mathematical, astronomical, and astrological scraps – partly in Latin' (Voigts and McVaugh 1984: 24; Rand Schmidt 2001: 41–5). MS 84/166 in the same collection shows a different pattern, with recipes, prognostications, herbals and a phlebotomy in Middle English, and a number of treatises by Galen, Avicenna and Walter of Agilon in Latin (Taavitsainen 1988: 170; Rand Schmidt 2001: 2–13). The trilingual London, British Library, Sloane MS 5, owned by a barber in the fifteenth century, comprises Middle English copies of Bernard of Gordon's *De prognosticiis*,

Gilbertus Anglicus's *Compendium medicinae* and the widely disseminated herbal text, *Macer floridus*. Latin and French texts in the codex include astrological and gynaecological treatises and Galen's *De sectis* (Voigts and McVaugh 1984: 18; Voigts and Kurtz 2000, hereafter *eVK*). A bilingual anthology extant in six fifteenth-century manuscripts related to the Sloane Group displays an equivalent use of Latin and English, containing, for example, texts on uroscopy, plague and a regimen of health (Voigts 1990: 31–3, 52–3; 1996: 822–3).[6] Polyglot *receptaria* are common. Two fourteenth-century codices containing mixed-language recipe collections are discussed by Hunt (2000: 133–6; ed. Hunt and Benskin 2001). In a compendium of 632 receipts in Oxford, Bodleian Library, Rawlinson MS C.814 (ff. 33v–73v), 34.3 per cent of the recipes are mainly in Latin and 65.7 per cent in Anglo-Norman, with sporadic use of English glosses. A compendium of 702 recipes in Cambridge, Corpus Christi College MS 388 (ff. 1ra–35vb) exhibits an unusually equal proportion of the three languages: 31.5 per cent Latin, 32.2 per cent English and 36 per cent French, with individual recipes containing a mixture of the languages. Voigts (1996: 821) also lists *receptaria* mixing Latin and English recipes apparently indiscriminately in several manuscripts, including Oxford, Bodleian Library, Ashmole MS 1452, Longleat House Library MS 176, and the National Library of Scotland Adv. MS 23.7.11.

While these examples mainly illustrate co-occurrence of discrete texts in different languages in a single manuscript, juxtaposition of languages is also common within individual texts. Again the combinations of languages and the patterns of switching vary. Several polyglot texts can be cited, for example, from the collections of Trinity College, Cambridge (see also Mooney 1995). MS R.14.52, a fifteenth-century codex comprising a variety of scientific and medical treatises mainly in Middle English, also contains texts incorporating some Latin and French. A lengthy Latin passage is found in the remedy section of a Middle English gynaecological treatise, falsely attributed to Trotula (ff. 131r–133r).[7] Latin and English occur side by side in a list of herbs and spices (ff. 201v–212r). Both Latin and French occur beside English in a trilingual list of the names of herbs, plants, trees and spices (ff. 175v–201r). Some headings and marginal comments in the codex are in Latin, and Latin terms and phrases occasionally appear elsewhere in the texts as well (see Pahta forthcoming; Tavormina forthcoming b, *passim*). A fifteenth-century compendium of 254 recipes in one scribal hand under the title *Liber medicamentorum* in MS R.14.39 (ff. 27v–68v) contains mostly English recipes, some with Latin headings. MS R.14.37 has instances of Latin recipes with English headings (f. 76v):

(1)   to albyssye ven*es*
       pone sal co*m*mune bene prep*ar*atum In vrina pueri et calisat cupriu*m* ad
       rubedinem . . .
       to purge lead & tyme
       R*ecipe* mell disspumati p*ar*tes duas salis communis mundi . . . (Mooney
       1995: 154)

MS O.1.65 has a recipe mixing French and English (f. 148r):

(2) Pour le piere
     Pour prendre le ewe de lekys & le greyne de geneste & le gromull stamper
     bien en vne morter & therynne putte water of lekys and warme it in the fire
     and drinke iiij sponfull þerof a morne an le pelle de peiun? of þe mawe & le
     pelle de peiun? & des gallines & de cheristons et bebeis en vyn blanke Et
     enoyntes vostre dos (Mooney 1995: 164)

The instances noted here serve as representative examples. Equally varied patterns of language mixing could be cited from the collections of numerous other
manuscript repositories.[8]

4.4   Code-switching

4.4.1 Approaches to code-switching

Code-switching, the alternation of languages in a single communicative event,
is regulated by a number of factors operating on different levels. Because of the
multifaceted nature of the phenomenon, explanations for switching have also
been sought on many levels, including syntax, language typology, psycholinguis-
tic processing, discourse, pragmatics, sociolinguistics, and anthropology. A great
deal of information about functional (social and pragmatic) and structural (syntactic and morphological) aspects of switching in various bilingual communities
has accumulated in research within different disciplines and theoretical frame-
works over the past few decades.[9] The emphasis in the analyses is on spoken
data, whereas patterns of switching characteristic of written texts are mostly
unexplored.[10] While functional analyses of switching have aimed at describing
and explaining the indexical values of specific codes in communication on social
and interpersonal levels (see below), structural analyses have mainly focused
on establishing either language-specific or universal constraints governing
switching in terms of possible switch sites and switched segments. It has become
evident that the same code-switching examples can be accounted for in various
ways, which is in accordance with the multileveled and polysemous nature of the
phenomenon. There is also a general consensus that constraints regulating code-
switching, whether functional or structural, work in terms of tendencies rather
than categorical rules. Recent research has further confirmed that full competence
in both languages is not an absolute prerequisite for code-switching, nor is code-
switching necessarily connected with inadequacy in one of the languages involved
(Franceschini 1998, Halmari 1997, Meeuwis and Blommaert 1998; Poplack 1982).

4.4.2 Functions of code-switching

The key issues in functional analysis of code-switching can be summarised in
the question 'who speaks [or writes] what language to whom and when' (Fishman

1979: 15). The communicative situation in which switching takes place is thus crucial in the analysis. It can be defined in terms of the setting (place and time of speech event), participants (who they are and what their relationship is), and purpose (topic or task of the conversation and the goals of the participants). In code-switching research, the communicative functions of switching are often divided into two basic types: situational vs. non-situational switching, also referred to as transactional vs. conversational or metaphorical switching (Romaine 1995: 161). Both types are almost always socially motivated and thus related to and indicative of group membership (Myers-Scotton 1993: 476). In both types a change of code can also coincide with a change in the communicative situation. Situational switching is generally related to community level norms and governed by relatively stable usage rules determined by the social context. It is especially common in diglossic communities, where distinct varieties are typically employed in different functions. In conversational switching, a change of code is in a more complex relation with social variables; the main concern in code selection is the communicative effect or interactional meaning of the utterance. As a communicative strategy, code-switching is known to have important discourse functions. It can be used to emphasise, elaborate or evaluate a point, to mark a reconstructed dialogue, reported speech or a quotation, to specify a particular addressee as the recipient of the message, to establish intimacy or social distance, or to negotiate social or interpersonal identities. Code-switching can have a metaphorical function as well, when a certain code is seen as associated with certain abstract notions, such as power or prestige. Switches can also be multifunctional, serving simultaneously both macrolevel social functions and/ or several microlevel interpersonal functions. (Gumperz 1982: 75–81; Romaine 1995: 161–5; Eastman 1995: 6–8; Halmari 1997; Bailey 2000: 166).

4.4.3 Analysing code-switching in medieval writing

The analysis of code-switching in medieval writings along the lines of modern theories is complicated by a number of methodological issues. Problems arise, on the one hand, in defining what constitutes a code and, on the other hand, in defining the communicative situation in which switching takes place. In addition, the special nature of written discourse as opposed to speech also needs to be taken into account, as the two media differ from each other in several respects and impose different functional and structural production constraints on switching.[11]

The systems of the languages in use in medieval England are not adequately described and not clearly separable, which complicates the definition of a 'code' and therefore inherently also the definition of 'switching' between 'codes' (Schendl 2000b: 71). There is great internal variation in the English, Latin and French used in medieval England. The limits between the languages are not watertight either, with words and morphemes that can be assigned to more than one of the languages (cf. e.g. Rothwell 2000; Wright 2000). Some contemporary documents, including multilingual glossaries, indicate that medieval authors themselves were not always certain about which language is which (Trotter 2000: 2).

A related difficulty is drawing the line between borrowing and switching – one of the most problematic and controversial issues in code-switching research in general. This problem is usually discussed in relation to the embedding of single lexical items, but it also applies to phrasal segments, such as professional terms consisting of more than one lexical element (see p. 82 below). Switching and borrowing can be seen as a continuum with development across time: at some point in the history of either individual or societal bilingualism a code-switch may become a fully accepted borrowing (Halmari 1997: 17–18). All code-switches do not, however, result in borrowing, nor do all borrowed items start out as switches (cf. Norri's chapter on medical terms, p. 100 below). The distinction between the two may seem straightforward in theory: switching involves the use of two languages in one utterance, whereas the term 'borrowing' is used of embedded elements that have been integrated into the host language. However, even in present-day spoken data this criterion yields mixed results and definitions of the degree of integration qualifying an item as a borrowing vary. Traditionally, borrowings are characterised as items that are syntactically, morphologically and phonologically integrated into the host language, and typically are both recurrent in the usage of an individual and widespread in the community (Poplack et al. 1989: 136; Boyd et al. 1997: 260–1). But structural accommodation alone does not seem to distinguish borrowed items from code-switches. Genuine code-switches too can be morphologically integrated into the host language, particularly when the host language relies heavily on inflectional morphology in the marking of grammatical relations (Halmari 1997: 176–81). Moreover, some switched segments are repeated often enough in a language to be regarded as habitual and are socially integrated into the language of the community, even though they may not be linguistically integrated (Poplack 1982: 245). Some scholars suggest that absolute frequency and relative frequency of occurrences provide more reliable criteria for differentiation than the degree of integration. It has also been pointed out that in dealing with contact-induced phenomena in regard to such an open system as the lexicon, one cannot expect that any statements will hold categorically (Myers-Scotton 1997: 163–4). Many scholars now share the view that attempts to distinguish borrowing and switching are doomed (cf. Eastman 1992).

In written medieval mixed-language texts, distinguishing between switching and borrowing is no less difficult. Applying criteria from research on present-day spoken data is not straightforward. As the linguistic integration of a lexical item is continuous rather than discrete, it is often impossible to determine the degree of the phonological or even morphological assimilation of a given item at a given point. The assessment is complicated by variation in medieval spelling habits. The use of abbreviations and suspensions in medieval handwriting suppresses recognisable inflections and blurs the distinction further (cf. Wright 1994, 2000: 155 and 2001: 370, 372). There are also items and inflections that can belong to more than one language. The maxim of recurrence or frequency does not provide a solid basis for classification either, since it is often difficult to define whether a particular word was frequent in the usage of an individual or widespread in the community at the time. In some cases where several of the criteria can be applied, the results are contradictory, for example items that are not unambiguously integrated into English qualify as borrowings on the basis of their frequency and wide distribution. Even though a clear differentiation between borrowing and switching is crucial for establishing the constraints which govern code-switching and for any statistical analysis, such a differentiation seems hardly possible in medieval mixed-language texts (cf. Schendl 2000b: 74; Hunt 2000; see also Norri, p. 106 below).

Although written texts can be seen as communicative events between producers and the projected audience, it is often impossible to define the communicative situation in which medieval texts were produced. As in the case of texts in focus here, there is little or often no information about the authors, audiences, genesis or function of the texts.[12] This complicates the analysis of code-switching as a sociolinguistic or pragmatic phenomenon. Also, in studying documents that may be several times removed by layers of copying from the original production, it is not always certain whose usage they reflect, and whether the features attested in the text can be assigned to one speaker/writer. Texts could be written by more than one scribe – a fact that can be concealed by modern printed editions of manuscript texts. Even in cases where a single scribe has written the text, he may have copied *litteratim* an exemplar written by more than one scribe, thus reproducing linguistic performance of several people from an underlying layer. It was also common that another person added the rubrics and subheadings to a text. Factors like these make it difficult to draw definite conclusions about changes of code in relation to bilingual performance or competence of individuals. Yet, even if we may not reach the level of an individual language speaker, we can gain information about the possible patterns in code-switching on a more general level and about the ways in which resources of different languages were exploited in text production in the new vernacular register.

4.5   Functions of Latin in vernacular medical texts

The social patterns of language distribution in medieval England are reflected in the material. Although macrolevel sociolinguistic factors do not determine code-selection completely, it is possible to discern two specific social domains where switches into Latin are frequent. Many switches are connected, on the one hand, with learned medical knowledge and, on the other hand, with religion; both are domains where Latin had a primary role. Switches pertaining to these domains include both prefabricated utterances, such as Latin titles of religious or medical works and quotations from Latin texts, and 'free' utterances of various structural types; the range is from technical terms consisting of single words to switched prayers extending over several sentences. In both domains, but especially in the case of medical tradition, switches are related to professional language use. Thus they simultaneously serve as indexicals of group membership in the discourse community.

The texts also contain switches that cannot be accounted for within the concept of domains, and thus other reasons for switching need to be sought. Some tendencies emerge through the analysis of textual structures. Switching frequently serves a text-organising function, separating texts or parts of a text, or text and metatext. In this function, Latin code-switched elements are often, though not always, formulaic and typical of the written medium. In addition, there are a large number of switches for which no overt discourse-functional explanation seems plausible.

In the following sections I will discuss the three main types of Latin code-switched elements and their subtypes in the material. I will begin with switches related to the special language of medicine, then proceed to switches connected with religious discourse, and to switches that have a text-organising function. There is some overlap between the categories, and for many switches multiple explanations are possible. The final sections of the analysis discuss switches that remain outside these distinct categories and fluctuation in code-selection.

4.5.1 Special language of medicine

Since Latin had been, and at the time still was, the prevailing language of medical science, it is not unexpected to find a large number of switches connected with medical knowledge even in vernacular writing. Two main types of switches can be identified within this domain: specialised terminology and indications of intertextuality, i.e. identifiable traces of earlier texts in the form of references and quotations. Both types of switches are related to issues of group membership. Sometimes the use of Latin may also have had an exclusive, secretive function and denied access to in-group knowledge from the outsiders; whether this was deliberate or not on the part of the writers can be debated. A small number of switches within this domain are connected with the notion of 'secrecy' on a different level, i.e. decorum or taboo. Many switches are multifunctional.

4.5.1.1 Medical terms: Switching or borrowing? In scientific and medical writing technical terms are important for creating a discourse of organised knowledge (Halliday and Martin 1993: 4). At the same time terms also function as index-icals of group membership, as they form an essential part of the special knowledge that the practitioners are expected to share in order to operate within the field. The writers of Middle English medical texts had to create the terminology for topics that in many cases had not been discussed in vernacular writing before. There were two basic methods to deal with the problem. The first one was to use the resources of the vernacular language: a technical source language term could be replaced by a more colloquial native word or a new equivalent could be coined from native elements. The other solution was to turn to the source language for help. Here again two methods were possible: to use the source language term as such, or to adapt it into the phonological and morphological structure of the target language, thus turning the original foreign term into an anglicised variant.

The term formation strategy that relied on the source language resulted in a continuum of lexical elements where the borderline between code-switching and borrowing is fuzzy.[13] The problem of distinguishing between the two phenomena, fundamental in code-switching research in general (see p. 79 above), is evident in the present material as well. My observations in this study, however, are based on terms that can be characterised unambiguously as switches as opposed to borrowings on the basis of formal or contextual criteria. A formal indication of a switch is provided by the retention of an original Latin inflectional ending (example 3), whereas contextual disambiguation is seen in cases where an explicit flag marks an item as a switch into Latin (example 4; see also Norri, p. 107 below).[14]

(3)   þe partie þat is hered, in þe whiche *membra animata*, þat is to seien, members þat haue soule (ed. Wallner 1995: 18)

(4)   Þe ouermest partie of þe eere hatte *pynnula* in latyn (ed. Seymour *et al.* 1975: 190)

Code-switched terms defined by these criteria occur primarily in treatises that stem from the learned tradition, with great variation between individual texts. All unambiguous switched terms are of limited currency; many occur only in one or two texts. They range from single lexical items to multi-word phrases and represent various lexical fields, for example body parts (5–7); sicknesses (8–9); medicines, ointments and powders, and their ingredients (10–11); and instruments (12).

(5)   It is alsa called *lactea porta* or *porta lactis* (mylk ȝete or mylk gate) for þis skyll (ed. Jasin 1983: 150)

(6)   þere ben also y-sett two oþere 'bonys' smale, þat is to witen on ech side verual boon oon, þe whiche ben y-callid *Ossa petrosa*, or ellis *Ossa mendosa* (ed. Grothé 1982: 20a–20b)

(7)   all þe remenawnt . . . descendith downe into a gut þat is kallid **in Latyne** *saccus ventris*, id est, anglice the wombe-sac (ed. Hanna 1994: 200)

(8)   gendrith in his jowis suche a passioun whiche is cald **in Greeke liqoides** **and in Latyne** *lupus*, that is to say stranglyng. (ed. Pahta 1998: 177)

(9)   Laborynge of efimera weche we sei *synocham inflativam*, mynusche (ed. Voigts and McVaugh 1984: 42)

(10)   in somer tyme j day aftyr hele it with *unguentum fuscum cirurgicum* or with *unguentum viride regeneratim* the wyche ar sayd afor. (ed. Beck 1974: 116)

(11)   after mynuschynge take electuary *frigidum & confortativum*. (ed. Voigts and McVaugh 1984: 47)

(12)   Iff thou will kutte it þan schalt þou take *acum rostratam* and putte it þur3 þe midde3 of þe lengþe of þe instrument þat is called *tendiculum*, bygynnyng at þe gretter ende. (ed. Power 1910: 23)

As the examples show, the code-switched terms are incorporated into the text in different ways. In examples (10) and (11) the switched element is 'used' by the writer to denote a concept in the flow of discourse so that it forms an integral part of communication that cannot be left out. In other cases, often connected with the naming of objects or medical concepts, the Latin term is 'mentioned' by the author in a metalinguistic comment (examples 6–8). Both types are common. In both types the switched element can also be accompanied by a vernacular synonym, which shows that the only function of Latin terms was not to fill gaps in English lexicon, although this must have been one of the factors motivating the use of Latin. The code-switched special terms contribute to the precision and specificity required of scientific discourse. The author may also use them for reasons of style or prestige, to give the text an air of technicality and learnedness. Sometimes the Latin term is clearly given for didactic or instructive purposes. Both stylistic and didactic motivations are also related to issues of group membership and the shared language of the discourse community.

Although the status of a term as a code-switch or a borrowing often remains ambiguous without an explicit indicator, there are also terms or genre-specific expressions, such as indications of measurement or quantity, that can be re-garded as genuine code-switches. These Latin terms and expressions, illustrated in examples (13–15), do not show any integration into English in their written manifestation and are not known to have been widespread in the language in general at the time; in the corpus data, too, most of them are infrequent.[15] Their distribution resembles that of the explicitly disambiguated switches: on average they are more frequently attested in specialised and surgical treatises, but can also be found in recipes and herbal texts. There is great variation between individual texts in all varieties of medical writing.

(13)   Also we sene vppon welle drye hille herbus growe þat bene moist of kinde, as þe herbis þat hatte *crassula*, *cimbalaria*, *vermicularia*, *irassula*, and oþir. (ed. Seymour *et al.* 1975: 138)

(14)   For *ignis sacer*. Medle rue iuus with oile roset (ed. Frisk 1949: 74)

(15)   [T]ake bugle pigle & senegle … þᵉ rote of mader peritorie burnete crispmall *omnia ana* bot of mader as mech os of all þᵉ oþer erbis (ed. Benskin 1985: 202)

Several texts also contain terms that escape unambiguous classification as a code-switch or borrowing. The term *colera* may serve as an example of the complexity of drawing the line between the two phenomena. In the corpus data the item *colera* occurs 60 times. In seven cases it occurs as a head in a Latin noun phrase, sometimes explicitly flagged, where it can be classified as a part of a code-switched Latin element (examples 16 and 17). In 53 instances the same item occurs in an English context either as an unmodified noun (18) or with modification (19); in this case there is no explicit indication of its status. The 60 occurrences are spread across four texts, although 88 per cent of the instances are found in one text alone – John Trevisa's translation of Bartholomaeus Anglicus' learned encyclopaedia, *De proprietatibus rerum* (cf. Taavitsainen, 'Transferring', p. 59 above). According to the *MED* and *OED*, the word, although rare, is also recorded in some other Middle English texts, including a copy of Chaucer's *Canterbury Tales*.

(16)   And in þis season arisith and encrecith melancoly, callid in Latin *Colera nigra* (ed. Manzalaoui 1977d: 7)

(17)   þan is ibred *citrina colera*, þat is lesse hoot (ed. Seymour *et al.* 1975: 158)

(18)   Þis pouder drunkyn with mulsa destroieþ þe *colera*. (ed. Frisk 1949: 101)

(19)   Þis blak *colera* is enemye of kynde (ed. Seymour *et al.* 1975: 161)

A related problem area is ambiguous 'sigils' that recur in scientific and medical texts of the period. They include weight and measurement specifications and other brevigraphs, and visual symbols representing planets or zodiacal signs. Although these extralinguistic symbols have their origin in Latin, they also occur in English and mixed-language texts and often cannot be assigned unambiguously to either Latin or English (see Voigts 1989a).

4.5.1.2 Expressions of intertextuality: References and quotations. In addition to special terms, switches connected with the learned medical tradition include expressions reflecting intertextuality, also characteristic of professional discourse (cf. Atkinson 1999). These switches mainly consist of prefabricated Latin utterances, such as references to medical works and quotations from them. References citing authoritative texts by their Latin title occur sporadically in treatises belonging to the learned traditions.

(20)   Yt is to wyt as seyþ Galien *in Metategni* þat if it owth to be done by apoferisim (ed. Voigts and McVaugh 1984: 39)

(21)   Of þe þridde part, þaᵗ is of þe emunctorijs, Galien telliþ, *libro de iuuamentis* in þe firste & in þe secunde chapitres (ed. Grothé 1982: 25a)

Latin references are frequent only in one of the translations of Guy de Chauliac's *Chirurgia magna* (examples 22–23) and John Trevisa's translation of *De proprietatibus rerum* (24–25). In both texts the titles are often accompanied by a more specific Latin reference to a particular section or chapter of the work. The reference can also be extended to a Latin metadiscursive comment clause (25), and have a text-organising function in separating the different sources of knowledge in the learned encyclopaedic compilation from each other (cf. Taav-itsainen, pp. 60–1).

(22)   Also Haly Abbas, .8.º sermone, prime partis libri disposicionis regalis demeþ þat which-euer of vlcere3, symple or componed, if it passe þe space of .40 daie3, it is called fro þens-forþ a fistule (ed. Wallner 1982: 11)

(23)   And þat it is to be bounden & no3t to be kutte, dredyng þe emorosogie after G in cerapeutica loco prealligato. (ed. Wallner 1964: 118)

(24)   If þis colera is corrupte in any partye of þe body, it brediþ ful euel pas-siouns, of þe whiche passiouns þise beþ þe general signes and tokenes, as Constantinus seiþ in Pantigny libro 9º capitulo 2º. (ed. Seymour et al. 1975: 159)

(25)   A litwhat of colera oþir of anoþir humour imedled with pure blood infectiþ þe blood and drawiþ him to the liknes of his owne qualite. Huc vsque Constantinus in Pantagni libro 24º capitulo 1º. Aristoteles in libro de animalibus 3º capitulo [setteþ] oþir propirtees of blood (ed. Seymour et al. 1975: 150)

Sometimes a reference is in Latin even though the actual title of the work is not repeated (26–27).

(26)   And super amphorismorum it is iseide þat a womman þat is wiþ a knaue childe if sodeinliche iclepid, sche meueþ first þe ri3t foot, and þat makeþ þe hote blood þat worchiþ at þe fulle in hire þat conceyueþ a knaue childe. Et in eodem libro it is seide þat blood is þe firste and principal mater of þe herte and of þe liuour. (ed. Seymour et al. 1975: 152)

(27)   And if blood rotuþ in any membres, but it be itake out by craft or by kynde, it turneþ into þe venym and scabbis. Huc vsque libro 3º. Et libro 12º he seiþ þat þe veines beþ þe vesselle of blood. (ed. Seymour et al. 1975: 151)

Latin quotations from medical works are found in several texts in the learned tradition, as the habit of quoting from earlier sources lies at the heart of both commentary and compilation traditions (see Taavitsainen, 'Transferring'). The use of Latin quotations is especially common in surgical treatises (28–29), but can occasionally be found in some other specialised texts as well (30):

(28)   ofte tymes we fynde þat an old wounde is clepid vulnus, as ypocras seiþ vulnera anua necesse est in eis os taliefieri ℰ cicatrices concauas fieri: þat is to seie, it is nedful þat þe boon in an oold wounde to be rotid & þe cicatrices to be hollow (ed. von Fleischhacker 1894: 31)

(29)   Wherfor fysyke sayes Omnus artifex tenetur scire suum subiectum in quo operatur alias operando erat. And a surgen ys a craftyous man for mannys

body ther for yt ys nedfull for hym to know the natur and the makynge of mannys body. (ed. Beck 1974: 109)

(30) As Ysodre sais, dies creticus þus is discryed of physiciens: *dies creticus est dies evasicuis ab infirmitate fine ad vitam, fine ad mortem*. Day of creticacion is þe day of skapynge fra þe melady, or to lyf or to dede. (ed. Jasin 1983: 134)

The code-switched quotations serve simultaneously multiple functions. In terms of professional discourse, quotations can be seen as part of professional rhetoric. The author may use a Latin quotation to show off, to emphasise his own prestige or to indicate his membership in the educated Latinate circles. Quotations can also be used to amplify the argument by bringing in another, often authoritative voice for support. At the same time they also serve as a text-organising device in separating different levels of text from each other (see p. 92 below). In a few cases a Latin quotation reiterates or summarises the contents of the preceding English passage, as in example (31), where the switch in fact extends the limits of the quotation and may have been triggered by the Latin name and title:

(31) ȝif þere is in þe body oþir in any partye þerof to moche moisture þat may not be ireuled of kynde, þan moisture is cause and mater of rotynge and of corrupcioun, and brediþ in þe body ful euel passiouns and sikenesses, as it is iseyne in apoplexia; in þe whiche euel superfluite of moisture occupieþ so alle þe chaumbres and dennes of þe brayne þat þe spirit þat hatte spiritus animalis may not passe by þe synowes of felinge to make þe body fele and meue, and so bynymeþ þe body þe soule his worchinge in þe body, and also it binymeþ þe body felinge and meuynge, and bringiþ in at þe laste stoffinge and deþ. So seiþ *Galienus in commento super amphorismos, exponens illud verbum Ypocratis: Soluere apoplexia[m] fortem impossibile est, debilem vero non facile*. (ed. Seymour et al. 1975: 144)

4.5.1.3 Secrecy: Code for exclusion and decorum. In addition to indicating membership in a certain group, code-switching can also have an exclusive function in denying access to that group from outsiders. The use of the vernacular for learned medieval medical writings in general can be understood as a process by which outsiders gained knowledge that had previously belonged to a small élite group of Latinate university-trained physicians. However, attitudes towards the use of the vernacular were still cautious, and it has been suggested that occasionally Latin was used even in vernacular texts to disclose the secrets of medical knowledge from the unlearned (see e.g. C. Jones 1998: 205). There is no direct evidence to support this view in the present material, except for the basic premise that the use of Latin as such must have automatically functioned also as a barrier for those who were not familiar with the language. However, writers of vernacular texts usually translated or paraphrased their Latin medical quotations and many also strove to explain in more familiar words the code-switched vocabulary that could have created a barrier to medical knowledge, which rather testifies to a non-exclusive attitude among them.

The concept of secrecy on another level is relevant in switches apparently motivated by decorum or taboo in connection with topics that were regarded as socially inappropriate. For example, John Trevisa's translation of *De proprietatibus rerum* twice switches to Latin to address 'women's secrets' (examples 32 and 62 below), and a code-switched comment on the effect of sexual intercourse on health occurs in the collection of remedies in the Thornton manuscript (33):

(32)   And in amphorismorum particula vi°. it is iseide: *mulieri deficientibus menstruis* it is good to blede atte nose. (ed. Seymour *et al.* 1975: 194)

(33)   For full many for defaute of gud gouernance in dietynge falles in þis sekenes, thare-fore þat tyme vse none excesse nor surfete in mete & drynke nor bathes nor swete noghte gretly þan, for all thies opyns þe pores of þe body & makes venemous ayere to entre & þat febles þe body, *et super omnia alia nocet coitus & accelerat ad hunc morbum quod maxime aperit poros & destruit spiritus vitales*, also vse littill froyte or none & ett littill or noghte of garleke or lekes and slyke þat brynges a man in-to a vnkyndely hete (ed. Ogden 1938: 51)

4.5.2 Religious discourse within medical writing

In medieval society Latin was the language of the Church and of religious ceremonies, where code-choice can also be seen as part of the ritual. Religious considerations were important in medieval healing, and instances of religious practice occur in medical texts of the period. The special connection of religion and healing can be seen in some of the religious code-switches in the material. Religious use of Latin is also more prominent in remedybooks than in surgical or specialised expository treatises. The switches can be divided into four main types. Only the first type, prayers, contains instances of 'free' discourse while the other categories consist of prefabricated chunks of Latin. Not all religious discourse in the material is in Latin, which shows that there is fluctuation in code-selection within the domain (see p. 96 below).

4.5.2.1 Prayers.

Code-switched religious passages contain prayers, illustrated in examples (34–35). The use of Latin in such passages can be interpreted in several ways. On a sociolinguistic level it can be seen as a preconditioned choice reflecting the diglossic situation in the community at large. On an interactional level it can be seen as a contextualised convention, where the switch into the language of religion also has a special, metaphorical meaning in aiming to heighten the power of the words. In many cases the change of code at the same time also has a text-organising function, as code-switched prayers often occur at the end of a treatise, where they also serve as a cue to signal that the text has come to its conclusion (see p. 90 below).

(34)   Now here I make an eende of þis tretis þat is clepid þe mooste & þe souereyneste secrete of alle secretis, and a passynge tresour þat may nouȝt fayle *O quantum malum foret, si hic liber perueniret ad manus hominum mundanorum, ad noticiam tirannorum, et ad seruicium reproborum ! quia, sicut sancti per hunc librum poterunt continuare opera vite christiani diucius et vehemencius, ita et reprobi possent peruerso vsi diucius perseuerare in malo. ego autem, quantum in me est, propter solos sanctos librum hunc constituo, et ipsum custod[iae] ihesu Christi commendo nunc et in eternum* (ed. Furnivall 1899: 25)

(35)   and thus endythe the cures of this sekenes. and use to every pocion or medecin to say thys oryson wiche holy saynt damyan used sayde & made. *Omnipotens eterne deus qui dedisti medicinam ad sanandas corporum humanorum infirmitates da benedictionem tuam sanctam de celo super hanc medicinam ut in cuius corpore introierit sanitatem mentis & corporis suscipere valeat per christum dominum nostrum amen.* (ed. Zimmermann 1937: 471)

4.5.2.2 Performatives and power words: Blessings and charms. Some Latin prefabricated utterances act as performatives, and have a 'doing-it-by-saying-it' effect.[16] As the performatives in the texts are connected with medicinal powers, they can also be seen as part of the special language of contemporary medical practice. Like in prayers, the function of the code is to enhance the power and efficacy of the words. Latin occurs in ritual blessings, as in example (36), where English is used in the metatextual introductory description.

(36)   Here begynnyth ye blyssyng wpon herbys whech is medycynabyll and rygth goode and holsome for all manere of grevows wowndys and sorys. *Deus qui in mundo primordia inter cetera olera virencia crescere & multiplicare precepisti te submissis humilimis precibus exoramus ut has herbas in usum medecinalem collectas in tuo sancto nomine + consecrares + & benedicas ut quicumque ex eis potamina gustantur vel unguenta perceperint sanitate cordis & corporis percipere mereantur qui vivis et regnas deus per omnia saecula saeculorum. . . . Sic vbicumque hec medicamenta sint egrotantibus in tuo nomine exhibita omnia expellantur vicia et tua gracia benedicantur per dominum nostrum Jesum Christum filium tuum & c.* (ed. Heffernan 1993: 309–10)

A related group of switches contains instances of Latin, sometimes combined with transliterated Greek or Hebrew, in religious charms for medical purposes. Charms are often embedded in recipes and occur in remedybooks.[17] In most cases there is a similar functional distribution of codes as in the above blessing: the instructions on how to compile and use the charm are given in English, while the actual power words are a code-switched prefabricated utterance (cf. p. 96 below).

(37) For woman þat haþe grete trauail in childes beryng
Do write þis writte in perchemyn of a calf and bynd to þe wombe: + *In nomine patris et filij spriritus sancti. Amen. + Sancta maria peperit et mater illa non doluit christum genuit qui nos suo sanguine redemit alpha + et O + Christus vincit + christus imperat +.* (ed. Braekman 1986b: 134)

(38) For þe man þat may noȝt sclepe.
Nim þe mures v ȝ and tempre it and drink þe jus and o/se/þe plastre and bind hit about his heued and he schal sclepe ¶ Oþer write þis letteris in þe letteris of goldeflowres and ley vp on þi heued þat þe hit wete noȝt *exmael exmael adiuro te angelum michaelem ut soporet homo ille* and ette alitil letuse oft (ed. Edmar 1967: 99–100)

(39) For þe demegreyn: Take sangdragon and tempere it with þe white of an eye wel-swonge, and make a plastir as brood as þe soor is. And þus do twies or thries til þou be hool. And in leyeng to of þe plastir and when it is plastrid, sey þis Colet in worship of Seynt Joon Baptist: *Perpetuis nos domine Sancti Iohannis Babtiste; tueri, presidere, etc.* (ed. Getz 1991: 5–6)

4.5.2.3 Quotations. A few quotations and reported passages in the material are from religious texts. The function of the religious quotations in these passages is to amplify the argument (see also p. 92).

(40) as it is seid deutronomium 28 in þis maner. '*Si audire nolueris vocem domini dei tui, ut custodias et facias omnia mandata eius, veniant super te omnes maledicciones; iste maledictus eris in ciuitate &c.*' *et infra;* '*ad-iungat tibi pestilenciam donec consumat te de terra, percuciat te dominus egestate, febre, et frigore, ardore et estu, et aere corrupto ac rubigine, et persequatur donec pereas*' *hec ibidem; et infra* '*percuciat te dominus vlcere egipti, et partem corporis per quam stercora egerantur. scabie quoque, et prurigine, ita ut curari nequeas; percuciat te dominus necessitate ac furore mentis*' Therfore a gret fool were he þat wolde presume to cure þese plagis of pestilence þat ben vncurable (ed. Furnivall 1899: 23–4)

(41) So seiþ Gregor super Iob 38° capitulo, *Quis posuit mari terminum,* 'who settiþ a bounde to þe see'. And Ieromye super Ieremiam seiþ þat same, *Posuit arenam terminum mari* 'a settiþ þe grauel a bounde to þe se'. (ed. Seymour et al. 1975: 137)

4.5.2.4 Titles and formulaic expressions. Other instances of switching related to religious discourse consist of short prefabricated expressions. They occur more frequently in remedybooks, but occasional instances can also be found in surgical texts and learned specialised treatises. They include formulaic pious wishes, which can also have a text-organising function in signalling the end of a treatise (example 42), and titles of familiar prayers or hymns (43–45). It is worth noting that in many cases the prayers and hymns are not referred to only in connection with religious practice: they also serve as indicators of time or measure and as such are related to the professional language of medicine.

(42)   And yff the cure tarye þat nature helpe not, yeve them fleshe of yong gootys gelded, soden and not rooste, tyll they be recouerede. *Deo gracias.* (ed. Eldredge 1996: 92)

(43)   let boyle hem to gedere by þe space of þis psalm. syng. *miserere mei deus.* and þanne do þi lycour in a vessel of pewter (ed. Edmar 1967: 104–5)

(44)   Stampe þe flour & temper it with warm wyn & gyf it hym to drynk & þer-whills þu & he bothe says ȝour *Pater noster* with *Credo in Deum* & *Aue Maria.* (ed. Ogden 1938: 60–1)

(45)   When it haþ boiled ynouȝ sette it fro þe fire and late it stande stille without mouyng by þe space of a *'pater noster '* – & *'aue maria',* þat þe litarge of þe lede þat is in it may descende to þe grounde (ed. Power 1910: 91)

4.5.3 Textual organisation

Code-switching is common as a text-organising device. In such cases a change of code occurs at a boundary between texts or different parts of a text. Within a text, a switch can indicate, for example, an embedded text representing a different genre, as in recipes containing an embedded charm (examples 37–39 above). A code-switch can also mark out the informationally distinct headline from the text, separate a reported passage or a direct quotation from the flow of discourse, or an author's comment from the actual text. There are also cases where a switch co-occurs with a change from the preface to the text (see Voigts 1996: 821). Many switch types belong to medieval scribal conventions that are common in other types of writing as well.

4.5.3.1 Textual boundaries.
Metatextual utterances that guide the reader or function as comments about the evolving text are frequently in a different code from the running text (cf. Taavitsainen 2000a; see also examples in Taavitsainen, pp. 54, 60 above). The recurrent use of Latin rubrics to mark boundaries between English texts is a case in point (46). Instead of actual rubrics, text boundaries are often indicated by Latin incipits or explicits (47).

(46)   *Liber Cophonis*
Here bygynnen þe Exprimentes of Cophon þe leche of Salerne For ache of heued þat comeþ of fleumatyk (ed. Fordyn 1983: 19)

(47)   . . . wont to dispose nature moche without reasoun in so moche.
Explicit Liber Cerebri (ed. Carrillo Linares 1993: 91)

In longer works, Latin subheadings, incipits and explicits are also used to mark boundaries between books or chapters (examples 48–49), to introduce a new topic (49–50), or a new text component (51–52).

(48)   Bod if it be gud it sais hele, myght, & vertew of kynd, as with grace of God I sall schew in þis 2 folowynge bukys, as autors spekys and techys. *Explicit liber primus uricrisiarum. Incipit secundus liber uricrisiarum, primum c[apitulum]*: of colours in generall & of nowmbre of þam. (ed. Jasin 1983: 119; see also Plate 3)

(49)   *De humani itaque corporis et parti[u]m eius proprietatibus tractaturi [ab] elementalibus qualitat[ibus] et humoribus ex quibus constat corpus e[s]t primitus inchoandum.*
To trete of þe propertees of mannes body and of þe parties þerof, we schul first biginne to trete of þe qualitees of þe elementis and of þe humoures of whiche þe body is maad.
De elementis. Capitulum primum.
Elementis beþ foure, and so beþ foure qualitees of elementis of þe whiche eueriche body þat haþ a soule is componed and imade as of matir (ed. Seymour et al. 1975: 129)

(50)   *Suffocacio matricis.* Suffocacyon of þe moder is when a womans hert, her lyghtes ben þrust to gedure be rysyng of þe moder (ed. Hallaert 1982: 49)

(51)   *Hic incipiunt bonas medicinas.* Here begynne medicinys þat good lechys haue made (ed. Henslow 1899: 139)

(52)   *Cura*: For to helpe women of these sekenesses ther be many diuerse mede- cynes as blode letyng (ed. Rowland 1981: 66)

In recipe collections, Latin rubrics frequently introduce English recipes:

(53)   *Pro passionibus stomachi.* Tak ache seed, lynseed and comyn ana, stampe hem to gedre wel, and ʒef þe seek wyþ hote watur. *Pro tumore in stomacho.* take fenel roote, ache rote ana, stampe hem to gedre, and tempre hem wyþ wyn, &~ ʒef þe sek to drinke. *Ad generandum appetitum.* Take centorie, and seþe hit in watur, &~ let þe seke drinke hit warme þre dayes, &~ he shal be hool; for þis medycyne purges þe stomak~ and eke þe breste. (ed. Heinrich 1896: 71)

Sometimes the beginning of a new recipe is only marked by the use of Latin *item* or *aliud* (54–55). In manuscript context the abbreviated Latin *recipe* 'take' at the beginning of a recipe also functions as a similar cue (cf. example 63).

(54)   *Contra fluxum sa[n]guinis ex naribus.*
Drynke the juce off weybrede and yt schall stawnch be goddys grace.
Item medyll bole with þe juce off sanguinary and draw yt in at thyn nosethyrlis.

Item medele bole with þe gleyr off an eye and with the juce off sa[n]guinary and make a playster þer-off and ley yt to hys tempyllis. (ed. Schöffler 1919: 197)

(55)   ffor ye mygrane
Also for to make thys Emplastyr good to hele a body of ye mygrane. Take ye juse . . .
Aliud
Also for ye mygrane a noythyr manere emplaystyr. (ed. Heffernan 1993: 315–16)

Some code-switched references and religious passages also have a text-organising function (see p. 84 and p. 89 above).

4.5.3.2 Emphasis and focus. Switching is common in recipes between the actual recipe and a metatextual closing remark in which the efficacy of the medicine or treatment is emphasised in a formulaic tag phrase (55–57). Efficacy phrases do not add any further information about the recipe; their function is simply to attest to its value (cf. C. Jones 1998: 199–202).

(56)   Take eufras and stampe it. Þen streyne it þoroughe a clooþ and lete it clere. And put in þe iȝe of þe clere duringe þre daies at eue and at morwe. And he shal be hole. *Probatum est.* (ed. Getz 1991: 53–4)

(57)   Take a lytyll off good aloes and medyl yt with the juce of fenell and put yt in a brasyn vessell V days in þe sunne and put þer-off in thyn eye; *probatum est.* (ed. Schöffler 1919: 193)

(58)   put þ~to halue a pynt of clarified hony and drynke þ~of first and last *& sanabitur* (ed. Dawson 1934a: 54)

Efficacy phrases, like other metatextual utterances, can also appear as marginal notes. When thus physically separated from the running text, marginal comments serve as visual cues for focusing the attention of the reader on particular points in the text (see Plates 3 and 6). For example in Cambridge, Trinity College MS R.14.52, Latin marginal comments in the hand of the original scribe are used with varying focus. In some theoretical texts they function as references and indicate passages citing authoritative sources of knowledge, in a recipe collection they indicate different remedies, and in a text on diagnosing and treating sicknesses the marginal comments point out good and evil signs of sicknesses (Pahta forthcoming).

4.5.3.3 Quotations. Quotations are frequently marked out from the flow of discourse by a change of code. The material contains some isolated examples of Latin religious quotations from the Bible or the church fathers' commentaries (see p. 89 above), but the majority of prefabricated utterances citing earlier work are derived from the canon of medical writings (cf. pp. 85–6 above). Some quotations provide more general guidance (59), and the code-switched passages also include quotations from various sources in verse form (60–61).

(59)   ffor the wise man seith, '*Sicut ad omne quod est mensuram ponere prodest, Sic sine mensura deperit omne quod est*': 'As it profiteth to putte mesure to al thing that is, So without mesure perissheþ all þing þat is.' Skorne he no man. ffor of that it is seid, '*Deridens alios non inderisus abibit*': 'He that skorneþ other men shal not go away vnskorned.' (ed. Power 1910: 4)

(60)   yt ys a token of mens deth in battelys, etcetera. Vnde this verse:
Mors furit, urbs rapitur,
Seuit mare, sol operitur,
Regnum mutatur, plebs peste fame cruciatur. (ed. Pickett 1994: 271)

(61)   as says þe vers: *qui bene degerit, ingerit, egerit, est homo sanus.* ʒyf yu wyll ete, defy, & schyte, yu art hale whare yu gas or sittys. (ed. Jasin 1983: 142)

As the examples show, the code-switched quotations are usually preceded by an English introductory clause, sometimes explicitly indicating the source of the quotation (cf. Taavitsainen, pp. 51 ff. above). An English translation or paraphrase also usually accompanies the quotation, except in the quotations from the Bible. Thus in most cases the switched passages are not significant for their semantic content, but rather it is the switch itself that is significant. In addition to serving a text-organising function, the switch can be seen as a way of giving more authority to what is being said, thus underlining typical scholastic reliance on book learning and authoritative knowledge. The semantic content of the quoted passage can, however, be important as well, for example in cases where Latin is used for reasons of decorum. In the lengthy passage on menstruation in example (62) the 'secret' topic appears to be more significant for the choice of code than the boundary between text categories, as Latin is retained throughout the passage containing quotations from Aristotle and Constantinus Africanus and the author's commentary:

(62)   And libro 9⁰ Aristotil seiþ: *menstruum in fine mensis in mulieribus maxime viget, et ideo tunc vtiliter expellitur talis sanguis. Et libro 16⁰ dicit quod sanguis menstrualis non habet certam temporis reuolucionem sed in maiori parte accidit in diminucione lune. Et hoc est rectum quia corporalia sunt tunc temporis frigidiora, quam in illo tempore aer est frigidior . . . Item oportet vt fluxus sanguinis menstrualis actualiter sit in corpore antequam mulier impregnetur, sicut dicit Aristoteles in libro 15⁰ et Constantinus, sicut oportet arborem primo florere quam fructus facere . . . superfluitas trancit in plumas et in pilos, vt dicit Aristotolus. Item dicit Constantinus super Rufus: mulieres nimis se excertentes et cepius mouentes non multum menstruant* (ed. Seymour et al. 1975: 154–5)

4.5.4   Other code-switched utterances

The switches that remain outside the above three main types form a heterogeneous group. The switched utterances vary in length and occur in texts from different traditions. In most cases no particular overt discursive function can be assigned to the switch. For example, there seems to be no special contextual reason for the lengthy code-switched passage in the gynaecological and obstetrical materials excerpted from Gilbertus Anglicus's *Compendium medicinae* (63), since the vernacular is otherwise used in the treatise for discussing similar topics on 'women's secrets'. The writer just seems to lapse into Latin in a set of recipes that contain long lists of medicinal ingredients, many of them in Latin (see also Green and Mooney forthcoming).

(63)   And þe same medecyns ben good for swellyng of a mannes fete oþer legges þat jorneyeth by the weyes.
Ad menstrua prouocanda: R$_x$: parsily rotes, fenell ana m. i, of isop leves, saueray, betonice, *foliorum lauri*, rosmarin, lauendre ana m. sem., nepte m. iii, dyptani, rute, arthemisie 3 ii & sem., *carui, pollipodi 3 iiii, vini albi lagenam i, tonsis & coctis ad medietatem & collatiis & iterum coctis cum croco . . . hoc tribus diebus mane, videlicet contra vomitum & fastidium tollit & dat appetitum comedenti & cetera. Probatum est de* Lyghtfote Gardener *quem vxor sua vocat pater, super quem* Gardener *probatum erat.*
Ad mulieres tantum: Fiat fleobotomia sub cauillis cum subfumigacione radicis yris. Fyrst ther must be made hyr a potage (ed. Rowland 1981: 152–62)

The texts also contain short insertional switches that cannot be assigned to any of the types discussed in the previous sections. In the majority of cases the switched element is an adverb or prepositional phrase functioning as an adverbial (64–67), but other sentence elements are also found (68–69). Many of the switched items are formulaic expressions that can be found in other types of medieval vernacular texts as well (examples 67 and 68). They reflect the writer's familiarity with Latin textual conventions and thus serve as indicators by which the writer, consciously or unconsciously, identifies himself as a member of the educated Latinate social strata.

(64)   tyme makeþ or doþ no þing *ad rumbum*; whatsom-euer tyme (ed. Wallner 1982: 5)

(65)   G. crieþ *per totum* þat no þing sharpeþ more (ed. Wallner 1982: 17)

(66)   ʒif þe uryn be mare thyn upward þan donward, it is takyn of lyf; ʒif it be *eiusmodi*, of deth. (ed. Jasin 1983: 146)

(67)   Tak Wormot & þe white of an egge *vt supra* for poudir for dede flesche. (ed. Ogden 1938: 76)

(68)   *Nota* that scabig etyn rowe purgyth the body (ed. Zimmermann 1937: 463)

(69)   oure 5. essence . . . makiþ a man liȝt, iocunde, glad, and merie, & puttiþ awey heuynesse, angre, melencoly, & wraþþe, þe whiche þat deuelis loue *et ideo nostra 5 essencia digne vocatur celum humanum* Also if a man be traueylid wiþ a feend, and may not be delyuerid fro him, lete him drinke a litil quantite of oure 5 essence (ed. Furnivall 1889: 19)

4.5.5   Fluctuation in code-selection

Although the majority of code-switched utterances detected in the material occur in certain contexts and can be seen to serve specific discourse functions, further analysis of similar contexts and discourse functions across the whole material shows that code-selection operates in terms of tendencies rather than rigid categories. English, or sometimes French, also occurs in the contexts and functions where Latin is employed, which suggests a certain neutrality between the codes. For example, the use of Latin code-switched elements as a text-organising device is not systematic or uniform: English texts can contain English rubrics, incipits or chapter headings, and English efficacy phrases, such as *it is proved*, are common (cf. C. Jones 1998). Outside the corpus data it is also possible to find texts with reversed patterns (see p. 76 above). There is fluctuation in the use of codes in quotations as well: examples (70–71) illustrate that all quotations, whether from learned medical texts or from more popular sources, are by no means consistently marked out by a change of code.

(70)   Auicen, forsoþ, seiþ, 'experience ouercomeþ reson'; and galien in pantegni seiþ, 'No man ow for to trust in reson al-oon but ȝit it be proued of experience.' (ed. Power 1910: 3)

(71)   And þis is þat G seid in de tumoribus preter naturam: And a fistule, forsoþ, is a streite & a longe sinus .i. lap or bosom like to oþer lappeȝ suffryng contraccioun & hardneȝ of þe inward partie (ed. Wallner 1982: 31)

English and Latin also occur side by side in passages rich in medical terms, although there is a distinct predilection towards Latin in the more specialised terminology; an extract from the list of contents in a fifteenth-century vernacular surgical book may serve as an example.

(72)   fo. 94 Capitulum xj of *ignis per sicus* or *meliarius*
       fo. 95 Capitulum xij of *prima albras*
       fo. 96 Capitulum xiij *de una & morbelis* in pokkes & meseles
       . . .
       fo. 118 Capitulum xlij apostume over the knes
       fo. 118 Capitulum xliij *mugo in calcaneo*
       . . .
       fo. 120 Capitulum *de ciatica passio* xlv
       . . .

fo. 120 Capitulum xlvj a gowt cald *podegra*
fo. 121 Capitulum xlvij a Gowt calyd *cyragra*
fo. 122 Capitulum xlviij *fistulata*
fo. 122 Capitulum xlix of the scab & yoke (ed. Beck 1974: 107)

Another example is provided by a passage listing terms for different colours of urine in Henry Daniel's *Liber uricrisiarum*; the majority of terms are in Latin and Greek, and only two in English (see Plate 3):

(73)   For all colors of uryn are comprehendyd in þis 20, & yu sall fynd na colour in þat it nes lyk to sum of þise 20 & are all de ordore, as autors puttys. þe fyrst is *niger*, 2) bla, 3) whyte, 4) *lacteus*, 5) *glaucus*, 6) *karopos*, 7) *pallidus*, 8) *subpallidus*, 9) *citrinus*, 10) *subcitrinus*, 11) *ruffus*, 12) *subruffus*, 13) *rubeus*, 14) *subrubeus*, 15) *rubicundus*, 16) *subrubicundus*, 17) *inopos*, 18) *kyanos*, 19) *veridis*, 20) *niger*. What all þis ben, & in Ynglyssh, & how þai suld be knowen, & what þai betakyn, see inward in þe capitles by & by. (ed. Jasin 1983: 120)

Compartmentalisation of languages is not complete in religious or ritual usage either, which shows that even within this domain code-selection is not determined purely by sociolinguistic preconditions or textual conventions. English is also employed in prayers (74–75), and, outside corpus material, French occurs in a prayer that forms part of a religious charm (76).

(74)   Cryst, þat made boþe est and west,
       Leue here soules haue good reste,
       Euere-more in ioye to be
       In heuen with God in trinitie.
       Amen, [amen] for Charitie.
                                     (ed. Henslow 1899: 126)

(75)   THe holi tr^inite þa^t is heed and welle of kunnynge, ȝeuere & grauntere of gr^ace to alle þo þa^t by her power tr^aueilen truly aboute science & kunnynge, þa^t is helpe & edifiynge to his peple, graunte ȝou gr^ace þa^t þis compilacioun schal haue so for to vsen & disposen þe fruyt of medicyns & of worchinge in it conteyned (ed. Grothé 1982: 1a)

(76)   ffor staunchynge of blode a gode medecyn.
       Take and drynke þe jus of smalache . . . Also sey þis orisoun Seint Marie le vergine et de son doulez sont quil spondist en hye croys et pur le mesme saint je vous emplerant esponditz estanches le sanc de cesty. say þis orisoun þries. (ed. Miller 1978: 56–7)

Further evidence of fluctuation in the use of languages is provided by a charm outside the corpus material in Cambridge, Trinity College MS O.1.57 (f. 126v), where the actual power words consisting of a lengthy prayer in English are preceded by instructions in Latin (see Mooney 1995: 156). On the other hand, many writers translated their Latin quotations from learned medical sources, which implies that they did not expect their projected audience to be fluent in medical Latin.

4.6   Conclusion

Although the wish to make contemporary medical knowledge available for an audience that was only literate in English must have been a major incentive for the vernacularisation of medical texts in medieval England, the discourse community of vernacular medicine was clearly not monolingual. Since Latin was the point of departure for the whole process, it is self-evident that at least some members of the discourse community had to have command of Latin. Similarly, the translators or compilers of texts based on French sources naturally had to know French. In many cases the projected audience of vernacular texts, too, must have been literate in other languages, as passages of varying length in Latin, and sometimes French, were frequently incorporated into vernacular materials. A large number of switches in the material consist of prefabricated utterances or formulaic expressions that cannot be taken as evidence of multilingualism in the proper sense of the word, but there are also examples of switching that requires fluency in both English and Latin from the audience as well.

Code-switches into Latin occur in different types of texts ranging from recipes and remedies (Plate 5) and other instructional materials to translations of learned surgeries (Plate 6) and specialised expository treatises (Plate 3). Some tendencies in the distribution of different types of switching can be discerned, although systematic patterns running across the whole data cannot be established. A number of switching strategies are shared by all varieties of medical writing, whereas some types are more characteristic of only some types of texts. There is also great variation between individual texts belonging to the same general tradition of writing: the writers' idiosyncratic linguistic propensities, conscious choices in translation strategies, habitual scribal practices, and assumptions about the projected audience must have played a part in text production. Although the majority of texts analysed in this study contain some degree of code-switching, there are also texts that can be characterised as truly monolingual. These tend to be placed at the theoretically less sophisticated end of the text spectrum. However, the learned tradition of writing does not automatically imply frequent switching, as some vernacular translations of learned special treatises contain practically no switches into Latin.

Three distinct discourse functions where switches into Latin are frequent can be discerned in the texts. The most prominent function is related to professional discourse. Switched specialised terms in particular occur in texts from all traditions, although all texts do not contain them. Another domain where switches are common is religious discourse. Religious code-switches tend to occur in remedybooks – a feature reflecting the importance of religion in healing. Code-switching is also frequent for text-organising functions. As a metadiscursive practice Latin occurs in texts belonging to all three varieties, with variation between individual texts in all traditions. Switching for quotations is most frequent in surgical texts, whereas in learned specialised texts Latin quotations are rare, and in recipe collections non-existent. There are also switches for which no external discourse function can be assigned; these switches rather seem to stem from the author's or scribe's idiolectal habits and may serve more immediate interpersonal functions. Many switches are multifunctional, serving simultaneously both macrolevel social or textual functions and microlevel interpersonal functions.

Notes

* I would like to thank Professor Outi Merisalo for sharing her expertise in Latin with me in the course of analysing this material.
1. I use the term 'French' in this study indiscriminately to refer to all varieties of French and Anglo-Norman. For the status and varieties of French in post-Conquest England, see e.g. Short (1980), Rothwell (1991), or Burnley (2001) and the references therein.
2. Among the best-known are John Capgrave (1393–1463), a prolific author in Latin and English, and John Gower (d. 1408), writing in Latin, French and English.
3. For code-switching in medieval medical texts, see also Voigts (1996), Hunt (2000) and Panta (2003). The mixture of codes in other types of texts written in medieval England has received attention, e.g., in studies by William Rothwell, Laura Wright, Siegfrid Wenzel, Tim William Machan, Herbert Schendl, and Hans-Jürgen Diller. For a state-of-the-art survey in historical code-switching research, see Schendl (2002b). See also Nurmi and Pahta (forthcoming).
4. For astrological and alchemical materials, see also e.g. Taavitsainen (1988: 112–15) and Voigts (1996).
5. E.g. John Arderne's original 'Latin' surgical text is in fact polyglot, with passages in French or Middle English inserted within Latin (London, British Library, Sloane MS 56). In at least one of the Middle English translations, some of the French passages were retained untranslated (P. M. Jones 1989: 68, 71).
6. For discussions of the Sloane Group in the present volume, see Jones, pp. 33–4, and Taavitsainen, p. 217.
7. This treatise, originally part of the *Compendium medicinae* by Gilbertus Anglicus, is extant in several copies. Rowland (1981) and Hallaert (1982) have previously edited two versions, and an edition of the Trinity copy is forthcoming by Green and Mooney.
8. Cf. the lists of macaronic texts in *IMEP* handlists. See also Voigts (1989a and b, 1996) and Hunt (2000).
9. For accounts, see e.g. Romaine (1995), Eastman (1995), Milroy and Muysken (1995) or Myers-Scotton (1997). For theories of code-switching, see also e.g. Gumperz (1982), Heller (1988), Halmari (1997), Auer (1998), Muysken (2000) and Myers-Scotton (2002).
10. The tendency to focus on spoken language is shared by modern sociolinguistic research in general. The few studies focusing on code-switching in present-day written texts include Stølen (1990, 1992), Myers-Scotton (1998) and Graedler (1999).
11. For differences between speech and writing, see e.g. Biber (1988) or Biber et al. (1999).

12. This is by no means true for all medieval writings. Materials that can be firmly anchored to their social, spatial and temporal context include e.g. many types of official documents and letters. For code-switching in medieval personal letters, see Schendl (2002a), and Nurmi and Pahta (forthcoming).
13. Cf. Norri (1998: 115 and p. 107 below), who points out in his analyses of medieval medical terms that any classification into anglicised or foreign, i.e. borrowed items or code-switches, 'would have to be largely intuitive and yield a multitude of borderline cases'.
14. In the examples, the relevant code-switched Latin items appear in italics and bold type. In some examples, other relevant passages, e.g. flags, appear in bold without italics.
15. For the distribution and frequency of medical terms, I have checked the number of their occurrences in *MEMT* and consulted the latest versions of the standard reference works: the online versions of the *Middle English Dictionary* (*MED*) and *Oxford English Dictionary* (*OED*), and the two volumes on Middle English medical vocabulary by Norri (1992, 1998).
16. For performatives, see e.g. Searle (1985: 16–20) and Palmer (1981: 161–2).
17. For the relation of recipes and charms, see Hunt (1990: 78–99) and Taavitsainen (2001c: 92).

5 Entrances and exits in English medical vocabulary, 1400–1550

JUHANI NORRI

5.1 Introduction

The earlier chapters have provided us with an account of how English emerged from the shadow of Latin and French as the language of medical writings in the late Middle English period, from *c.* 1375 onwards. The advent of printing in England in 1476 had no immediate effect upon the contents of medical works, English medical books, until about the middle of the sixteenth century, mostly reproducing material that was already available in manuscript during the preceding centuries. These averments raise a number of important questions concerning the history and development of medical vocabulary in English. To what extent were writers and translators in late medieval England able to rely on already existing vernacular medical terminology? When there was no earlier model available, what alternatives did they have for expressing a particular meaning? What was the survival rate of the new coinages and adoptions from foreign languages? Is the close affinity between the contents of the earlier sixteenth-century works and fifteenth-century manuscripts also reflected in their vocabulary? It is the purpose of the present chapter to formulate some tentative answers.

Historical linguists and lexicologists have traditionally emphasised the central role of the sixteenth century in the development of scientific and medical terminology in English. Knowles (1997: 69), for instance, says that by that time there was a growing demand for books in English and that the scholarly writers had to 'find words to express concepts which had no conventional English equivalents'. The solutions, adopting a foreign word or coining a new one, were 'the same as those used in the fifteenth century by the Lollards and their opponents'. Knowles further states that 'now it was on a bigger scale, in both the number of words, and the range of texts'. According to Görlach, the Early Modern English period, in particular the decades between 1530 and 1660, witnessed the fastest increase of vocabulary in the history of the English language. The sixteenth-century lexical accrual, he observes, was due to two main factors, one being 'the objective need to express new ideas in English (mainly in fields that had been reserved to, or dominated by, Latin)', and the other 'the subjective desire to enrich the rhetorical potential of the vernacular' (Görlach 1993: 137–8). Schäfer is another scholar who stresses the significance of the sixteenth century for the development of scientific terminologies, being rather dismissive of any pre-1500 progress in this area:

> Around 1500 English was incapable of providing a linguistic medium for traditional scholarship and for the rapidly developing scientific disciplines since it lacked the necessary terminologies. This deficiency was remedied during the sixteenth century by a steady flow of translations, primarily from Latin, and by the publication of increasingly sophisticated, specialised handbooks, which ultimately supplanted medieval encyclopaedic lore. Appropriate vocabulary was supplied for fields as disparate as geometry and rhetoric, and by 1600 there was virtually no field of traditional or new learning which could not be studied in the vernacular. (Schäfer 1989b: 1)

Statements such as the above may be valid for some disciplines, but in the case of medicine we must tread more carefully. The importance accorded to the sixteenth century must not be allowed to overshadow the major developments that had taken place in the vernacular medical vocabulary during the preceding 125 years. In a recent book, McConchie examines the vocabularies in thirteen medical works published between 1547 and 1612, drawing attention to the treatment of the words therein by the compilers of the first edition of the *Oxford English Dictionary* (*OED* 1933). The author rightly states that as far as the history of the early sixteenth-century vernacular medical book is concerned, 'it now seems safe to say that English was well established and perhaps felt to be comparable with Latin by this time, having been in use for over a century for such purposes' (McConchie 1997: 16). In what follows, a main argument will be that the period 1375–1500, besides pioneering the use of the vernacular even in the most technical kinds of medical writing, also laid a solid foundation upon which the relevant lexical fields would be constructed in the centuries to come. It is noteworthy that McConchie's lists of antedatings and unrecorded terms contain a large number of words and phrases already present in Middle English medical manuscripts.[1]

The lexical material analysed for the sections below consists of the 1,188 names of sicknesses and the 1,176 names of body parts that I collected for Norri (1992) and (1998), respectively. Examination of the aggregate 2,364 lexemes will shed light on the general developments that took place in English medical vocabulary at a time when the vernacular was gradually gaining a firm foothold in medical writings alongside Latin and French. The treatises from which the medical terms were gathered represent the three main categories of Middle English medical writing (see Pahta and Taavitsainen, p. 14 above), comprising as they do fourteen remedybooks, nine surgical treatises, and ten academic treatises.[2] Altogether, the material covers close to 7,000 pages from manuscripts and early printed books.

Many of the surgical works referred to are translations from Latin, including Middle English versions of treatises by Guy de Chauliac, Lanfrank, Roger of Salerno, Teodorico Borgognoni of Lucca, and John of Arderne.[3] In the sixteenth century, Joannes de Vigo's *Practica in arte chirurgica compendiosa*, published in 1517, was also translated into English, with the title *The Most Excellent Workes of Chirurgerye* (1543). The translator, Bartholomew Traheron, appended a glossary of foreign terms.[4] One of the nine surgical works goes back to a German original: Hieronymus von Braunschweig's *Buch der Chirurgia* was published in Strasbourg in 1497, but our text, *The Noble Experyence of the Vertuous Handywarke of Surgeri* (1525), was translated into English from Dutch.[5] Besides translations, the surgical treatises studied comprise two manuscripts that are compilations from the works of the most famous ancient and medieval authorities. Of particular interest is the first known surgical compendium in English that is not a direct translation from Latin, put together in 1392 by an anonymous London surgeon, who drew especially upon Lanfrank and Henry de Mondeville.[6] A longer list of sources is given at the beginning of another Middle English manuscript, said to derive from 'Ypocras, Galyen, Auicen, Henricus de Amondavilla, Willelmus de Saliceto, Lamffrank, Tederyk, Brune, Rogeryn, and other auctoris the whiche were expert surgenes'.[7]

Middle English renderings of Latin originals among the academic treatises examined include translations of Bernard of Gordon's *Lilium medicinae*, Gilbertus Anglicus's *Compendium medicinae* and Bartholomaeus Anglicus's *De proprietatibus rerum*. In Bartholomaeus's encyclopaedia, the English version of which was completed by John Trevisa in 1398, the fifth and seventh of the nineteen 'books' deal respectively with body parts and sicknesses.[8] Somewhat misleadingly, the vernacular translation of the Latin *De humana natura*, an anonymous survey of topics relating to anatomy and generation, begins with the words 'Incipit Liber Cerebri'.[9] Two Middle English works of a more original nature, but still primarily relying on material from earlier sources, are the texts written by a so far unidentified 'Austyn' for his 'dere gossip Thomas Plawdon citiseyn & barbour of London',[10] and the urinary compiled from 'þe bokes of meny auctoures' by Henry Daniel, a Dominican friar. Daniel wrote the *Liber uricrisiarum* at the request of a certain 'Walter Turnour of Ketoun', who had asked him to compose a urinary in English.[11] We know that Daniel was writing the treatise in 1378, because at one point he states that 'we ar now in þe 1378 ȝere of Criste'.[12] The academic works studied embrace four further texts, each of them a book printed in the sixteenth century. According to Hibbott (1990: 68), Andrew Boorde's *Breuiary of Helthe*, first published in 1547,[13] is 'the first medical book by a medical man to be originally written and printed in English'. Boorde, a Carthusian, was dispensed from his religious vows at his own wish so that he could devote his time to studying medicine, but there is no evidence that he completed a university degree in medicine.[14] It seems that Sir Thomas Elyot, who based his *Castel of Helthe* (1541) on 'the moste princypall wrytars in phisicke',[15] also lacked a university training, his erudition stemming from private study of famous classical works. Unlike Boorde and Elyot, Christopher Langton, author of *A Uery Brefe Treatise, Ordrely Declaring the Principal Partes of Phisick, that is to Saye: Thynges Natural, Thynges not Naturall, Thynges Agaynst Nature* (1547), is known to have possessed an M.D. degree.[16] In the category of academic treatises there is finally an anonymous compilation said to derive from the works of renowned medical authorities, entitled *Prognosticacion Drawen out of the Bookes of Ipocras, Auicen, and Other Notable Auctours of Physycke, Shewynge the Daunger of Dyuers Syckenesses, that is to Say, Whether Peryll of Death be in them or not, the Pleasure of Almyghtye God Reserued* (1554). A passage on apoplexy suggests that the writer may have had a formal medical training.[17]

Medieval remedybooks are characterised by a tradition of gradual modification and accretion, the compilers borrowing freely from sources which they usually do not indicate. Only exceptionally is there any information about the identity of the writer. Such rare instances in the material here studied include the sixteenth-century remedybook in Oxford, Bodleian Library, Ashmole MS 1389.I, pp. 1–256, where the remark 'probatum est per me W Aderston' is appended to a recipe on p. 28. This is possibly a reference to William Altoftes of Atherstone (Adderston), surgeon to Henry VII (Talbot and Hammond 1965: 380–1; Beck 1974: 153). Even here, however, it is possible that the prescription mentioning 'W Aderston' was simply copied from some other source, the person indicated having no significant role in the putting together of the collection.[18] The lengthy title of one printed remedybook that is attributed to a particular author begins: *This is the Myrour or Glasse of Helthe, Necessary and Nedefull for Euery Person to Loke in that Wyll Kepe Theyr Body from the Syckenes of the Pestylence.* The author is identified on f. B1r as 'Thomas Moulton, Douctour of Diuinite of the ordre of the frere prechours'.[19] Sometimes there seems little justification for such attributions as there are. The title 'Experimenta Dinamidiorum libri Galieni' stands at the beginning of a fifteenth-century remedybook in London, British Library, Additional MS 34111, ff. 114v–167v, but the contents of the manuscript bear no resemblance to the 'Galenic' *Dinamidia*, an examination of various classes of medicines, together with descriptions of specific medicinal substances (MacKinney 1936: 408–14). Likewise, although the Middle English collection of remedies in Oxford, Bodleian Library, Rawlinson MS D.251, ff. 72v–113r (ed. Schöffler 1919), begins with the words 'Incipiunt practica phisicalia Magistri Johannis de Burgundia', it seems that the name of Johannes de Burgundia, a professor of medicine in Liège from about 1330 to 1370, was attached to the treatise just to lend it authority. In the matter of simple copying, we know that the scribe of one of the Middle English manuscripts examined, i.e. the *Liber de diversis medicinis* in Lincoln Cathedral, MS A 5.2, ff. 280r–314v (ed. Ogden 1969), was Robert Thornton, lord of East Newton in the North Riding of Yorkshire.[20] In the remaining nine remedybooks, no similar pointers to particular authors or scribes are to be found, although classical medical authorities and contemporary doctors are from time to time mentioned in individual recipes.[21]

The delimitation of the two lexical fields, names of sicknesses and names of parts of the body, calls for some further comment. It is often difficult to decide with any certainty whether a given word should be assigned to a particular lexical field, and in this matter the present study is no exception. The reader may wonder, moreover, why *sickness* rather than *disease* is used in classifying the terms collected. The decision was taken because in the medieval period the latter word had a much less specific meaning than today. The latest edition of *Dorland's Illustrated Medical Dictionary* (Anderson *et al*. 2000) defines *disease* as 'any deviation from or interruption of the normal structure or function of a part, organ, or system of the body as manifested by characteristic symptoms and signs'. *Symptom*, in turn, is stated to mean 'any subjective evidence of disease or of a patient's condition, i.e., such evidence as perceived by the patient; a noticeable change in a patient's condition indicative of some bodily or mental state', whereas *sign* is said to designate 'an indication of the existence of something; any objective evidence of a disease, i.e., such evidence as is perceptible to the examining physician, as opposed to the subjective sensations (symptoms) of the patient'. This threefold classification did not exist in the English language between 1400 and 1550, as is shown by the entry for *disease* (i.e. lack of ease) in the *Middle English Dictionary* (*MED*), where the general sense 'trouble, misfortune, misery' covers both 'bodily discomfort, suffering, or pain' and 'bodily infirmity or disability; sickness, illness, disease'. The modern distinction between disease, on the one hand, and its symptoms and signs, on the other, was made only vaguely, if at all, in medieval medical treatises, where 'the description of particular diseases often amounted to no more than a list of the symptoms with which it was associated' (P. M. Jones 1984: 58). The name of the disorder was used for what would now be considered a set of symptoms, not for the underlying invasive entity (Siraisi 1990: 117). According to Rawcliffe (1995: 46), 'little or no distinction was made between the symptoms of a disease and the actual ailment itself, since the practitioner regarded both as the products of humoral imbalance, which he had to rectify'. There are thus ample grounds for avoiding the word *disease* when discussing the terms assembled from the texts examined. By using it, one might evoke misleading associations between the medieval and modern meanings of the word.

In present-day English, *sickness*, except in combinations like *caisson sickness* and *sleeping sickness*, has a more general meaning than *disease*, coming close to the Middle English senses 'an abnormal or a special state of physical health' and 'a specific physical or mental disorder' (*MED* s.v.). In studies of Middle English vocabulary, it is therefore more accurate to talk about a lexical field of sickness, rather than one of disease. It must be noted, however, that the word *sickness* was in Middle English commonly used of injuries (cf. Norri 1992: 88), and therefore terms like *fracture*, *lesion*, *puncture*, and *wound* must for our purposes also be consigned to this lexical field.

The delimitation of the lexical field of body parts is an equally complex matter. A natural starting-point is the way in which the word *part* is used in descriptions of the human body in those manuscripts and books examined. The following passage from Christopher Langton's *A Uery Brefe Treatise* adduces the binary classification of body parts commonly used in the Middle Ages:

The ix chapter, of the partes of mannes body. The firste diuision of partes of mannes body is of those that ye Latten men call SIMILARES & DIS-SIMILARES, whiche in Englishe may be called lyke and vnlike. For SIM-ILARES be such partes as be lyke vnto themselues in all thinges, which when they be diuided or parted in sonder, the leste of them kepeth the same name that the hole dothe whereof it is part. And DISSIMILARES be such as are vnlyke themselfes in all thinges, which whan they be deuided or parted asunder, none of them can be called by the name that the hole is, as in example no part of the head can (yf it be separat & parted from the head) be called an head. No more can any part of the hand be named an hand, nor of ye foote a foote, nor of the eye an eye. Yet euery parte of water is called water, and euery part of bloud is called bloude, and euerye parte of bone bone, and euery part of flesh is called fleshe. Therfore these last rehersed be such as the Laten men call SIMILARES and the other be the selfe same that be called DISSIMILARES or INSTRUMENTALES. Galien sayeth that the same partes which the Latyns call SIMILARES be the first elementes and begynners of mannes bodye, although the selfe same be common to brute beastes also, for ther is nether oxe, horse ne dogge but they haue pulses, vaynes, senewes, tiinges, gristilles, skinnes and fleshe . . . Of these, the other which be called DISSIMILARES or IN-STRUMENTALES be made, as hed, handes, feet & such lyke. (Langton, ff. D2v–D3v; *pulses*: 'arteries', *tiinges*: 'ligaments')

Langton, like many another medieval medical author, thus regarded *like parts* or *similares* as the basic components of *unlike parts* or *dissimilares* (*instrumentales*). The former had a fairly homogeneous composition, and the same name could be applied to both the whole structure and parts of it. Langton gives water, blood, bone, artery, vein, nerve, ligament, gristle, skin and flesh as examples of such parts, also described as *like members, simple members, single members, common members, universal members, consimile members*, and *consimilia* in the treatises examined (cf. Norri 1998: 64–6). To cite another writer, 'Austyn' in Cambridge, Gonville and Caius MS 176/97 mentions bones as belonging to the category of *consimilia*, because 'a litel parti of a bon ys as meche in name as þe hole substaunce of it berith' (p. 47). *Unlike parts*, for which we also find the terms *compound members, composed members*, and *membra heterogenia*, could not be divided so that their parts would still have the name of the whole. Head, hands and feet are instanced by Christopher Langton.

The question of what counts as a lexeme denoting a body part in Middle English and Early Modern English medical works is, however, more complicated than the above might suggest. *Part* and *member*, as shown by the phrases cited, appear to be equivalent terms in the present material. Medieval lists of 'things natural', i.e. basic concepts concerning the composition of the human body and its functions, usually include *members* as one category and accord with the in-ventory given by Thomas Elyot: 'Thynges naturall be vii in number: Elementes, complexions, humours, members, powers, operations, and spirites' (f. 1r). According to Siraisi (1990: 101), in these lists *humours* were 'body fluids', *members* 'parts of the body'. Langton, however, mentions water (an element) and blood (a humour) as examples of *like parts*, which suggests that for him at least, *part* had a wider meaning than *member* in the sevenfold classification. For my study of the names of body parts, I selected only those words and phrases that met the requirements of *members* as used by Thomas Elyot, but passages like the one in Langton's book give grounds for thinking that more extensive culling could be justified.[22] Adams, who has studied anatomical terminology in Latin, states that '*bilis* . . . does not strictly indicate a part of the body' (1980: 53), a reminder that the names for body fluids should not, however, be placed at the centre of the lexical field of body parts.

When linguists discuss lexical fields they usually prefer to study single words or idioms and eliminate compounds and phrases from their analysis. Anthropologists, on the other hand, when investigating folk taxonomies have adopted a different approach, including also complex constructions in their inventory of terms for particular phenomena (Lehrer 1974: 19). Not all lexicologists restrict the concept of lexical field to simple lexemes only, and Lipka (1990: 152) for one makes a distinction between a *word-field*, 'exclusively containing morphologically simple items', and a *lexical field*, 'consisting of simple or complex lexemes'. In my studies of the names of sicknesses and body parts, I have understood *lexical field* in the same way as Lipka and thus included combinations such as *tertian fever*, *head ache*, *iliaca passio*, *little finger*, *optic nerve* and *shoulder joint* in the list of lexemes gathered from the medical treatises. Such designations are examples of what Sager *et al.* (1980: 233) call 'extended terminological units', each of which represents a separate and specific concept.

Before considering the results of the lexical analysis, one final issue must be addressed, namely the degree of anglicisation of terms of foreign origin. When studying a Middle English or Early Modern English medical treatise, one frequently comes across a previously unattested lexeme of a highly technical character which has been adopted from a foreign language. Whether such terms were ever really an established part of the English language is a moot point. Pahta's article in the present volume provides us with an examination of the relationship between code-switching and borrowing (see pp. 79, 81–84 above), and only the lexicographical aspect of the matter will be commented upon here. Historical dictionaries tend to be somewhat inconsistent when it comes to listing technical words of foreign origin, and sometimes do not indicate any criteria for their inclusion or omission. In *MED*, for example, the reader finds an entry for *favose* 'a kind of ringworm', but not for *acorose*, another variety of ringworm, although in one of the *MED* citations s.v. *favose* the two terms occur cheek by jowl in the same sentence ('Anoþer [medicine] expert to acorose & fauose').[23] At least in the case of Middle English and Early Modern English medical treatises, frequency of occurrence can hardly be considered a valid criterion for deciding about inclusion in a lexicon. Too few texts have been studied so far to ascertain which lexemes in contemporary treatises were common, which unusual, and any classification, especially considering the profusion of borderline cases, would have to be largely intuitive. When collecting the names of sicknesses and body parts, I have therefore thought it wiser to record *all* the relevant words and phrases occurring in a basically English-language context,[24] with two exceptions only. First, medieval writers often explain that a sickness or body part is called this or that in Latin, French, Greek or Arabic. Typical examples of such constructions, also discussed in Pahta's article (p. 86 above), are 'men in arabie clepen it albarec' (ed. von Fleischhacker 1894: 193), 'called in Latine caroli' (Vigo 1543: f. 72ra), and 'the foot hatte *pees* in latyn' (ed. Seymour *et al.* 1975: 269). Passages attributing the word or phrase to a foreign language should not be ignored by lexicologists and lexicographers, because they often contain information that clarifies the meaning of the term in some other context. Citations such as the above would, however, seem out of place in a dictionary of *English*, unless their special status was somehow indicated, for instance by the use of brackets, which is the policy adopted by *OED*. In my studies of the names of sicknesses (Norri 1992: 389–97) and body parts (Norri 1998: 418–24), an inventory of terms indicated as foreign was given in an appendix, independent of the main lexicon.

The second group of lexemes listed separately consists of a handful of foreign terms which only occur in a Latin form other than the nominative in an English-language context (cf. Pahta, p. 82 above). There is often some further indication of their foreignness, as in the quotations below (italics mine):

> Auycen forsoþe . . . saide *spinam* to be made of a kyndely colre . . . (ed. Ogden 1971: 104)

> But congelacion þat þat Galien clepiþ *catalexim* comyþ of colde & drye. (Oxford, Bodleian Library, Ashmole MS 1505, f. 69r)

The Latin case-ending in these examples shows that the word has been taken over unchanged from the original and retains its foreign character. The Middle English translation of Guy de Chauliac's surgery edited by Ogden (1971) contains a relevant comment on the 'English' forms of Latin technical terms. The translator explains the policy he has adopted as follows:

> Afterward clense it wiþ vnguentum apostolorum (It myghte be saide wiþ vnguento apostolorum in þis translacioun, and þat were more sewynge the fourme and congruyte of gramer, but alle suche termes of Latyn schal be schewed in þis Englisshynge in þe nomynatyf case, for-why þe Latyn of þe nominatyf case is most vsed among Englisshe termes. And also it is so beste to be vnderstonden in commune langage, and most esy, namely to men þat can but þe comune langage.) or wiþ vnguentum Egipciacum. (ed. Ogden 1971: 290)

The form *spinam* in the earlier citation from the same text does not, however, conform to this principle, being a mere copying of the word *spinam* in the Latin original.[25]

Table 5.1. *Chronological layers of medical terms*

	Sicknesses	Body parts	Total
OE (before 1100)	51	125	176
12th century	6	8	14
13th century	29	14	43
14th century	279	260	539
15th century	686	627	1,313
1500–1550	137	142	279
TOTAL	1,188	1,176	2,364

5.2   Chronological layers of medical words

The magnitude of the challenge that medical vocabulary posed to writers and translators in late medieval England can be gauged by examining the chronology of the 2,364 words and phrases collected from the material studied. For this purpose, the lexemes were divided into six different groups according to the period when they are first recorded in written English: Old English (before 1100), twelfth, thirteenth, fourteenth, and fifteenth century, and 1500–1550. When establishing the dates, historical dictionaries of English, in particular *MED* and *OED*, were consulted for each term. The information given in these volumes was complemented by analysis of the 33 treatises, which in fact contained a large number of words not listed in any of the dictionaries of English at present available. In the chronological classification, the date of the manuscript or the year of the printed edition were the primary criteria. Unfortunately, there is some disagreement among scholars concerning the date of Oxford, Bodleian Library, Ashmole MS 1396, which contains an English translation of Lanfrank's *Chirurgia magna*. The editor, von Fleischhacker, estimates that the manuscript was written *c.* 1380. The *MED* dating 'a1400' (*Plan and Bibliography*, p. 51) places the text in the last quarter of the fourteenth century. Keiser (1998: 3646), however, thinks that the translation was made in the fifteenth century. In the present article, as in my 1992 and 1998 studies, the earlier date has been used when analysing the chronology of individual terms, but the effects of a later dating will be indicated whenever relevant.

Although the vocabularies of only a small section of surviving Middle English and Early Modern English medical works have so far been investigated and a good deal of work remains to be done, some general tendencies can already be discerned in the development of the terminology. Etymological study of the names of sicknesses and body parts yields an interesting pattern with respect to the number of lexemes in the different chronological layers. The stratification of the vocabulary is set out in Table 5.1.

Many of the medical terms in the manuscripts and books studied had a long history, reaching back as far as the Old English period. The 176 words and phrases in the oldest layer account for some 7 per cent of the total inventory. The Old English stratum contains a considerably larger number of terms for body parts (11 per cent) than for sicknesses (4 per cent), but in both areas the terms already found in pre-1100 manuscripts belong to the core vocabulary. Generally speaking, they signify common ailments (e.g. *ache, blain, boil, itch, sore, swelling, wart*) or familiar organs and limbs (e.g. *arm, back, bladder, brain, foot, hand, heart, mouth, nail, shoulder, side*).[26]

In marked contrast to the Old English period, only a handful of our lexemes are first recorded in the twelfth century. Among the fourteen terms in this chronological layer we find for example *paralisi, pricking, smart, skin, reins*, and *stone* 'testicle'. The paucity of words and phrases dating from 1100–1200 no doubt partly reflects the predominance of Latin and French as the languages of medicine and the scarcity of vernacular medical texts at that time. In medical contexts, English continued to be outshone by the two foreign languages for the hundred years that followed, and, although the number of new lexical items rises from fourteen to 43, that is still a far cry from the Old English figure. Some examples of the words in the thirteenth-century layer are *dropsy, fallinge evill, lepre, malady, scab, belly, face, front, skull*, and *spleen*.

As has been pointed out in the earlier chapters of this volume, there was a great increase in English medical writing from *c.* 1350 onwards, and the range of subjects dealt with in the vernacular became wider. The proliferation of medical treatises in English had a radical effect on the terminology for sickness and body parts. The number of words and phrases first attested in the fourteenth century that survived into the fifteenth is 539, which accounts for 23 per cent of the entire lexical inventory. The earliest known written occurrence of hundreds of central medical terms dates from this period, some examples being *ague, gout, fester, infirmity, s(c)iatica, bowels, cartilage, ligament, palate*, and *temple*. The greater part of the lexical expansion takes place between 1375 and 1400, when 256 names for sicknesses and 207 names for body parts are first found in written texts. Together they make up no less than 86 per cent of the chronological layer, which suggests that the last quarter of the fourteenth century witnessed a veritable invasion of new words and phrases. The complexities mentioned concerning the dating of Lanfrank's *Science of Cirurgie* in Oxford, Bodleian Library, Ashmole MS 1396 may at first sight lead one to query this statement, because as many as 341 of the terms collected are first recorded in that treatise. That the enormous accretion of medical vocabulary actually began around 1375 is, however, beyond doubt, for reasons that will emerge when we look at the next chronological layer.

The number of terms making their first appearance in the fifteenth century, namely 1,313, is remarkable, since it is more than twice as many as in the preceding century. As explained in the description of the material studied, three of the fifteenth-century manuscripts examined are known to transmit texts written in about the years 1378 (Henry Daniel's *Liber uricrisiarum*), 1392 (the treatise by the anonymous London surgeon), and 1398 (Trevisa's translation of Bartholomaeus Anglicus's *De proprietatibus rerum*). It is instructive to see what

Table 5.2. *Chronological layers of medical terms (dating according to the date of the original)*

	Sicknesses	Body parts	Total
OE (before 1100)	51	125	176
12th century	6	8	14
13th century	29	14	43
14th century	536	613	1,149
15th century	429	274	703
1500–1550	137	142	279
TOTAL	1,188	1,176	2,364

effect the alternative way of dating, i.e. according to the date of the original, would have on the figures presented in the previous table. Table 5.2 shows the chronological stratification of the vocabulary when the latter criterion is used.

Medieval medical manuscripts in English are known to contain miscopied words due either to the scribe's inattentiveness or his failure to understand the original (e.g. Müller 1929b; Keiser 1978; Norri 1988a and b). It is usually impossible to say exactly when the corrupt forms arose. Sometimes a scribe may have replaced a term in the original with one that was more familiar to him. Such uncertainties have been something of a headache to lexicologists classifying words and phrases according to chronology.[27] The *MED* lexicographers have adopted a policy whereby, for example, the treatise by an anonymous London surgeon in Wellcome MS 564 is dated 'c1475(1392)', the year when the original was written appearing in brackets after the date of the manuscript. Even allowing for slight changes in the vocabularies of different manuscripts of the same work, the figures presented in Table 5.2 clearly indicate that a huge augmentation of medical terminology had already begun during the last quarter of the fourteenth century. The influx of hundreds of new words and phrases continued in the following century, when for example *contusion, corn* (on the toe), *inflammation, priapisme, ringworm, lacuna, mam(m)ille, membrane, noddill,* and *rumpe* are first recorded in writing, all of them in manuscripts with no known fourteenth-century original.

It seems that the basis for the development of an English medical vocabulary was indeed laid between 1375 and 1500. During the first fifty years of the sixteenth century, only 279 new lexemes are to be found in the treatises studied. This is a relatively low figure, considering that nine medical works from these decades, comprising approximately 2,000 manuscript and book pages, were examined. The accrual from 1500–1550 is some 12 per cent of the total lexical stock. The new arrivals recognisable to present-day readers include terms such as *cutte, falling sicknes, smal(l) pockes, tension, vitiligo, hymen, intestinum rectum, nipple, uretere,* and *wind pipe.*

In the course of the five or six centuries that have passed since our writers and translators completed their task, there has been a vast increase in medical knowledge and the theoretical framework of medicine is now entirely different from that in the late medieval period. Medical vocabulary has grown steadily over time, together with a better understanding of the nature of sicknesses and corporal structures. The fundamental importance of the late Middle English period, in particular 1375–1500, for the shaping of medical terminology in English is, however, obvious even from a glance at present-day medical dictionaries. These works often list a host of phrases built around a particular headword and signifying a very specific concept, one that would most likely not have appeared in medieval medicine. The headword itself, however, is in many instances familiar to readers of Middle English medical manuscripts. Thus, in *Dorland's Illustrated Medical Dictionary* (Anderson *et al.* 2000), we find 19, 45, and 114 phrases explained s.vv. *herpes*, *sclerosis*, and *hernia*, respectively. All three lexemes first appear in written English during the period 1375–1500, when they also managed to establish themselves as part of the vernacular medical vocabulary, being commonly used especially in academic and surgical treatises (Norri 1992: 338–9, 368).[28] In the lexical field of anatomy, examples of such terms are *artery*, *muscle*, and *nerve* (Norri 1998: 316, 372, 374), each of which will be followed by a plethora of phrases in modern medical dictionaries.

5.3   Sources of new medical words

The authors and translators of medical works in late medieval England often faced the challenge of finding a term for a particular illness or body part where no earlier vernacular designation existed. The following paragraphs present an appraisal of the possibilities available to the writers of the 33 treatises studied in their search for a word or phrase to carry a particular medical meaning. All of the lexemes cited, unless otherwise stated, are first recorded in written English during the last quarter of the fourteenth century, or later. The three linguistic techniques used to meet the need for a new term, discussed in turn, are: (1) adopting a foreign word, (2) modifying the meaning of a non-medical word, and (3) coining a new term.

5.3.1   Terms of foreign origin

Of foreign languages, it was French and Latin that had the most profound influence on the development of English medical vocabulary during the period investigated. It is well known that one of the main difficulties in etymological studies of Middle English words is the uncertainty as to whether certain lexemes came into English via French or Latin. Three criteria point to an indisputably French origin. First, some of the words are attested in French only, with no Latin equivalent (e.g. *blister*, *cramp*, *croupe* 'buttocks'). Second, there are adoptions whose Latin etymon has undergone a sound-change typical of French. Thus, Latin *fistula* first developed into *fistle* in French as the penultimate vowels became slurred. When the unfamiliar consonantal group was modified, this yielded Old French *festre*, which passed into English *c.* 1400.[29] Third, besides changes in sounds, other types of modification took place in French to assimilate medical terms of classical origin. Medieval Latin *malum mortuum*, for instance, became Old French *mormal* or *mort mal*. In Middle French *demigraine*, the first element only of Latin *hemicrania* has been translated into French. It is obvious that Middle English *mormal* and *demigrein* were taken over from French rather than Latin.

By the time our writers started their work, French influence on English medical vocabulary had already passed its peak. The purely French element among the fifteenth-century additions to the lexical stock is less prominent than in the preceding century. For the names of body parts to be found in academic treatises, for example, the number of exclusively French imports drops from 24 in the fourteenth century to a mere nine in the fifteenth, the corresponding figures for surgical manuals being 25 vs. 16, for remedybooks 19 vs. 3 (Norri 1998: 190, 262, 292). The dwindling of purely French adoptions continues in the first half of the sixteenth century, during which period only ten such, descriptive of either sicknesses or body parts, make their appearance. These findings accord with those of Jespersen (1972: 86–7), who made a statistical study of 1,000 words passing from French to English between 1050 and 1900. Nearly half of the words that Jespersen collected from *OED* belong to the years 1251–1400, the heyday of French influence. More recently, Coleman (1995) has studied the chronology of terms belonging to the lexical fields of hate, love, sex and marriage in English. She makes a distinction between a 'new form', i.e. adoption of a word from the original language, and a 'new sense', i.e. a semantic development within English. Her findings parallel my own; Coleman notes that, as far as French influence is concerned, the transition from the fourteenth to the fifteenth century marks a radical decrease in the number of both new forms and new senses (Coleman 1995: 105, 111).

Some further examples of adoptions from French first recorded around 1400 or later are *corn* (on the toe), *felon* 'sore, boil', *foine* 'wound made by thrust', *froncle* 'boil, furuncle', *glet* 'congestion of phlegm or mucus', *gravel* 'urinary crystals in the bladder', *maile* 'pustule in the eye', *rage* 'pain', and *ruby* 'red pimple'. From anatomy, we have, among others, *coffre* 'thorax', *fillette* 'filament of muscle', *fourche* 'the two collar bones as a unit', *gisere* 'liver', *loines, secretes* 'genitals', *uretere*, and *vesie* 'urinary bladder'. The frequency of words taken from French during this period varies greatly: ten of the lexemes cited are found in one treatise only, but there are also terms that are quite common in contemporary medical writings, basic names of sicknesses and body parts like *cramp, fester* and *loines*. In general, many of the French borrowings found in the books and manuscripts studied had already gained a firm foothold in English medical vocabulary during the preceding centuries. Most of the newly adopted terms were not apparently regarded as having a particularly foreign flavour, because the 'called in French' formula occurs only six times in connection with sickness and body part terminology in the material examined.[30]

Many of the relevant lexemes in Middle English and Early Modern English medical treatises have equivalents in both French and Latin, and it is often impossible to state with any certainty which language was the immediate source. Thus, *ulceration* and *palate*, both first recorded in English *c.* 1400, may have been adopted from French (*ulceration, palat*) or Latin (*ulceration-em, palatum*), and there exists the possibility of influence from both sources.[31] Although late Middle English *soda* 'headache' and *orobus* 'caecum, first part of the large intestine' look Latin enough, they are also to be found in the French translation of Guy de Chauliac's surgical *magnum opus* as early as 1370, beside the acclimatised versions *sode* and *orobe* (Sigurs 1965: 211, 215). According to Sigurs (1964: 65), the latter work contains a large number of words retaining their Latin or Greek form, further examples from his list being *noli me tangere* 'erosive ulceration of the face', *sclirosis, herpes, cistis fellis* 'gall bladder', *peritoneum*, and *rectum*, each of which appear in late Middle English texts in identical form. Ellenberger (1974: 150) has argued forcefully in favour of a Latin etymology for Middle English *mots savants*, claiming that '[a]s the medieval libraries of England contained mainly Latin books and school curricula concentrated on Latin texts, learned words borrowed into French from written Latin sources would be more likely also to have entered English from those same sources than through French'. In the light of Sigurs's findings, and considering that the translation of learned medicine into French began a full century before such works started appearing in English (Voigts 1984: 326–7), one must be very cautious, at least where medical vocabulary is concerned.

Terms of possibly dual origin, French and Latin, are the largest single group of foreign adoptions in all three text traditions, i.e. academic treatises, surgical works, and remedybooks.[32] Both languages lie behind *catarr(h)e, colik, exulceration, fracture, indigestioun, inflammation, lientery, priapisme, quotidian* 'quotidian fever', *tension, ventositie* 'flatulence', and *vitiligo*, among others. In the vocabulary for body parts, the terms traceable to both French and Latin include *carotides* 'carotid arteries', *extremites, hymen, lard, mam(m)ille* 'breast', *mandible, membrane, organ, tendon*, and *testicle*, to mention but a few. As in the case of purely French adoptions, the frequency of individual words varies quite considerably. Thus, for instance, citations for *colik, fracture, ventosit(i)e, lard*, and *testicle* are not difficult to find, whereas *membrane*, although recorded as early as the first quarter of the fifteenth century, had not, apparently, managed to establish itself as part of anatomical vocabulary by 1550, as it occurs in only two of the 33 treatises studied.[33]

The general character of the next category of foreign adoptions, words stemming directly from Medieval or Classical Latin, differs from that of the two previous groups. Many of the exclusively Latin imports were evidently technical terms of limited currency, being used in one or two texts only. For instance, the average number of treatises in which particular (Medieval) Latin anatomical designations occur is 1.23, the corresponding figure for the French adoptions being 3.74, for the combined French and (Medieval) Latin adoptions 2.64 (Norri 1998: 152). The following are typical examples of words for sickness that were, it seems, taken over from Latin only, there being no attested occurrences in French: *aliahar* 'ability to see at night but not in daylight', *anelitus* 'difficulty in exhaling', *emfraxis* 'obstruction preventing the free flow of humours', *melanchitone* 'jaundice with severe discoloration of the skin', *rixis* 'rupture of a blood vessel'. The Latin adoptions in the field of anatomy also tend to be technical in nature, as can be seen from terms like *alohosos* 'lower end of backbone, coccyx', *aruina* 'fat surrounding internal organs', *cristal(l)idos* 'lens of the eye', *clavalia* 'temporal bone, especially its tympanic and petrous parts', and *lacuna* 'hole thought to transport excess cerebral fluids to the nasopharynx' (also called *infundibulum*). But alongside the highly specialised words and phrases that require profound medical knowledge before they can be understood, the writers occasionally use a Latin word instead of the common native word for the same referent. *Epar*, for instance, occurs many times in Henry Daniel's *Liber uricrisiarum*, where it is, perhaps for stylistic purposes, used more or less interchangeably with the more familiar *liver*:

> And when sanguis dominatur, þan is epar heile & sounde and in gode temperour and þat is cause and token of gode helthe and nurisshinge of lif, for in helþe of þe lyuer stant helþe of þe blode and in helþe of þe blode stant helth of þe body principaly. (London, British Library, Royal MS 17.D.I, f. 23vb)[34]

Of the foreign languages that between *c.* 1400 and 1550 were to supply English with names for sicknesses and body parts, French and Latin are by far the most important. Among the handful of adoptions from other sources are some words from Old Norse that are first attested during this period, including *gulsuffe* 'jaundice', *rumpe* 'buttocks', and *thombeltoo* 'big toe'. Middle Dutch contributed *speckel* 'small spot on the skin' and perhaps *sprot*, with the same meaning, although for the latter a Middle Low German provenance is also possible. The Dutch original of Hieronymus von Braunschweig's surgical treatise has clearly influenced the vocabulary of the English translation, one example being *bult* 'protuberance; hump on the back', which goes back to Middle Dutch *bulte* (*MNW* s.v.):

> Somtymes is the dysmembrynge in the vndermoost parte or spondyles, somtymes in that myddyl, than maketh a bult on the bake. (von Braunschweig 1525, f. Q2ra; *dysmembrynge* 'dislocation', *spondyles* 'vertebrae')

Little need be said about Greek influence on English medical vocabulary in the same period. Adoptions from Greek without intervenient Latin are very rare, but there may be a number of such terms in the glossary appended to Vigo's surgical book (1543), including *mesareon/mesenterion* (< Gr *mesaraion, mesenterion*) for the mesentery:

> That parte whych is sette in the myddeste of the entrayles and is tied to the backe is called mesenterion or mesareon. (de Vigo 1543, p. 15b)

5.3.2 Modification of non-medical words

A second technique for meeting the need of a new medical term was to take a non-medical word and use it to describe the malady or structure in question. This often meant the use of a metaphor, which, as is evident in many of the comparisons implied in the English, Latin and Greek names of sicknesses and body parts, has from earliest times been invaluable for the creation of new medical terms. Dirckx (1983: 24–5, 33–5, 47–8, 52, 60–1) cites a host of examples from present-day medical English and André (1991: 249–53) lists 105 anatomical metaphors found in Classical Latin texts. Except for the toes (*daktylos*), all the individual Greek terms for the bones of the foot are metaphors (Michler 1961: 219). Galen told his readers that the molars (*mylai*) were so called because their function resembles that of mills (*myloi*) grinding corn (Singer 1948: 771).

The names of sicknesses first recorded in written English between *c*. 1400 and 1550 include many metaphors, each of them highlighting some singularity of the disorder in question. The term *blast*, for instance, used by Andrew Boorde for an unspecified eye condition which began suddenly, like a gust of wind, well expresses the manner in which the affliction fell on the patient. The following passage suggests that the old Anglo-Saxon belief in 'flying venoms' that blew about in the air, each giving rise to a different ailment (Bonser 1963: 41; Rubin 1974: 63), may also have had something to do with the naming of the eye trouble:

> XROPHTHALMIA is the Greke worde. In Englysh it is named a blast or an impediment in the eye, the which may come certeyne wayes . . . This impediment doth come of an euyl wynde or els of some contagiouse heat or of an euyl humour or suche lyke, for the eye wyll neither swell nor water nor droppe. (Boorde 1547, f. 140v)[35]

The abruptness of the affliction also explains why *schot(h)e*, recorded as early as Old English in the sense of 'sudden sharp pain', came to be used of an onrush of blood into the eye. The suddenness is evident also when Henry Daniel employs the same word as an equivalent of *cramp*: 'if on haue þe schote or the cramp and þer come a feuer, it is curable' (f. 85va). Several animal metaphors were used to describe the course of a consuming or corroding sickness. Cancer of the rectum remains unnoticed for a long time, and its furtive character was compared to the behaviour of an owl in the day-time:

> The owle is a postem þat is withinne þe fundement growynge in langaone with grete duresse but it hath but lytyll sorowe ne ache þerwith, þat is to seye tofore þe vlceracion. Þe weche is no þinge ellys but a canker hydde þat may not be knowen be þe syghte of þe ye in his begynnynge, for he hydeþ hymselff all withinne þe fundement & þerfore it is callyd þe owle, for as þe owle is a beest kepynge derk places so is þis syknesse hyde hymselff withinne þe fundement at his begynnynge. (Cambridge, Emmanuel College MS 69, f. 102r; *fundement*: 'anus', *langaone*: 'rectum')

Cancer, or perhaps gangrene, in the thighs or legs was called the *wolf* on account of its fierce and consuming nature:

> The cankre is a perlows evill þat commyth to a man throwʒ malyncoly and [hath] but one hole large and blake and euer stynkyng. For þat at commyth in thyes or in legges ys callede þe woolfe. (London, British Library, Sloane MS 240, f. 106v)

Various swellings and growths were compared to familiar objects of the same shape. A hail-like growth on the eyelid was called a *hail*, a stye or a pustule on the eye was known as a *corn*, and many other words associated with the idea of a 'knot' or a 'knob' – *knap*, *knot*, *knorre*, *knarle*, *knorle* – came to be used of rotund excrescences and swellings. Yet another word descriptive of shape is *nail*, which may have meant a pterygium, a wing-like structure extending from the conjunctiva to the cornea.[36] Further examples of disorders interfering with vision are *web*, *cloth*, and *cloud*, all difficult to identify in modern terms, but cataract seems one possibility.[37]

When searching for a word to express the feeling of pain or discomfort associated with a malady, the writers of the texts studied often resort to a colourful metaphor. Christopher Langton, for instance, talks about 'many frettes and pinchinges both in the belly & also in the mouth of the mawe' (f. H2r). *Thorne*, another name for *erisipila*, a condition characterised by 'gnawynge akþe and prikkynge' (ed. Ogden 1971: 102), reminds us of the excruciating pain felt by the patient. The recipe entitled 'For þe stake in þe syde' in the *Liber de diversis medicinis* (ed. Ogden 1969: 35) tells us how to alleviate a stitch in the side, the feeling of pain being identified with the effect of a pointed stake piercing the side.

In Middle English and Early Modern English anatomical vocabulary metaphor is also commonplace. A body part is often compared to some familiar object of similar shape. The pupil, supposed to be a globular solid body,[38] was known as the *apple* of the eye as early as the Old English period. In late Middle English medical treatises, *ball* conveys the same idea: 'The cataracte is a manere spotte of the pannycles wiþynne the eyʒe afore þe pupille (i. þe balle) of þe eyʒe' (ed. Ogden 1971: 459; *pannycles*: 'membranes'). The cartilages of the windpipe were likened to a *ring*, the tunicae of the eye to a *rind*, and the upper surface of the liver to a *hill*. Among the most frequent anatomical terms in the manuscripts and books studied are *cod* 'scrotum', a metaphorical use of *cod* 'bag, pod of a plant', and *yard* 'penis', so called because of its resemblance to a twig or a rod, both earlier meanings of *yard* (*OED* s.v. *yard* n.2). Position, as well as shape, probably occasioned the designation *tail* for the coccyx, or lowermost part of the spinal column.

Some of the anatomical metaphors are based on the function of the body part in question. The nurturing or protective roles of the uterus and the cerebral meninges are reflected in the term applied to both, i.e. *mother*:

The modir in a womman is a singuler membre disposid as a bladdre, and
kynde haþ ordeyned þat membre to fonge and resseyue þe humour semynal.
(ed. Seymour *et al.* 1975: 263)

To defende þe brayn tweye wedes ben nedeful þat ben iclepid þe modres
of þe brayn. (ed. Seymour *et al.* 1975: 174; *wedes*: 'membranes')

Mother 'cerebral meninx' goes back ultimately to an Arabic metaphor that emphasised the enwrapping function of the membrane. In the twelfth century,
William of Conches suggested rather fancifully that all nerves have their origins
in the meninges, and said that this explains the name (O'Neill 1993: 96). In the
Chauliac manuscript studied, the thorax is called *ovene*, an image which, according to French (1979: 101), is based on the idea of the chest as 'a rigid, hollow
structure containing the heat-producing heart'.

Of course, other functions than protection and nurture underlie anatomical
metaphors, a good example being *wellis* 'salivary glands' in the sentence: 'In þe
þrote [read: rote] of þe tunge ben .ij. wellis þat spotil is gaderid þeron, & holdiþ
alwey þe tunge moist' (ed. von Fleischhacker 1894: 261). The metaphor *diche* can
only be understood in the light of medieval medical theory, signifying as it does
an orifice once thought to exist in the ethmoid bone, draining off excess fluids of
the brain:

Thanne a litil aforn þese two additamentis [olfactory lobes] is a diche or
concauite, which þat is callid Colatorium of summen, & is bitwene þe
tweyne y3en vndir þe vppere extremite of þe nose. (ed. Grothé 1982: 65)

The essence of some metaphorical denotations of body parts goes beyond resemblances of shape, position or function. In the English version of Hieronymus von
Braunschweig's surgical treatise, for example, the lobes of the lungs are compared to a feather, partly perhaps because of the lightness of the organ, but also
no doubt the structure: 'The longues hath.v. lobos or feders, .iij. in the right syde
and .ij. in the left syde' (f. B4ra).

Quite a large number of the Middle English and Early Modern English
metaphors for sicknesses and body parts are the result of copying a Latin model.
Medieval Latin *ungula*, besides its basic meaning 'finger-nail', also came to signify 'tumour in the eye' (*RMLW* s.v.), and the English word *nail*, as shown above,
simply imitated this Latin usage. *Mother*, both in the sense 'uterus' and 'cerebral
meninx', is likewise a translation of Medieval Latin: in the former case *matrix*
'womb', in the latter *mater* 'meninx'. In Table 5.3 I give some further examples of
this practice, known as 'semantic borrowing' or 'loan shift', from the two lexical
fields investigated.

Metonymy, a transfer of meaning founded on the nearness in space or time of
things or activities, is also manifest in the material examined, although its role is
not as prominent as that of metaphor. Metonymy tends to give abstract words a
concrete meaning, for example by extending the name of an action to its result
(Ullmann 1977: 220). *Breach* is first recorded in Old English in the sense of 'the

Table 5.3. *Some examples of semantic borrowing among Middle English medical terms*

English term	Latin counterpart
Cloth	ML *pannus* 'piece of cloth', 'film over the eye' (*RMLW* s.v. *pannus* 2)
Hail	ML *grando* 'hail', 'stye on the eyelid' (*DML* s.v.)
Web	ML *tela* 'web', 'spot in the eye' (*RMLW* s.v.)
Ovene	ML *clibanus* 'oven', 'thorax' (French 1979: 101)
Ring	ML *anulus* 'ring', 'segment of the trachea' (*DML* s.v.)
Yard	ML *virga* 'twig', 'penis' (*RMLW* s.v.)

act of breaking something' (*OED* s.v. *breach* sb.), and later developed the meaning of 'an injury (a wound, fracture, hernia, etc.)'. Similarly, *stroke* 'the act of striking' came to mean also the mark or injury left by a blow, as seen from the heading 'Pronosticacion of woundes, strokes, and strypes' in the book on *Prognosticacion* (?1554, f. B3r).

In one type of metonymy, the so-called *pars pro toto*, a salient part of some thing comes to represent the whole. A good example is *pock(e)s*, the plural of *pocke* 'a pustule, pimple or spot'. *Pock(e)s* or *poxe* also began to signify the condition provoking such eruptions, especially syphilis. In Boorde's book, it is stated that 'a man doth abreuiate his lyfe . . . by takyng the pockes with women' (1547, f. 7r).

Among the lexemes studied, there is only one metonym based on nearness in time, the rather curious *nighte* that occurs in the Chauliac manuscript:

> Of pymples and of blaynes and of swetynges and of the ny3tes (þe whiche ben smale clostres in a membre of mykel swetynge) and of knottynesses in the flesshe comynge with ycchinge when þat a man is right hote and claweþ hym while he sweteth. (ed. Ogden 1971: 399)

In the Latin version of Chauliac edited by McVaugh (1997: 297) we find *planta noctis* in the corresponding passage. Sudhoff (1910) observes that Medieval Latin *planta noctis* is actually a mistranslation of the Arabic, which meant 'daughter' of the night, not 'plant' of the night. According to Avicenna's *Canon*, the pimples are so called because they multiply most at night (*ibid.*).

In the lexical field of anatomy, only a handful of terms appear to have been derived metonymically from non-anatomical words between *c.* 1400 and 1550. *Si3t* 'pupil of the eye' and *stappis* 'soles of the feet' manifest a semantic development whereby the meaning is extended from an action, seeing or stepping, to the part of the body involved:

> 3if þou frotyst þe sy3t of þyn y3e wiþ þyn honde þe schal seme þat þe ly3t daunsiþ & lepiþ vpward & adounward & nere & fere. (Oxford, Bodleian Library, Ashmole MS 1505, f. 107v)

So seiþ Basilius *super illud verbum in Exameron*: He schal bruse þine heed, and þou schalt ligge awaite vpon his helis and stappis, *Genesis 3º*. (ed. Seymour *et al.* 1975: 210)

In another kind of metonymic shift, the name of a quality comes to denote the person or object exhibiting it (Ullmann 1977: 220). The *black* of the eye 'pupil' is a black hole in the middle of the organ, the parts surrounding the iris being the *white* of the eye. The latter word could also signify aqueous humour, the watery fluid between the cornea and the crystalline lens: 'The thyrde humour or substance is the white of the eye' (Boorde 1547, f. 100v).

In some cases, the semantic shift that yields the medical term is neither metaphor nor metonymy. Rather, what we have is an everyday word finding its way into the language of medicine, where it comes to be applied to a special *type* of the condition or structure in question. OE *fitt* meant 'a conflict, struggle' (*OED* s.v. *fit* sb.2), but the use for a recurrent attack of a sickness, especially fever, is not recorded until about 1450. A whole group of words for a stain or crack proved useful for denoting similar marks on the human body. An ocular scar that obstructed vision was in late Middle English known as a *mole*, which goes back to OE *mal* 'a spot, blemish': 'If it [ophthalmia] is euel ikept þerof leueþ a litil mole and infeccioun' (ed. Seymour *et al.* 1975: 361). As well as 'spots' in the human eye, the Middle English word signified discolouring marks on the skin, thus being equivalent to *speck*: 'Also in þe body beþ diuers speckes, nowe red, now blak, now wanne, now pale' (ed. Seymour *et al.* 1975: 424). The vocabulary for fissures and chaps in the skin is multifold, including terms like *chine*, *chink*, *clift*, and *cracke*.

In anatomy, this way of augmenting terminology is represented for example by *bande* 'ligament', which refers to a special type of 'band', one linking together two bones at a joint. Among the names for the joint itself, we find *bought* 'bend, curve', as in *bouȝte of þe elbowe* (ed. Grothé 1982: 91) and *boowghte of þe knee* (Cambridge, Emmanuel College MS 69, f. 172v). The cleavage between the buttocks is called the *clift of þe buttockes* (ed. Seymour *et al.* 1975: 266), and the same word is also found in the senses of 'cranial suture' and 'vulva':

One ioynynge [of bones] is as it were a sawe, as in þe commyssures or cliftes of þe brayne panne. (ed. Ogden 1971: 350; *commyssures*: 'sutures', *brayne panne*: 'skull')

The matrix or moder . . . hath a cleft namyd vulua. (von Braunschweig 1525, f. C1ra)[39]

5.3.3 Coinages

A third main technique for meeting the need of a new term is coinage, i.e. creating a new name for a sickness or body part, especially by affixation or compounding. The writers of the works examined employ suffixation, almost always with a native suffix, much more often than prefixation. Marchand (1969: 210–11) states that it took some time before suffixes of French and/or Latin origin resulted in new English words. This is because users of English had to familiarise themselves with the French or Latin syntagma before they could adopt the foreign pattern in native formations. This is more demanding than adding a native suffix to a foreign adoption, since in the latter case there is no comparable assimilation of a structural pattern.

For the names of sicknesses, the commonest suffix by far in the present material is *-ing*, mostly used in the sense of 'the action of – ' or 'a particular instance of – '. *Fainting, fest(e)ring, putrefying, vomiting*, and *wasting* are examples that even present-day readers would recognise. The word sometimes closely reflects contemporary medical theory, denoting a disturbance of the four humours, often attributed to excessive heat (*boiling, chaufing, heting, incending, inflaming, scalding, seething*) in the body. The coagulation or *congealing* of humours also upset the system. The verbal root may involve metaphor or specialisation of meaning. Numbness in the limbs, for instance, was called the *sleping* of the hands or feet: 'And if þe ston is in þe reynes, hit is iknowe by slepinge of þe fote and in þe ioyntes of þe lift side' (ed. Seymour *et al.* 1975: 409). Besides indicating an action, the suffix *-ing* may denote its result, as in *biting* 'a bite', *breaking* 'a fracture', *cutting* 'a cut', *disjoining* 'a dislocation', *poisoning*, and *wresting* 'spraining of an ankle'. In some of the above instances (e.g. *fest(e)ring, poisoning*), because an identical substantival and verbal form pre-existed the suffixed word, it is almost impossible to say which is the root. Only seldom, however, does the formation appear to be indubitably de-nominal in origin. Such rarities include *fistuling, ulcering, syncoping* (from *syncope* 'fainting'), and *scabbing*. The small number of de-nominal forms can no doubt partly be explained by the fact that the suffix adds little or nothing to the meaning of the root.

After *-ing*, the commonest suffix in the names of sicknesses is *-ness*, which mainly forms de-adjectival nouns expressing the condition referred to by the adjective. Some fifteenth- and early sixteenth-century examples are *bareinesse* 'sterility', *franticnes* 'insanity', *lothsomnes* 'nausea', *stonines* 'hardening of tissues', and *goggeliȝednes* 'squinting of the eyes'. The adjective is sometimes transparently metaphorical, as in the two terms for numbness, *ded(e)nesse* and *slepinesse*:

> dedenesse in a mannys fete þat cometh of colde (Oxford, Bodleian Library, Ashmole MS 1505, f. 46v)

> a slepynesse in his legges, with a lyttell feuer (Elyot 1541, f. 90v)

Nominal roots only occasionally attract the suffix *-ness*, but there are formations like *anguishnes* 'pain, sickness', *potagrenes* 'podagra, gout in the feet', *rot(e)nes* 'putrefaction, suppuration; tooth decay', and *scabnes* 'a scabby condition of the skin'. As with *-ing*, the paucity of de-nominal coinages is partly due to the suffix adding little or nothing to the root noun. The suffix *-ness* preponderates, almost completely, over the other two native suffixes of similar applicability, namely *-head* and *-ship*. For most of the latter formations there is also a commoner alternative with -*ness*. This is true of *bareinhede*, *defhed*, *horeshed*, *rot(t)enhed*, *sorehed*, *blereship (of the eyes)*, *narewship (of the breast)*, and *rotschipe*. Suffixes of foreign origin are hardly ever used in the coining of new terms for sicknesses. It has been suggested that *hicket* is the noun *hick* 'hiccup', plus the originally Old French diminutive suffix -*et* (*OED* s.v. *hicket*). No direct Latin or French origin has as yet been found for *aborcement* 'miscarriage', *astonis(s)hement* 'paralysis, numbness', and *obtalmicacioun* 'ophthalmia, ocular inflammation'. In all three instances, however, the English writer apparently simply altered the form of the foreign word: *aborcement* seems to be a blend of Medieval Latin *aborsus* and Old French *avortement*; *astonisshement* has the same meaning as Middle French *estonnement* 'apoplexy'; and the term corresponding to *obtalmicacioun* (ed. Ogden 1971: 443) in the Latin Guy de Chauliac is *obtalmiacione* (ed. McVaugh 1997: 328).

There appear to be very few English names of sicknesses formed by prefixation in late Middle English and Early Modern English medical treatises. In the material examined, *misturning* 'contortion of the face due to an apoplectic or epileptic fit' has both prefix and suffix: 'And mysturnyng of þe face, also falling dovne to grounde, is a grete token' (ed. Getz 1991: 28). *Unfeling* 'numbness', *unjointing* 'dislocation', *unbursting* 'fracture', and *unhelling* 'loss of skin' (from *helen* 'cover') render Medieval Latin *insensibilitas*, *dislocatio*, *disruptio*, and *excoriatio*, respectively. Prefixation only is present in *distemperature* and *mistemperure*, both of which mean 'an upset state of the bodily humours'. No French or Latin etymon has so far been found for those two words.

Derivation is on the whole much less frequent among Middle English and Early Modern English anatomical terms than in the names of sicknesses from the same period. Suffixation, almost always with a native suffix, is again far more frequent than prefixation. The suffix -*ing* occurs in *binding* and *tiing* 'ligament', which emphasise the linking function of the ligaments, as well as in designations for the various bends and curves in the human body, including *bending*, *bowing*, *croking*, and *folding*. Latin *panniculus* 'membrane' is rendered as *cloþing*. The processes, or thin projections, of bones are called *eching*, a term deriving from the verb *echen* 'increase, supplement':

And in þe ioynte half it [shoulder blade] is somwhat long and rounde in the manere of an hefte, wiþ þre echynges in þe ende. (ed. Ogden 1971: 50; *hefte*: 'handle, hilt')

The suffix -*er* is found in a number of names of body parts, among them *grinders* 'molars', *kervers* 'incisors', *roller of þe kne* 'kneecap', and *helpers* 'bones of the upper arms, humeri', a translation of Medieval Latin *adjutorii*.[40] The agentive -*er* is also the final element in *hyngers* 'testicles', seen as the 'hanging parts':

For hym þat will not be dronken . . . strenkill hym ofte with calde water or laye his hyngers in calde water. (ed. Ogden 1969: 37)

Two diminutive suffixes, *-ette* and *-ling* (*-lin*), make their appearance in the inventory of coinages first recorded around 1400 or later. *Lappette* 'lobe of liver or lungs' consists of *lap(pe)* 'lobe' and the suffix *-ette*. It is not quite clear why a diminutive suffix should have been added to a word that already signified the structure in question. Whatever the reason, however, such mutations are by no means rare in anatomical terminology. Sournia (1976: 103) draws attention to the phenomenon, instancing Latin doublets like *auris/auricula* 'ear' and *umbilicus/umbiliculus* 'navel'. The suffix *-ling* (*-lin*) has been grafted on to *poke* 'pouch' in the phrase *pokelyn of the galle* 'gall bladder'.

Fatnes and *fathed* 'fat' are unusual forms, nouns ending in *-ness* and *-hood/ -head* only seldom having a concrete referent (Marchand 1969: 293, 336). Another concrete noun with *-ness* is *wyitnesse*, given as an equivalent of *albugineus* 'aqueous humour of the eye' in the translation of the surgical work by Teodorico Borgognoni of Lucca (London, British Library, Sloane MS 389, f. 59r). The suffix *-ly* occurs only in *bodely* 'median cubital vein', third epithet in the verbose designation 'mediana, þe myddel veyne or þe bodely' (ed. Ogden 1971: 51). *Bodely* is a translation of Medieval Latin *corporalis*, the vessel being so called because venesection from it was thought to alleviate maladies in many different organs (Hyrtl 1879: 171).

Suffixes of foreign origin are hardly used at all to coin new English names for body parts. In the *Liber cerebri* (ed. Carrillo Linares 1993: 55), the first cell of the brain is called *fantastical*, the Latin version in London, British Library, Sloane MS 2454, f. 84vb, having *fantasticam* in the corresponding sentence. The translator of the Middle English version of John of Arderne's treatise here studied appears to have been responsible for the *-ive* ending in *extremitives* 'hands and feet, extremities', since the Medieval Latin text has *extremitas* or *extremitates* in these passages:[41]

> It is to be vnderstande þat a woman beeinge in þis passyoun behoueþ furste to haue stronge rubbynge in þe extremytyffes, þat is to seye in þe feet & in þe handes with salt & vinegre. (Cambridge, Emmanuel College MS 69, f. 162r)

MED s.v. *spiritualtive* suggests that the author, an anonymous London surgeon, may have produced a hybrid from Latin *spiritualis* and Medieval Latin *spiritivus*, when he informs the reader that 'þe mydrif departiþ bitwene þe nutritiues & þe spiritualtiues' (ed. Grothé 1982: 22; *mydrif:* 'diaphragm').[42]

Only a few names of body parts were formed by prefixation in late Middle English and Early Modern English. *Fore-* is the first component in *forefinger, forehande* 'forearm', *foreskinne* 'prepuce', and *forekitters* 'incisor teeth'. Another prefix with a locative meaning, *mid-*, occurs in *mid vein* 'median cubital vein'.

In addition to affixation, compounding was a common way of coining new words. Making a distinction between compounds and syntactic phrases is difficult in medieval texts. Compounds and phrases should perhaps be thought of as a continuum, with combinations where the composite parts have lost their formal or semantic identity at one extreme and those in which the components preserve their individual character at the other. The degree to which the two parts have fused will then become apparent, but it is not necessary to make any strict distinctions. Four main groups can be established for both names of sicknesses and names of body parts.

In the first type of combination, the elements are structurally fused. The construction of the lexical item differs either phonologically or morphologically from the corresponding free phrase. The term may, for example, lack an inflectional ending between the two components. In *gogle eye* 'squint' the first part is the verb *gog(e)len* 'stagger, wander' (*MED* s.v.), minus the participial ending. In *apegalle* 'inflammation of the penis', *ape* is probably an implied genitive, as the form *apes galle* is also recorded in *MED* s.v. *ape-galle*. The second part is *galle* 'a sore on the skin' (*MED* s.v. *galle* n.2). The painful condition may cause ulceration:

> Pro le scaldynge virge quod vocatur apegalle. Take lynnen clooþ, þat is clene wasshen, & brenne hyt, and make þer of poudre, & take oyle of egges, & anoynt þe sore, & put þe poudre in to þe holes, when þey beoþ anoynted, and þat shal hele eny pyntelle, þat is skalded or sore. (ed. Heinrich 1896: 76)

As for the origin of the term, the association of the ape with lubricity may have played a part. Quadrumanous mammals, the ape among them, are regularly associated with sensuality or lechery in the plays of Shakespeare (de Vries 1974 s.vv. *ape, baboon, monkey*).

In other instances of structural fusion, the elements of the corresponding syntactic phrase may be in a different order, perhaps accompanied by a preposition. The names of sicknesses combining a verbal form and an organ or limb usually consist of a gerund followed by an *of*-phrase (e.g. *bleeding of the nose*). Sometimes, however, the part of the body figures as a premodifier of the gerund, as in *nosebleding, heed swiming* 'vertigo', and *herte brenning* 'heartburn'. In anatomical vocabulary, instead of a postmodifying *of*-phrase there is a premodifier for example in *lunge pipes* 'bronchi', *eyȝe appul* 'pupil', *yȝe hoole* 'socket of the eye, orbit', and *wombe ȝate* 'vulva'. Sometimes it is difficult to know why a translator should have chosen a particular rendering of the Latin. *Erebowys* in the English version of Bartholomaeus Anglicus corresponds to *tympora* in the Latin original,[43] but the reason for calling the temples 'bows of the ears' is not clear:

> The oþir [nerve of the fifth pair of cranial nerves] comeþ by þe erebowys to þe chekes, and sperediþ and helpiþ þe worchinge of membres þereaboute. (ed. Seymour et al. 1975: 278)

Some of the structurally fused combinations have a locative particle as the first part. Compounds with *up* denote digestive disorders, in particular vomiting (*upspewing*) or nausea (*uppesething, upwelming*), but the same element also appears in *upblowing* 'swelling'. It seems that the particle is mostly emphatic in such formations, since *spewing, welming,* and *blowing* alone would convey the basal meaning. Marchand (1969: 121) states that *up* in Middle English verbs is often a translation of Latin *ex-*, *e-*. It is certainly possible that Latin *euomo* 'to vomit or spew out' from *ex-* 'out, away' and *uomo* 'to be sick, vomit' (*OLD* s.v.) is the origin of the terms for an upset stomach.

Besides *up*, the particle *out* is used to express the idea of protrusion or swelling. Excrescences, distensions and growths are called *outgoinges*, *out(e)growinges* and *outseminges* in one of the English translations of Guy de Chauliac's work:

> Smale apostemes, after Auicen, ben outsemynges and bleynes and smale ploukes apperynge in þe skyn. (ed. Ogden 1971: 74; *plouke*: 'a pustule', 'a pimple')

> Kyttynge and fretynge away of suche outegrowynges [scrophules] is mykel to drede aboute þe wombe. (ed. Ogden 1971: 116; *wombe*: 'stomach')

> And he [Albucasis] comaundeth to take scrophules and soche tretable outgoynges wiþ fyngres and kytte ham. (ed. Ogden 1971: 121)

In these cases, the particle is clearly a translation of the Latin prefix *ex-*, *e-*, since the Latin original has *excrescencia* or *eminencia* in the corresponding passages (ed. McVaugh 1997: 58, 89, 92).

In the English version of von Braunschweig's surgical book, the reader comes across two more particles occurring as the first part of a compound, namely *in* and *to*. *Inbowing* was a fracture in which the bones were stove in: 'Of the inbowynge of the heed, as a ketyll is inbowed whanne it falleth, or is cast downe' (f. A3ra). Middle Dutch *toeval*, defined as 'a symptom' in *MNW* s.v., is evidently the origin of *tofallinge*, a term for a sickness following or accompanying another sickness:

> If ye hele it [the wound] vp or the payne be passyd and gone, it is to be feared that an impostume and swellynge with great hete shall stryke to the wounde, and of that tofallynge it fortuneth somtyme the losse of a lymme or dethe. (von Braunschweig 1525, f. C4va)[44]

The locative particles *in* and *over* are used for coining new names of body parts during the period 1400–1550. *Inkitters* 'incisor teeth', a translation of Medieval Latin *incisores*, is only attested in the English version of Bartholomaeus Anglicus (ed. Seymour *et al.* 1975: 202), and the same manuscript contains the unique occurrence of *ouerliddes*: 'The browis ben iclepid *supercilia* "þe ouerliddes"; for þey ben isette aboue þe yӡeliddes' (ed. Seymour *et al.* 1975: 187). Just why the arched upper side of the foot should be called an *instep* remains a mystery (*OED* s.v. *instep* 1).

Some of the examples quoted above exhibit semantic integration as well as structural fusion. In *gogle eye*, *apegalle*, and *eyӡe appul*, for instance, one of the elements is a metaphor, the combination forming an idiomatic unity.

The second main category of compounds and phrases comprises items that are characterised by semantic integration only. The best examples of this group of coinages are those in which neither element alone signifies a sickness or a part of the body. Many of these combinations are translations of Medieval Latin, including *lions property* 'leprosy with gross disfigurement' (< ML *leonina*; see quot.), *canine (dogges, houndes) appetit* 'bulimia' or 'insatiable appetite' (< ML *caninus appetitus*; DML s.v. *caninus*), and *rauenes byle* 'coracoic process, a curved process of the scapula overhanging the shoulder joint':[45]

> LEONINA is the Greke worde. In Englyshe it is named the lyons propertie, for this worde is deriued out of LEO, LEONIS, whiche is in Englyshe a lyon. (Boorde 1547, f. 81r)

> There be .ii. kyndes of this infyrmyte [canyne/dogges appetyde] . . . Yf it do come of a melancoly humour, a man shal haue a rauinyng stomake to eate whatsoeuer he can get. And whan the stomake is ful repleted, than it is trobled, and than the pacyent is prouoked to vomytinge. And after that the stomake is so euacuated or empty than the pacyent doth fall to eatynge agayne, and so consequently to vomytynge againe. There is another canyne appetyde, whiche is whan a man is euer hyngry and is neuer satisfyed, nor is nat well but whan he is eatynge or drynkynge. (Boorde 1547, f. 29r)

> Þe twiseled forkes ben nedeful to bynde þe schuldres and to departe ham fro þe brest. Þe boones þerof ben rounde withoute, ibounde to þe tendirnesse of þe brest and behynde to þe rauenes byle. (ed. Seymour *et al.* 1975: 219; *twiseled forkes*: 'collar bone')

There are many other semantically integrated combinations where neither part is a medical term. *Elf cake* is defined as an enlargement of the spleen caused by elves in *MED* s.v. *elf*, sense 2.a, but the spleen was not the only organ affected:

> Whoso hath an yuyll on his liuere þat men clepen þe elff cake. Grynde wormode & make þerof a plastre & ley it to þe yuyll on þe same syde of man or of womman. (London, British Library, Sloane MS 1764, f. 11v)

Henry Daniel calls the middle finger *mikel man* (f. 48va), which connotes the size of the digit. One of the names for the index finger, *lic-pot*, refers, we may suppose, to the habit of scouring or 'licking' the pot clean after a meal. In the *Liber cerebri*, the taboo surrounding the literal mention of the anus is evident in the terms *secret cercle*, *shamefast cercle*, and *shamefast compas* (ed. Carrillo Linares 1993: 74, 83), all translations of Medieval Latin *pudicus circulus*.

Occasionally, combinations in which one of the elements is a medical word assume a unit-like character. *Dronken mannes coughe* 'hiccups' in Boorde's book (1547, f. 123r) involves the comparison of one ailment with another. Close semantic unity may lead to phonological reshaping, which obscures one or both of the original components. Obfuscation of one of the composite parts has led to the form *white blowe* in the second part of Boorde's 1547 book, called *Extrauagantes* and foliated separately:

> In Englyshe it [redimie] is named a white blowe, or a white flawe, the which doth grow about the rote of the nayle. (Boorde 1547, *Extrauagantes*, f. 18v)

The more common form in the treatises studied is *whit(e)flawe*. Various conjectures have been made as to the provenance of the word, a precursor of modern *whitlow* 'a painful inflammation or suppuration on the finger'. *OED* proposes that *white* and *flaw* 'a fissure' were combined. As shown by the passage from Boorde, there were at least two versions of the term in Early Modern English.

In the third category of compounds and phrases we find a very general word meaning 'sickness' or 'body part' used as the second element. In the names of sicknesses, the semantic relationship between the components varies considerably. *Falling sicknes* 'epilepsy' causes the patient to fall, *slepinge ivel* 'lethargy' to feel drowsy. *Oliphant sicknes* made the patient's legs and joints thick like those of an elephant, which brings to mind the condition now known as *elephantiasis*. *Yelow evel* 'jaundice' involved a discoloration of the patient's skin, as did *grene sicknes*, which may have been a variety of jaundice that made the skin a greenish colour.

Reasons other than the visible effects of a sickness underlie, for example, *children ivel*, a term for epilepsy: 'Also it [epilencia] hatte children yuel, for often children haueþ þat yuel' (ed. Seymour *et al.* 1975: 353). The possible cure for an affliction appears from the appellation *kinges evill*. Barlow (1980) has examined the complicated sense-development of *morbus regius* in detail. Classical Latin *morbus regius*, he says, denoted jaundice, but later, in ecclesiastical Latin, the phrase began to be used also of leprosy. Further confusion arose when *morbus regius* became associated with swellings, eruptions, and other wasting diseases besides leprosy (Barlow 1980: 4–5). The royal touch as a cure for scrofula seems to have become established in France around 1250 and in England between 1259 and 1272 (Barlow 1980: 24–5). Boorde refers to the confusion arising from the careless use of the term:

> For as muche as some men doth iudge diuers tymes a fystle or a French pocke to be the kynges euyll, in such matters it behoueth nat a kynge to medle withal except it be thorow and of his bountiful goodnes to geue his pytyful and gracious counsell. (Boorde 1547, f. 94r)

Elyot clearly has scrofula in mind when he mentions 'swellinges in the neck full of matter, called the kinges euyll' (Elyot 1541, f. 90r).

Many anatomical compounds and phrases have a latter element meaning just 'body part'. In constructions with *member* as the latter part, the premodifier often indicates the function of the organ, as in *fedinge membres, breþinge membres, generatif membris*, and *understandinge membres*. The heart and the lungs were jointly called *spiritual membres* because of their central importance in the production of vital spirit, the carrier of the life-maintaining virtue (Norri 1998: 70). Another important type of anatomical combination in the third category is constituted by manifold general designations for the genitals, all of which contain an adjective emphasising the private nature of this region of human anatomy. The following is a selection of such terms from late Middle English and Early Modern English: *prevay lemes, privy members, secret members, privy partes, secret partes, schameliche parties, privy places, secret places*. Mention may also be made of the highly expressive phrase *tikelinge places* 'armpits' (ed. Ogden 1971: 345, 355), a translation of Medieval Latin *titillicis* or *titillicum* (ed. McVaugh 1997: 258, 266).

In the fourth category of compounds and phrases, the head noun has a more specific meaning than just 'sickness' or 'body part'. Hundreds of such formations are to be found in the manuscripts and books studied, and only a small selection of examples can be given here to indicate the complexity of the criteria involved in classifying maladies and anatomical structures. In late Middle English and Early Modern English medical terminology, *hernia* signified a variety of swellings or protuberances. Conditions that are even today classified as varieties of hernia include *hernia ventralis* 'umbilical hernia' and *hernia intestinalis* 'inguinal hernia'. In medieval times, *hernia* was also used of other protrusions and swellings, especially those in the scrotum. *Watery hernia* (*hernia aquosa*) was a hydrocele, *windy hernia* (*hernia ventosa*) inflammation of the testes, *fleschy hernia* (*hernia carnosa*) a fleshy growth around the testis, and *hernia varicosa* varicocele, dilated veins in the spermatic cord:

> Or þer falliþ watir into þe same place [scrotum] as it were a dropesie, & þan it is clepid hernia aquosa. Ouiþir þer comeþ wijnd into þe same place, & þan it is clepid hernia ventosa. And sumtyme þer wexiþ fleisch aboute & is greet, & þan it is clepid hernia carnosa. And sumtyme þer ben veynes þereaboute ful of malancolious blood & wele be gret as it were notis, & þan it is clepid hernia varicosa. (ed. von Fleischhacker 1894: 269)

Further light is thrown on the reach of the term by the mention in one surgical manuscript of 'a dissese in þe nekke in maner of a gret enpostume þe whiche ys cleped bocium in gula othir hernia guttures' (London, British Library, Sloane MS 2463, f. 98r). *Hernia guttures* was probably goitre.

Gout is another word that was often modified to coin new names of sicknesses. *Gout* figures as a head noun in formations signifying ailments due to the 'dropping' of morbid humours on the part affected. *Artetik goute* was a pain 'whiche doth ronne all the iointes and partes of a mannes body' (Boorde 1547, *Extrauagantes*, f. 11r). In *rede gout, rody gout* or *rosy goute*, the patient suffered from 'an infeccion of þe nose withoutenforþ of moche reednes' (ed. Getz 1991: 86). The recipe for 'the gowte festre that maketh many holis' in London, British Library, Sloane MS 2463, f. 67r, gives instructions for treating fistulae, likewise attributed to an effluence of humours.[46] In the Middle English version of John of Arderne studied, a fistula is called *blody goute* (Cambridge, Emmanuel College MS 69, f. 22v). Epilepsy was thought to be caused by humours blocking the passages in the brain, hence the name *falling gout*, equivalent of Medieval Latin *gutta cadiva* (*DML* s.v. *gutta* 2, sense 6.b).

The modifiers had many other shades of meaning besides those already instanced. *Small pockes* was so called to distinguish the condition from the 'great' pox, syphilis (Dirckx 1983: 26). When syphilis first came to England, the English blamed the disease on the French, who in turn accused the Spaniards (Dirckx 1983: 77). Boorde explains that in his youth *French poxe* was also known as

Spanishe pockes (1547, f. 94r). *Saint Anthonies fire* 'erysipelas or ergotism' expresses, for example, the redness, the pain felt by the patient, and the belief that the hermit saint could cure the disease (Thurston and Attwater 1956, 1: 109). In the translation of Guy de Chauliac studied, we find *fire of Seint Marcial* given as an equivalent, rendering into English the original *ignis sancti Marcialis* (ed. Ogden 1971: 97; ed. McVaugh 1997: 75). St Marcial (or Martial), who was bishop of Limoges in the third century, is represented in art as extinguishing fire with his crozier (Roeder 1955: 158).

Late Middle English and Early Modern English anatomical terminology contains a large number of compounds and phrases where the head noun has a more precise sense than just 'part of the body'. Dozens of names for various bones are first recorded during the period 1400–1550, among them *ancle bone*, *buttocke bone* 'ischium', *flank bone* 'haunch bone, ilium', *heele bone* 'heel bone, calcaneus', *nose boon, skulle boon, tailboon* and the equivalent *rumpe bone* 'coccyx', and *temple bon*. Ancient and medieval authorities considered the tympanic parts of the temporal bones to be particularly hard, their purpose being to protect the ear and its chambers from injury and excessive noise. *Stony bone* appears in a description of the ear in the English version of Bartholomaeus Anglicus:

> Þese holes [auditory meatuses] ben isette in þe stony boon in þe whiche synewes ben ipiȝt þat comeþ fro þe brayn and bryngeþ to þe eeren felinge and meuynge, and bringiþ lyknes of þe voyce þat is isonge in þe hooles to þe dome of þe soule. (ed. Seymour *et al.* 1975: 190)[47]

The vocabulary for blood vessels is plentiful, most of the terms having *vein* as the head noun. *Vein* does not, however, always signify a vein. Henry Daniel's *pouse vein* (f. 78va; *pouse*: 'pulse'), for instance, refers to an artery, his *vena visibilis* (f. 31vb) to the optic nerve. Further terms for arteries include *beatinge veine*, *pulse veine*, *pulsing veine*, *vena pulsatilis*, and the intriguing *arterie veyne*:

> Basilica sittiþ adoun aforȝens þe elbowe, vndir þe arme, & þis veine sittiþ ful nyȝ þe gret arterie: & þerfore a man mote be wel war þat he touche not þe arterie veyne. (ed. von Fleischhacker 1894: 300; *aforȝens*: 'against')

Of the veins proper, some of the commonest for venesection were the cephalic vein (*cephalic vein*), the basilic vein (*vena basilica*, *epaticke vein*), the median cubital vein (*cardiaca veine*), and the metacarpal vein between ring finger and little finger (*splenetica vena*). All four had additional names in which the Latin adjectival modifier was Englished or otherwise 'naturalised', the result being things like *head vein, base veine, liver vein, hert vein*, and *splene vein*. The much less numerous phrases with *artery* as the head noun do not always denote vessels considered arteries in modern medicine. The pulmonary vein, which like the arteries was thought to carry pneuma (Norri 1998: 70), is referred to as *arteria venalis*, *veinie arterie*, or *venosa arteria*. The Greeks originally applied the word *arteria* only to the windpipe and bronchi, and Middle English / Early Modern English *artery* is also recorded in this sense. Sometimes a clarifying modifier is added, as in *trachea arteria* and *þroteful arterie*.

Mention may be made here of another group of anatomical compounds and phrases, namely the terms for the different segments of the alimentary system. The estimated length of the duodenum, twelve finger-breadths, gives us *12 bowel* (ed. Carrillo Linares 1993: 73). The segment next to the duodenum, the jejunum, was found to be empty in dead bodies, hence the description of it as the 'fasting' gut in Greek and Latin manuscripts (Skinner 1949 s.v. *jejunum*). We find the same image in Middle English medical treatises:

> ieiunium, ieiune or fastand gut . . . Þis is þe skil whi it is callede ieiunium for when he haþe soken vp al þe iouse, þe humidite, to epar be certeyn veyns and sent it to epar, os Y saide, right as it were in maner of a swete for it haþe none issue where þe iows and þe moysture may gone oute, it is as it were fastande and voide and empty. (London, British Library, Royal MS 17.D.I, f. 7va; *skil*: 'reason')

Caecum, a blind-ended pouch at the junction of the small and large intestines, is referred to as *blinde gut* and *one-eyȝed gutte*. Andrew Boorde points out that at 'dyuers tymes the longacion, which is the ars gut, doth fal out of the body' (1547, f. 18r), and we notice how words for the genitals and the rectal area tend to take on smutty overtones with the passing of time. Three other terms, *strait gutte*, *even gutte*, and *intestinum rectum*, are in fact misnomers, because the rectum is not particularly straight. It is possible that those who gave the rectum its name had been studying simian anatomy (Singer 1959: 6).

As can be seen from the above, the sources of new medical terms in fifteenth- and early sixteenth-century English are many and varied. On the one hand, writers freely borrowed words from Latin and French, assuming that their readers would understand them. On the other hand, a vast array of new names for sicknesses and body parts was being created by extending the meanings of non-medical words and by using various techniques of word-formation. Analysis of different translations of the same Latin original may lead to lexical inventories that are far from identical. Peter Jones's (1989) examination of the four independent Middle English translations of John of Arderne shows how the translators of these four versions used different techniques when dealing with Medieval Latin technical terms. The possibilities include retaining the Latin word as such, modifying its form, and producing a vernacular translation. Wallner (1964b: xxviii–xxx; 1991) has compared two of the three independent Middle English translations of the entire text of Guy de Chauliac's treatise. According to him, the New York Academy of Medicine MS 12 adheres to the Latin more closely than the Paris MS (Bibliothèque Nationale, MS Anglais 25) edited by Ogden, which is an attempt to render the text in a more thoroughly English manner.

5.4   Loss of medical words

As we have seen above, hundreds of new lexemes entered English medical vocabulary during the period investigated. Many of them, however, proved fairly short-lived, there being no record of them after the middle of the sixteenth

Table 5.4. *Chronological layers of lexical loss in medical terminology*

	Sicknesses	Body parts	Total	Per cent
OE (before 1100)	4	11	15	9
12th century	–	–	–	0
13th century	3	2	5	12
14th century	55	80	135	25
15th century	352	387	739	56
1500–1550	58	93	151	54
TOTAL	472	573	1045	44

century. In order to gauge the extent of lexical loss, the post-1550 history of each of the 2,364 words and phrases was checked in *OED*. Possible entries for these terms in various books supplementing *OED* were also examined. The most important additional source of information was McConchie (1997), who in his study of thirteen medical works published between 1547 and 1612 discovered 3,985 new items of data for inclusion in *OED*, including 2,558 antedatings, 246 new senses, 1,089 unrecorded lexemes, and 92 postdatings (p. 145). Schäfer (1989a) provides an alphabetical inventory of all the lemmas to be found in monolingual glossaries and dictionaries of English printed between 1475 and 1640. In another volume, the author lists some 6,000 additions and corrections to *OED* based on that material and other Early Modern English works (Schäfer 1989b). Before Schäfer, Bailey (1978) had already published a compilation of approximately 4,400 previously discovered Early Modern English citations, which will, or should, necessitate revision of existing *OED* data, or the drafting of entirely new entries.

Judging from the information that we now have about the subsequent history of the words and phrases collected, one feature of late Middle English and Early Modern English medical vocabulary was its impermanence. Table 5.4, presenting the lexical material in chronological layers according to the date of the manuscript or book (cf. section 5.2), indicates the number of terms that have not been attested in written English after 1550. Thus, for instance, four names of sicknesses and eleven names of body parts first recorded in Old English manuscripts apparently failed to survive beyond 1550. Also given is the percentage of lexical 'loss' from the total chronological layer in question.

As can be seen, almost half of the words and phrases collected (44 per cent) seem to have become obsolete before the terminal point of the investigation. There are, however, great differences between the chronological layers concerning the persistence of the lexemes. The earlier strata of the vocabulary, from Old English to the thirteenth century, contain mainly basic words which continued to be used for a long time, even after 1550. Terms begin to fall away more abruptly from the fourteenth-century layer onwards. More than half of the lexical items in the fifteenth- and early sixteenth-century layers have not been recorded since the middle of the sixteenth century. This 'death' of vocabulary concerned especially technical words taken over unchanged from Latin originals, many of which never really caught on and perhaps occur in one medical treatise only. Some examples of names of sicknesses recorded between 1400 and 1550 but not thereafter are *anelitus* 'breathing disorder', *anostropha* 'upset stomach involving vomiting and diarrhoea', *pedicoun* 'epilepsy', *clavis* 'corn on the toe', *ruonia* 'swelling of the face', *rixis* 'rupture of a blood vessel', and *gahen* 'tearing of a ligament'. Among the names of body parts that had apparently fallen into disuse before 1550, we find *uritides* 'ureters', *mappa ventris* 'diaphragm', *tentigo* 'clitoris', *quadrupli* 'lateral incisor teeth', *clavalia* 'temporal bones', *poplitica* 'popliteal vein', and *cristal(l)idos* 'lens of the eye'. Many native coinages, including literal translations of Latin terms, also seem to have become obsolete or obsolescent some time between 1400 and 1550, including *oliphant sicknes* 'elephantiasis' (< L *elephantia*), *lions property* 'form of leprosy' (< ML *leonina*), *misdede* 'impotence' (< ML *malefactio*), *clere droppe* 'blindness' (< ML *gutta serena*), *lousenes* 'infestation with lice', *water springe* 'dropsy', and *outcoming* 'dislocation'. The following anatomical coinages, among others, met a similar fate: *childes sak* 'membranes enclosing embryo' (< ML *saccus infantis*), *milke ʒate* 'jejunum' (< ML *porta lactis*), *wome ʒate tunge* 'clitoris' (< ML *lingula vulue*), *fether* 'lobe of lung' (< ML *penna*), *one-eyʒed gutte* 'caecum' (< ML *monoculus*), *water gates* 'ureters', *arme pipe* 'humerus', and *tiinge* 'ligament'.

The rate of disappearance from view of terms dating from the first half of the sixteenth century (54 per cent) is close to that of the preceding century (56 per cent). This suggests that it was just as difficult for new medical lexemes to gain a foothold during the first fifty years of the Early Modern English period as it had been in late Middle English.

The alternative way of dating words and phrases, according to the year when the original version of the treatise is known to have been written, causes no radical change in the above general picture. The figures would then be as in Table 5.5.

The rate of lexical eclipse is still more than 50 per cent in the fifteenth-century and early sixteenth-century layers. The main difference when compared with Table 5.4 is that we now have a much higher figure, 41 per cent, for the fourteenth century. This indicates that the enormous increase in English medical vocabulary that started around 1375 was accompanied by the simultaneous rapid loss of many of the new adoptions and coinages.

It is usually impossible to say with any degree of certainty why a particular name of sickness or body part failed to establish itself. Why, for instance, should *sebel* 'eye condition characterised by tear-shedding, itching, and veins engorged with blood', at one time frequent in surgical treatises, only be recorded between *c.* 1400 and 1543? The words *gibbe* and *zima*, denoting respectively the upper and lower surface of the liver, are only found in medical works dated *c.* 1375–*c.* 1460. In a number of cases, however, it is possible to suggest linguistic factors that may have hastened the dying out of a word or phrase. *Wlatinge, wlatnesse, wlatfulnesse,* and *wlatsomnes,* four terms signifying 'nausea', as well as *wlaffinge* 'stammering',

Table 5.5. *Chronological layers of lexical loss in medical terminology (dating according to the date of the original)*

	Sicknesses	Body parts	Total	Per cent
OE (before 1100)	4	11	15	9
12th century	–	–	–	0
13th century	3	2	5	12
14th century	182	294	476	41
15th century	225	173	398	57
1500–1550	58	93	151	54
TOTAL	472	573	1045	44

became extinct in the course of the fifteenth century. The likely reason for the disappearance is phonetic: the consonant group *wl-* in word-initial position had fallen away by the sixteenth century (Horn and Lehnert 1954: 1072). The last citations for words beginning with *wl-* in *OED*, with two exceptions, date from the Middle English period. Another initial group, *fn-*, became *sn-* in the fifteenth century (Dobson 1968: 956), which explains why we do not find *fnesing* 'sneezing' after 1475, the form *snesing* taking over *c.* 1460.

In his book on linguistic evolution, Samuels (1972: 69–71) states that 'the pressure of homonymy should be regarded as potential in some area of most semantic fields, always present to combine with other factors to cause redistributions within that field, and irrespective of whether it eventually causes obsolescence or not'. When it comes to the shaping of English medical vocabulary in the late medieval period, it seems that there are only a few instances where homonymy was a factor in a medical word's failure to survive. The second element in *yelow alde* 'jaundice', only to be found in Schöffler (1919: 216) in the material studied, derives from OE *adl* 'illness, ailment'. The word gradually became rarer after the Old English period, five of the seven *MED* examples dating from *c.* 1200 or earlier (*MED* s.v. *adle* n.). *OED* gives no citations of *adle* after *c.* 1200. It has been suggested that the word died out because of a homonymic clash with *addle* 'filth' (Palmer 1936: 111). Homonymy may indeed have played a role here, since the concepts of 'illness' and 'filth' are both part of the semantic field of medicine.[48] In today's special languages, because of the danger of ambiguity, there is a general tendency to avoid homonymy in one and the same subject.[49]

In Middle English and Early Modern English, the native word *corn* was applied to a variety of tumefactions. In the remedybook edited by Müller (1929a: 127), it is said of a medicinal preparation that 'þe scrophilis, cornes, and postemys it dissoluyth with-owtyn fyuer' (*scrophilis*: 'scrofulas'; *postemys*: 'swellings'). An ocular ulcer, according to Lanfrank, is preceded by 'a reed poynt or a corn' (ed. von Fleischhacker 1894: 246). Andrew Boorde (1547) is another writer who uses the word in the latter sense (f. 108r: 'pusshes or whyte cornes vpon the eye').

These metaphorical applications of a native word seem to have vanished by the middle of the sixteenth century, possibly because of the adoption of the Anglo-Norman word *corn* (< OF *cor* < L *cornu*) 'corn on the toe or foot' into English, where it is first recorded *c.* 1425. It is not difficult to think of contexts where *corn* might have signified either 'swelling' or 'corn', the reader not being certain which meaning was intended.

It may well be that some words and phrases failed to gain a foothold in English medical vocabulary for homonymic or related reasons. The translator of our Middle English version of Chauliac uses *eyȝe sterne* (*sterne of þe eyȝe*) when rendering Medieval Latin *cornea* (first example) or *pupilla* (second example):

> Of brekynge of þe eyȝe sterne and of goyng out of þe humour. But if the sterne of þe eyȝe be broken and þe humour comeþ oute so þat þere folwe areryng vp, it is an open token, after Galien, vbi supra. (ed. Ogden 1971: 307; *areryng vp*: 'swelling')

> Neuerþelatter he shall firste be examyned if he be dede or alyue in touchinge his pulse, in clepynge hym, in drawynge hym by þe heres and by þe nose and in byholdynge þe sternes of þe eyȝen if þai be movede . . . (ed. Ogden 1971: 406; *clepynge*: 'calling')[50]

MED comments on the above two uses of the word s.v. *stern(e)* n.2 'stern of a ship'. The cornea and the pupil, however, are not at the back of the eye, quite the contrary. It seems more likely that the actual source of the anatomical term is the word *sterne* n.1 'star'. Perhaps the origin is clarified by the anonymous London surgeon who wrote that 'tunica cornea . . . schineþ as a schynynge horn' (ed. Grothé 1982: 61).[51] Readers who took the origin of the metaphor to be the stern of a ship no doubt found it difficult to perceive any connection between the nautical and anatomical senses.

Many of the medical lexemes that apparently failed to survive beyond the middle of the sixteenth century are very close in form to commoner terms for the same referent, and derived from the same root. Croft (2000: 176), who cites examples like *grammaticalization* versus *grammaticization*, states that in a linguistic community 'there is a strong tendency to avoid complete synonymy, that is, multiple forms with the same meaning and the same social (community) value'. If such pairs of words do emerge, he explains that the situation can be remedied in three different ways: by employing the two or more forms in distinct meanings, by reserving them to distinct groups within the community (e.g. occupational, age, or gender groups), and by increasingly selecting one form over the other. The last-mentioned situation will eventually lead to the extinction of the alternative form (Croft 2000: 177–8). The list of medical terms not recorded after 1550 includes many lexical items which seem to have been jettisoned simply through selection. For example, *acue, demigrein, febre, forne hede, leeste fingir*, and *arme pottes* apparently never managed to challenge the established *ague, migreine, fever, for(e)hede*, *littill finger*, and *armpittis*, respectively, and were lost from view before the terminal date of the present investigation. *Distempera(u)nce, distempere, distemperure*, and *distempering* all denoted an imbalance of bodily humours in late Middle English, but only the first two words have been attested in Early Modern English texts. The dominant and highly productive suffix *-ness* seems to have weakened the potential of formations with the suffix *-head*. According to Marchand (1969: 293), *-head* is 'an unexplained by-form' of *-hood*, which in de-adjectival derivatives like *false-hood* and *likelihood* 'is no longer productive and has never been strong'. The list of medical lexemes that have not been recorded after 1550 contains many coinages with the suffix *-head*, alternative forms in *-ness* surviving much longer. Examples of such pairs include *bareinhede/bareinesse, defhed/deafnes, horeshed/hoarsnes, rothed/rot(e)nes, sorehede/sorenes, streithede/straitnes (of the breast)* 'difficulty in breathing', *windihed/windines* 'flatulence; noise in the ears', *woodhede/woodnes* 'insanity', and *fathed/fatnes* 'body fat'.

In many other cases of lexical equivalence, the two or more words do not share a common root. The propensities described by Croft are also evident in these instances. As noted in the previous section, *epar, cor,* and *pulmo* appear side by side with the respective native words *liver, heart,* and *lunges* in Henry Daniel's *Liber uricrisiarum*. Daniel is, furthermore, the only author who occasionally uses *fel* for *gall, lumbi* for *loines,* and *pilus* for *her*. In the works by some other writers and translators, *capillus, caro,* and *dentes* are used instead of the usual *her, fles(s)he,* and *teeth,* respectively. The foreign adoptions from Latin were never really as-similated and occur in only a few of the medical treatises studied. No doubt their spread was partly hindered by the existence of an extremely common native word of identical meaning. The pairs cited remind one of Baugh and Cable's (1993: 221) statement that '[t]he most convincing reason for the failure of a new word to take hold is that it was not needed'.

Some of the coinages, including a number of translations from Latin, were semantically untoward, and this too may have contributed to their disappearance from English medical vocabulary. Readers of the Chauliac manuscript must have found *dede apple* a rather peculiar term for scabbiness of the feet or gangrene:

> A man myght saye many þinges of þe mormale or dede appel, but it is generally cured as þe scabbe, of þe whiche it is saide tofore, when þat it is noght elles but a stynkynge and drye scabbe. (ed. Ogden 1971: 532)

Dede apple is a mistranslation of Medieval Latin *malum mortuum*.[52] The translator has understood *malum* as 'apple' instead of 'evil, sickness'. The neuter of *malus* 'bad', which denotes various bad and negative phenomena in Medieval Latin, has the same form as the singular of *malum, -i* 'an apple'. In the same manuscript, *lauerok bone* 'occipital bone' is likely to have puzzled many readers, because there is no evident connection between the bone and a lark, *lauerok* being one of the spelling variants of Middle English *lark(e)* (*MED* s.v.):

Of þe whiche it semeth þat William and Lamfranque and also Henry sawe euel þe anothomye, for þey seien þe bone paxillare to be vnder þe lauerok bone and be one of þe bones of þe nekke. (ed. Ogden 1971: 40; *bone paxillare*: 'sphenoid bone, large bone forming the base of the skull')

The corresponding term in the Latin Chauliac is *osse laude*.[53] The form *lauerok bone* is evidently due to confusion between Medieval Latin *lauda* (from *landa*, altered form of *lambda*), the name for the bone based on its shape, and *alauda* 'lark'. Faulty translation has also occasioned *slepinge bone* 'temporal bone' in von Braunschweig (1525, f. G3va). In Middle Dutch, from which the book was translated, *slaep* meant both 'temple of the head' and 'sleep' (*MNW* s.v.). Yet another odd-sounding phrase, *wrecchyd veines*, is to be found in the English version of John of Arderne:

> After Auicennam alle þe intrayles of a mannes wombe ben contynually with þe wrecchyd veynes saff longaonem. (Cambridge, Emmanuel College MS 69, f. 40v; *wombe*: 'stomach', *saff*: 'except', *longaonem*: 'rectum')

The Latin Arderne has *venis meseraicis* in the corresponding passage.[54] It seems that the translator has here confused *meseraicis* with *miserabilis* 'wretched'. The ordinary term for the mesenteric veins in Middle English and Early Modern English was *miseraike veines*.

Sometimes the English translator has chosen a phrase that confounds the original image. In John of Trevisa's translation of Bartholomaeus Anglicus's encyclopaedia, *þe leues of þe longen* (ed. Seymour *et al.* 1975: 211) rather misses the point, as a rendering of Medieval Latin *folliculo pulmonis*.[55] The term in the English version plainly derives from confusion between Medieval Latin *folium* 'leaf' and *folliculus* 'bag, bladder, follicle' (*DML* s.v.). The compound *herte-rote* in the compilation by the anonymous London surgeon displays a complete failure to understand the Latin original. The writer describes the course of the vena cava as follows: 'and sche, passynge from þe caussula of þe herte-rote, entriþ þe pannicle on his riȝt side' (ed. Grothé 1982: 93–4; *caussula*: 'pericardium', *pannicle*: 'membrane'). In a Medieval Latin version of Henry de Mondeville's treatise, the corresponding passage reads: 'et transiens infra dictam casulam mittit ad cor ramum magnum, dextrum ejus ventriculum subintrantem' (ed. Mory 1977: 207; ed. Pagel 1892: 42). The English translation, including the coinage *herte-rote*, simply does not make sense.

In some other instances, what looks like an English translator's, or scribe's, error is in fact nothing of the kind, the corresponding Latin original being equally bungled. *Pori uritides* was a fairly common term for renal veins and ureters in late Middle English and Early Modern English (Norri 1998: 385). In the *Liber cerebri*, we find the name Englished as *greene canals* or *greene pores*, in an irredeemably corrupt passage (ed. Carrillo Linares 1993: 75–6). At first sight, *greene* seems to derive from the translator's mistaking the anatomical noun *uritides* for the adjective *viridis*. The two English phrases do, however, translate respectively *canales virides* and *virides pori* in the Latin version in London, British Library, Sloane MS 2454, f. 85va. As a matter of fact, forms like this are not infrequent in Medieval Latin texts (Hyrtl 1879: 39; Fonahn 1922 s.v. *porus viridis*).

Some of the anatomical designations that seem to have fallen into disuse before 1550 are tautological in nature. In the following citations, containing the only instances of *heed brayne* and *heed-scolle* in the material studied, the two compounds have a superfluous modifier, the latter element alone being the usual term for the anatomical structure in question:

> The fyrste token as whan the shot is in the heed brayne, so suffer the pacyent greate payne wherby the scome auoyde out of the mouth and at the wounde. (von Braunschweig 1525, f. D4ra)

> The noumbre of þe bonys of þe heed-scolle is seid diuers, of diuers men by diuers consideracioun. (ed. Grothé 1982: 37)

Further examples of anatomical terms with an element of reduplication about them include *ballok codde* 'scrotum', used by four writers but more commonly called just *cod*, and *blode vein*, the latter appearing only in the English translation of von Braunschweig's treatise (f. D1ra).[56] Sometimes the suffix attached to a word may be superfluous, as in *extremitives* 'hands and feet, extremities' in the Arderne manuscript (cf. section 5.3). Similar examples from the lexical field of sickness are *pestilence evel* 'the plague' and *lepre evell* 'leprosy', where *evel(l)* is used in the sense of 'sickness' and adds nothing to the meaning. The suffixation in *obtalmicacioun*, *syncopacion/syncoping*, *potagrenesse*, and *tisiknesse* hardly adds anything significant to *ophthalmia* 'inflammation of the eye', *syncope* 'fainting', *podagra* 'gout in the feet, podagra', and *tisik* 'pulmonary tuberculosis', respectively.

A further possibility is that some of the medical lexemes never gained wider currency because there was uncertainty as to their exact meaning. Thus, for instance, all we know about *verdigenet* on the basis of the quotation below is that the condition was supposed to affect the eyelids:

> Folwyngly it is to be saide of þe sekenesses of þe parties of þe ey3e, bygynnynge at the scabbe and at the sekenesses of þe ey3e liddes, the whiche ben nombrede 24. Thoghe þat the sekenesses of þe ey3en ben nombrede manye, neuerþelatter þai falle togidre into one, as we schall saie of yche, of brennynge, of redenesse, of heuynesse, of bolnynge, of verdi-genet, ... of vlceracioun and of soche oþere. (ed. Ogden 1971: 443; *bolnynge*: 'swelling')

Verdigenet, also in the Latin original (ed. McVaugh 1997: 328), does not appear anywhere else in the Chauliac manuscript, nor in any of the other treatises studied. A reader who only came across the word in the above passage would evidently have been unable to form any clear idea about the meaning of the term, and was therefore hardly likely to use it in his own writings. In the same work (ed. Ogden 1971: 389; cf. ed. McVaugh 1997: 290), the unique *algada* and *algasen* occur in a long list of 'spotty infecciouns of þe skyn', but no more information is given about the nature of the conditions so called.[57] Lexicographers writing entries for rare words appearing in rather general contexts are faced with many difficulties when drafting the definition: *MED* defines both *algada* and *algasen* simply as 'a skin disease', but for some reason there is no entry for *verdigenet*.

Occasionally a form found in only one treatise may quite simply be a mistake. In Boorde's book, *mussulages* appears in the sense of 'muscles', although the explanation is somewhat bizarre:

MUSCILAGO, MUSCULI, or MUSSULAGINES be the Latyn wordes. In Englysh it is named muscles or mussulages, the which be lytle straynes descendynge from the heed to the necke and face and other partes, and they be compounde of synewye fylmes and ligamentes and pannycles, and some saye that they be lytle grystley bones. (Boorde 1547, f. 96v)

OED s.v. *mussulage*, only recorded in Boorde's book, puts forward the idea that what we have here might be a combination of *muscle* and *-age*. This seems to me unlikely. Middle English *muscilage* (< ML *muscilago*), the etymon of Modern English *mucilage*, meant a 'thick, gelatinous substance obtained from certain plants', one of the spelling variants being *mussillage* (*MED* s.v. *muscilage*). One wonders whether in fact Boorde wrongly associated *muscilago* with *muscle*. There are many other instances in the material studied where miscopying or misunder-standing of the original may have led to an inexplicable formation.[58]

5.5   Concluding remarks

During the period investigated in this chapter, those composing medical works in English as well as the translators of Latin medical treatises were faced with the challenge of creating an English medical vocabulary as, for this purpose, the vernacular emerged ever more assertively from the shadow of Latin and French. Hundreds of previously unrecorded names of sicknesses and body parts make their appearance in written English between *c.* 1400 and 1550. Many lexicologists have emphasised the paramount contribution of the sixteenth century to the for-mation of English scientific vocabularies, but at least in the sphere of medicine, a vast accretion of new terms had already been going on during the last quarter of the fourteenth century. The meanings of the medical lexemes first attested in late Middle English or Early Modern English run the gamut from very general to highly technical and erudite. Today, we associate the language of medicine with a lavish sprinkling of Latin and Greek, many of the new terms being put together of components from the two classical languages. In the 33 manuscripts and books studied here, the sources of the terminology are more varied, the lexical inventory including adoptions from a number of foreign languages, extensions in the application of a non-medical word through metaphor, metonymy or specialisation of meaning, not to mention entirely new coinages made by the writer or translator. The survival rate of the names of sicknesses and body parts in the material examined may seem low: out of the altogether 2,364 words and phrases collected, only 1,319, i.e. some 56 per cent, have been recorded in texts written after 1550. This, however, does not in any way diminish the importance of especially the late Middle English period for the future development of medical terminology in English, since hundreds of the lexemes that did survive were to become the standard designations for particular conditions and anatomical structures. In modern medical dictionaries, such terms often appear as the head word in a multitude of phrases signifying related phenomena.

The present survey has only dealt with 33 medical treatises dating from 1400 to 1550, and there are hundreds more in the libraries around the world. When further manuscripts and books from this period are studied, many new lexemes will no doubt be discovered. Recent work on the cataloguing of Old English and Middle English scientific and medical texts, as well as the increasing number of editions of these manuscripts, provides vital material for lexicographers interested in the history of English medical vocabulary. Technology is now opening up all kinds of possibilities that could earlier only be dreamt of and it is to be hoped that before very long a computerised database will be available to supplement the traditional dictionary of late Middle English and/or Early Modern English medical terms. In any case, there are many interesting subjects for lexical research besides the names of sicknesses and body parts, for example those of medicines and instruments. There is still much work to be done and many avenues unexplored.

Notes

1. Some examples of McConchie's antedatings found as early as the Middle English period are: *accession, achor, apostemation, contraction, contusion, eminence, mola, morbilli, relaxation, talpa* (names of sicknesses), *basilica, crus, false rib, great artery, hollow vein, os sacrum, pleura, seat, table, tibia* (names of body parts). Of the terms unrecorded in *OED*, the following, among others, crop up in Middle English medical treatises: *ascachilos, bothor, branchus, diaria, hernia aquosa, hernia ventosa, lupia, morbus comitialis, talparia, vndimia* (names of sicknesses), *aranea, arteria magna, casula cordis, cephalica, concava, focile minus, monoculus, nodus gutturis, sagittalis, zirbus* (names of body parts). For Middle English occurrences of these lexemes, see the lexicons in Norri (1992) and (1998).
2. One of the academic treatises (ed. Carrillo Linares 1993) was analysed only for the book on body parts.
3. The manuscripts containing the Middle English versions studied were the following: Paris, Bibliothèque Nationale MS Anglais 25, ff. 2r–191v (Guy de Chauliac; ed. Ogden 1971), London, British Library, Additional MS 12056, ff. 31r–86v, and Oxford, Bodleian Library, Ashmole MS 1396, ff. 1r–272v (Lanfrank; ed. von Fleischhacker

1894), London, British Library, Sloane MS 240, ff. 1r–137r (Roger of Salerno), British Library, Sloane MS 389, ff. 2r–77r (Teodorico Borgognoni of Lucca), and Cambridge, Emmanuel College MS 69, ff. 1r–196v (John of Arderne).

4. 24720 in *STC*. Published as a facsimile edition in 1968 (Amsterdam and New York: Da Capo Press and Theatrvm Orbis Terrarvm).

5. 13434 in *STC*.

6. London, Wellcome Library MS 564, ff. 10r–128r (ed. Grothé 1982).

7. London, British Library, Sloane MS 2463, ff. 53r–151v.

8. The manuscripts containing the Middle English versions studied were the following: Oxford, Bodleian Library, Ashmole MS 1505, ff. 4r–244v (Bernard of Gordon), London, Wellcome Library MS 537, ff. 48r–310v (Gilbertus Anglicus; ed. Getz 1991), and London, British Library, Additional MS 27944, ff. 2r–330v (Bartholomaeus Anglicus; ed. Seymour *et al.* 1975).

9. Cambridge, Trinity College MS R.14.52, ff. 40v–44r (ed. Carrillo Linares 1993 and forthcoming).

10. Cambridge, Gonville and Caius College MS 176/97, pp. 37–228.

11. London, British Library, Royal MS 17.D.I, ff. 4r–118v. Quotations from f. 4ra.

12. F. 47vb.

13. 3373.5 in *STC*.

14. See the Foreword to Furnivall (1981) and the *Dictionary of National Biography* (ed. Stephen and Lee) s.v. *Boorde or Borde, Andrew.*

15. 7644 in *STC*, which also lists editions from 1537? and 1539, stating that in the 1541 edition 'a new preface replaces the dedic[ation] to Cromwell'. Quotation from f. A4v.

16. Langton's book is number 15205 in *STC*. For Langton's studies and career, see the *Dictionary of National Biography* (ed. Stephen and Lee) s.v. *Langton, Christopher.*

17. The book is number 13522 in *STC*, which also lists a previous edition from *c.* 1545. The passage on apoplexy reads: 'Pronosticacion of appoplexie. After Ipocras and Auicen dyd pronostike. I saye that I sawe many that had that dysease, but of trueth I neuer sawe any escape it.'

18. It is noteworthy, however, that 'W Aderston' had patients in the highest positions in society, including 'Ser Wyllyam Schynglyngton' (p. 210), 'Scheryff of Brystowe' (p. 221), 'Ser Wyllyam Elueden' and 'þe Mayer of Notyngun' (p. 222).

19. Getz (1990a: 10–12) and Keiser (1998: 3664–5) note that a plague treatise attributed to Moulton, later incorporated into *The Myrour or Glasse of Helthe*, already existed in a fifteenth-century manuscript. The book is number 18214a in *STC*, which dates it 'bef. 1531'.

20. Keiser (1998: 3656) observes that the history of the *Liber de diversis medicinis* extends from the late fourteenth to the early sixteenth century. According to him, '[b]ecause the scribe was often confused by the technical language of his exemplar, the Thornton text is one of the least accurate'.

21. The nine other remedybooks examined for the lexical analysis are the following: Medical Society of London MS 136, ff. 1r–95v (ed. Dawson 1934); London, British Library, Additional MS 33996, ff. 76v–148v (ed. Heinrich 1896); Stockholm, Royal Library MS X.90, pp. 1–155 (ed. Müller 1929a); London, British Library, Sloane MS 1764, ff. 7r–29v; British Library, Sloane MS 73, ff. 106r–127v and 176r–194v; Cambridge, Trinity College MS O.8.35, ff. 1r–112r; Cambridge, Trinity College MS R.14.51, ff. 1r–45r (all 15th c.); Oxford, Bodleian Library, Ashmole MS 1405,

ff. 1r–45v (16th c.). For a more detailed description of the authors and contents of the 33 treatises mentioned, see Norri (1992: 68–82) and (1998: 98–103).

22. The complex semantics of the matter are well illustrated by Siraisi's (1990: 101) comment that 'humors, that is, body fluids; and members, that is, parts of the body' were both 'physically perceptible bodily parts'. Siraisi also observes that when it denoted the substance flowing in the veins, *blood* meant 'a sanguineous mass consisting of a mixture of the pure humour blood with a lesser portion of the other three humours' (1990: 105–6). Perhaps it was in this sense that Christopher Langton regarded blood as a *part*?

23. Similarly, there is an entry for *aurigo* 'jaundice', but not for *peganicis* 'green jaundice' or *melanchitone* 'black jaundice', although the three terms appear in the same passage in the English translation of Bartholomaeus Anglicus's *De proprietatibus rerum*:

> And þere beþ þre maner of iaundes, as it is iseide in Platearius: ʒolouh þat comeþ of kynde colera, grene, and blacke. The firste hatte aurigo, for it makeþ a man ʒolouh as golde. And secund hatte somtyme peganicis, þat is to menynge 'grene', for þe body is imade grene wiþ grene colera. þe þridde hatte melanchitone, þat is 'blak', for it comeþ of blak colera ibrend. (ed. Seymour *et al.* 1975: 406)

Schäfer (1989b: 5) has observed something similar in *OED*, where, according to him, '[w]ords of comparable lexical status – whether found in a writer's text or in a dictionary – were sometimes included, sometimes omitted'. McConchie (1997: 201) notes that in its treatment of encysts, i.e. words which retain their non-English form, *OED* manifests 'a cacophony of indecision'.

24. Schäfer (1989b: 26) writes about Early Modern English lexicography and states that 'extraneous criteria, such as the frequency of words or their survival into the nineteenth and twentieth centuries, provide no valid basis for a historical study of the Early Modern English period . . . Only exhaustive coverage can do justice to the prolific lexical creativity of the period and reflect the resulting linguistic and stylistic uncertainty.' Schäfer's comments apply also to Middle English lexicography.

25. The corresponding passage in the Latin version reads as follows: 'Avicenna vero . . . a colera naturali . . . dixit fieri spinam' (ed. McVaugh 1997: 80). For the meaning of *spina*, see McVaugh and Ogden (1997), notes 59/22–24 and 77/11–12. Also cf. *thorn*, sense 4.c, in *MED*.

26. The forms given in the text, unless otherwise stated, are the same as the head entries in the lexicons of Norri (1992) and (1998).

27. In her book on foreign adoptions in English, Serjeantson (1935: 84) comments on her policy with respect to *Ancrene Riwle* as follows:

> The most important prose work of Early Middle English is the *Ancrene Riwle* or *Rule of Recluses*. It is almost certainly a product of the twelfth century, but although it is extant in a number of manuscripts none of these is earlier than the first quarter of the thirteenth century. The only one which has yet been printed is of about 1220–1230, and since it is at present uncertain how far the vocabulary of this agrees with the original, it is dealt with here as a thirteenth-century text.

28. The medieval meanings of the terms that survive in modern medicine were, however, often far more general than today. In late Middle English and Early Modern English, *hernia*, for instance, was used of any swollen condition of the scrotum or testes,

including hernia proper, hydrocele, varicocele, and growth in the testes (Norri 1992: 338).

29. See Pope (1966: 228–30) for the sound-changes involved.

30. For a complete list of occurrences of the 'called in X' formula in connection with the names of sicknesses and body parts, see respectively Norri (1992: 393–7) and (1998: 419–24). The terms stated to come from French in those lists are *cloroupis*, *flankis*, *landie*, *malum nostre domine*, *reins*, and *werbles*.

31. Historical dictionaries seem to vary in their policies with respect to words having an equivalent in both French and Latin. According to Coleman (1995: 109), *MED* gives many more twofold etymologies than *OED*, which 'tends to choose either French or Latin as the source language rather than giving them as equally valid alternatives'. In his articles of 1964 and 1969, Wallner argued that in both dictionaries the possibility of French influence had so far been overlooked in many of the entries for medical words.

32. For the number of the names of sicknesses and body parts in this category, see respectively Norri (1992: 101, 185, 241) and (1998: 120, 205, 274).

33. In *OED*, the first example of the word being used in the anatomical sense dates from 1615, but McConchie (1997: 244, 270, 361, 382) has found four earlier instances from between 1574 and 1612.

34. Similarly, Daniel uses *cor* and *pulmo* alongside the more familiar *heart* and *lunges*. For a discussion of the reasons why medieval medical writers resorted to foreign words in their texts, see also Pahta's article on code-switching in the present volume.

35. The modern *xerophthalmia* is defined as 'dryness of the conjunctiva and cornea due to vitamin A deficiency' in *Dorland's Illustrated Medical Dictionary* (Anderson *et al.* 2000).

36. The word *nail* may be important for deciphering the etymology of another Middle English term for an eye complaint, namely *haw (in the eye)*, which presumably denoted some kind of ocular excrescence. *MED* s.v. *haue* n.1 suggests two possible origins, namely *haue* n.2 'a hawthorn berry' and *hove*, a variant of *hof* n.1 'a hoof; a horny growth, a calculus'. The use of *nail* for a sickness of the eye lends some support to the latter theory.

37. *Cloth* and *web* were also used of discolouring infections of the face, as in the instruction 'to remeve þe webbe or clooþ and dede blood and wannesse in þe face' (ed. Ogden 1971: 22).

38. *OED* s.v. *apple*, sense 7.

39. Terms that already had a medical application were also subject to metaphor, metonymy, and specialisation of meaning, especially in anatomy. Thus, for instance, urethral meatus was called the *eye of þe ȝerde*, nipple the *heed of þe pappe*, and the vagina was known as the *neck of the matrice*. Some examples of metonymical extensions of names of body parts are *thigh* for 'thigh bone', *cod* for 'testicle; ovary', and *back-bone* for 'vertebra'. In the treatises examined, *epiglottis* appears in no fewer than six senses, namely, 'epiglottis', 'larynx', 'pharynx', 'Adam's apple', 'uvula', and 'trachea'. Specialisation of meaning is exemplified by *broke* 'open sore; boil', which goes back to OE *broc* 'affliction, trouble, misery'. The earliest meaning recorded in Middle English is 'disease, infirmity', *c.* 1150, and it is not until the fifteenth century that the more specialised medical senses are attested (*OED* s.v. *broke* sb., *MED* s.v. *brok* n.4). For occurrences of these terms, see the lexicons in Norri (1992) and (1998).

40. *OED* s.v. *adjutory* a. and n., sense A, states that the bone was so called because it assists in the raising of the hand.

41. Information from Dr Peter Jones.

42. The definition in *MED*, i.e. 'respiratory organ', is inaccurate, because the medieval term also included the heart.

43. Bartholomaeus Anglicus (1485) *Liber de proprietatibus rerum Bartholomei Anglici.* Strasbourg: Argentine. F. H3ra.

44. Both the Middle Dutch and the Early Modern English term parallel Latin *accidens* 'a contingent circumstance', present participle of the verb *accido* 'happen to, be the lot of, befall' (*OLD* s.vv.).

45. The corresponding term in the Latin Bartholomaeus (see note 43) is *corui rostro* (f. F4ra).

46. Guy de Chauliac informs us that 'þe humours þat renne oute and roten the place ben worse in a fistle þan yn an holwe vlcer' (ed. Ogden 1971: 295).

47. The terms *naily bones* and *petrouse bones* are also applied to the temporal bones in some of the texts.

48. Cf. the senses 'natural discharges of the body of man or beast' (2a) and 'morbid discharges of the body; purulent matter, pus' (2b) s.v. *filth* in *MED*.

49. In different subjects, or different branches of the same subject, however, a particular form is in fact quite often used for entirely different concepts (Sager 1990: 59, 72; Cabré 1999: 108, 111).

50. The corresponding passages in the Latin Chauliac read as follows:

> De ruptura cornee et exitu uvee. Sed si propter corrosionem rumpatur cornea et procidat extra uvea, ita quod sequatur elevacio, manifestum est, secundum Galienum ubi supra . . .

> Examinandum tamen prius est si est mortuus vel vivus: tangendo pulsum, vocando eum, trahendo pilos et nares, respiciendo pupillas oculorum si moventur . . . (ed. McVaugh 1997: 230, 302)

51. Cf. also the citation from John of Gaddesden's *Rosa medicinae* in *DML* s.v. *corneus*, sense 2, where the cornea is described as follows: 'tunica . . alia cornea . . , in qua est translucencia sicut in cornu lucido translucenti'.

52. The corresponding passage in the Latin Chauliac reads as follows:

> De malo mortuo posset homo dicere filatarias multas, sed generaliter curatur sicut scabies, de qua dictum est supra, cum nichil sit quam feda et arida scabies. (ed. McVaugh 1997: 390)

53. The passage reads as follows:

> Ex quibus apparet quod Guillelmus et Lanfrancus et eciam Henricus male viderunt anathomiam, quia dicunt os passillare esse sub osse laude et esse unum de ossibus colli. (ed. McVaugh 1997: 33)

54. Hunter MS 112, f. 22. Information from Dr Peter Jones.

55. F. F2rb in the printed book (cf. note 43).

56. *OED* gives *blood-vein* only in the sense of 'a kind of moth' s.v. *blood* n., sense 21.

57. For further examples of names of sicknesses occurring in contexts unfavourable to clarity of meaning, see *epith*, *ermosia*, *herberde*, *selertes*, and *sernac* in the lexicon of Norri (1992) s.vv.

58. Other possibly corrupt forms among the names of body parts include *cardiacle* and *lacirria* (Norri 1998 s.vv.), among the names of sicknesses *dissincla*, *grounde*, *lurlys*, *momplus*, and *scores* (Norri 1992 s.vv.).

6 Herbal recipes and recipes in herbals – intertextuality in early English medical writing

MARTTI MÄKINEN

6.1 Introduction

Herbals are manuals of medicinal plants with descriptions of their physical qualities and their virtues, i.e. their medical properties and uses in line with humoral medicine. In addition to description and virtues, which seem to be the minimum requirements for a text to be identified as a herbal, there are other, optional components in the genre. Recipes are among the most frequent and most important of such components (Mäkinen 2002b: 230–1). 'Herbal recipes' are understood in this article simply as recipes including one or more herbal ingredients; this simple definition will act as the basis of the text retrieval method described later. Recipes in herbals in this chapter are kept separate from the term 'herbal recipes'.

The textual tradition of recipes in medieval Western medicine derives almost solely from the Greek medical writings of antiquity, albeit with the help of Arabic translators. Consequently, medieval medical recipes form a close-knit textual 'population' (cf. Carroll in this volume), with few original texts. Evidence of intertextuality is inevitable. This chapter is based on data from edited and published manuscripts, and a closed set of keywords, hence the relations between texts are presented rather as intertextual links than as textual transmission lines in the history of medicine.

6.2 Aim and method

Middle English herbal recipes and their parallels and paraphrases in other contemporary medical writing are the subject of this chapter. The aim is to find out to what extent the recipes in medical texts containing herbal materials coincide with recipes in herbals.

Herbals originated as part of the *materia medica* literature which also included pharmacology, lapidaries and bestiaries; thus the early stages of the genre blend with other genres, and there is little reason to separate one from another. *Materia medica* literature evolved from a few source texts to distinct genres by the work of copyists and compilers who set the genres apart from each other.[1] The fields

144

of other medical writing were also dominated by a few influential source texts. The scarcity of sources lead to a dense network of interconnected vernacular versions. Within the scope of this chapter it is assumed that English herbals contain recipes with similar components and the same sources as other types of vernacular medicine. Recipes can be found in all traditions of medieval medical writing: in specialised tracts, surgical treatises, and remedybooks including *materia medica* (see Pahta and Taavitsainen in this volume, p. 14). The majority of medical recipes list herbal ingredients.

The textual network formed by medieval medical writings in England makes it possible to observe the relations between separate texts through an extensive text corpus. In this study I have used a corpus of herbal texts from Middle English to Early Modern English, and for parallels in other medical writing the *Corpus of Middle English Medical Texts (MEMT)*.[2] I have not pre-selected the material in the corpora in any way, i.e. the textual searches have been carried out to include all the texts written between the years 1375 and 1500, irrespective of genre. The program used for text retrieval is *Corpus Presenter*.[3] In order to focus my research and to limit the amount of output data, I have chosen three herbs as cues to herbal recipes, viz. betony (*Betonica officinalis* or *Stachys officinalis*), rue (*Ruta graveolens*), and rosemary (*Rosmarinus officinalis*). Betony and rosemary both had the reputation of being a panacea; rue seems to have been an ingredient in almost any medicine imaginable, thus all of these herbs as search terms yield plenty of hits. I have first generated word-lists of the texts, then chosen the different spelling variants for the names of the herbs, and used these lemmata as input lists for the searches. I have then used the text output as the material for qualitative analysis of the content: I have compared the cotext of the herb names in herbals and in other medical writing, and after verifying the cotext as a recipe I have included it to the final output data, which has then been used to find parallelisms and variants of recipes.

I have also used classifications of recipes by their type and content in order to distinguish between the recipes, as form and content seem to be relevant in some of the intertextual links. The ordering of information within the recipes provided a means to compare between them and to find patterns in the manifestations of intertextuality. This method bears a resemblance to Taavitsainen's (1988: 130–2).

6.3   Classification of recipes

6.3.1   *Types and contents*

Middle English medical writing contains various kinds of recipes. The types are *receptaria*, *antidotaria*, and *experimenta* recipes. A distinction can also be made between simples and *composita* recipes. The first three types are classified according to the textual tradition and internal conventions, and the last two according to the contents and complexity of recipes, i.e. how many ingredients are needed for a recipe. As a consequence, an individual recipe may be simultaneously classified, for example, as a *receptaria* type recipe, and a simple.

A fourth 'recipe type', a parallel to *antidotaria*, *receptaria* and *experimenta*, has been taken into consideration in the course of this study. 'Recipe paraphrases' are a co-occurrence pattern of features embedded in the text component called virtues. The paraphrases use covert instruction,[4] inanimate subjects, and conditional clauses. Functionally, this text-type can often be perceived as a recipe, both by the intention and the content. It is consequently regarded as a recipe paraphrase, and included in the study.

6.3.2 Ordering of information in recipes

Medieval recipes in general have earlier been said to contain six different kinds of information (*Fachinformation*) (Stannard 1982: 60–5). The six types are (as modified for the objectives of this study):

A   purpose,
B   ingredients (including equipment needed),
C   procedure,
D   administration of medicine,
E   justification, and
F   additional information.

The first four kinds of information are deemed necessary for a given text to be categorised as a recipe. Justification, or the evidence presented in a recipe to prove its potency, as well as additional information, such as efficacy phrases and cases treated with the medicine, may be omitted, and they often are. The information types are used to point out differences and similarities in the ordering of information in recipes.

6.3.3 Antidotaria/full recipes

Antidotaria recipes form the main body of *antidotaria* texts. They can also be called full recipes, as the ingredients are often numerous, the procedures described highly detailed, and there is often a comment on the use and the effect of the medicine. Full recipes are often given a proper name, such as *beve de Antioche* 'drink of Antioch', and they are described as *antidota*, a Greek word for remedies or medicine given against a disease or an ailment (Becela-Deller 1998: 74–5).

Purpose, ingredients, procedure and administration are always present in *antidota*, whereas justification (the arguments for the potency of the medicine) is an optional element, even in full recipes. Additional information is often included.

6.3.4 Receptaria/*short recipes*

Short recipes are characteristic of *receptaria* collections. They seldom have a name, and are often recognised by their purpose, for example *Medicamentum ad . . .* or *another medecyne for . . .* or just simply *for . . .* , followed by the name of the ailment. Comments on their administration or efficacy are rarer than in full recipes, and they are not as detailed in their procedure description (Becela-Deller 1998: 74–5). They do fulfil, however, the first three prerequisites of a recipe: purpose, ingredients, and procedure. The example following here presents the pattern BCBA, according to the types of *Fachinformation* defined in 6.3.2:

(1) Also take veruayne / betayne / & saxfrage and of euery of them lyke moche and stampe the~ & tempre them with whyte wyne / and this is good for them that haue the stone. (*Herbal*, ed. Larkey and Pyles 1941: I ii)

The recipe starts with the ingredients (B), continues with the description of the medicine preparing procedure (C), returns shortly to the ingredients (B; *whyte wyne*), and finishes off with a purpose (A) indicating sequence, i.e. the treatment of gallstones. More often in recipes than in herbals the purpose seems to be given at the end of the recipe; the reasons for this will be addressed in the section on recipe paraphrases.

Ingredients and procedure are essential parts of a recipe, though in short recipes they are often reduced to the minimum: for example *betony drunk* should give the reader the idea of processing a certain herb into a potable form. This strategy may be due to shared, or assumed knowledge between the author and the audience, the regular procedures of preparing medicines were probably well known to medical professionals and laity alike (Stannard 1982: 62).

In short recipes, the fourth prerequisite of recipes, administration, is not always fulfilled. Again, the concepts of internal/external medicines and the ways to administer the end product of a medical recipe were certainly no secrets among the people who practised medicine, thus this component may be omitted.

6.3.5 Experimenta

Experimenta recipes can rarely be found anywhere else but in commonplace books written *ad usum proprium*. Their roots are often not in the texts written by the ancient authors, but were passed down by word of mouth: *experimenta* were jotted down after hearing them from a colleague or an acquaintance who had proved the efficacy of the recipe in practice (P. M. Jones 1995: 49; see Taavitsainen 'Transferring' and Jones in this volume). *Experimenta* are not attested in my data.

6.3.6 Recipe paraphrases

(2)   Also hys flowrys mengte wyth hony & etyn fastande suffren no folons ne pestilens sorys to bredyn in mannys body (*Rosemary*, ed. Mäkinen 2002a: 316)

Example (2) has five parts, including all the four prerequisites of a recipe, forming the pattern BCDA. The components in order are ingredients (B; *hys flowrys, hony*), procedure (C; *mengte*), administration (D; *etyn fastande*), and purpose (A; *suffren no folons ne pestilens sorys . . .*). This text-type is often used in the virtues component in herbals. It usually presents precise descriptions of procedures in order to come up with an end product that can be called a medicine. For this reason I have come to regard this part of herbals as a paraphrase of a recipe, and I have included it in my analysis of the retrieved data. The distinguishable linguistic pattern of virtues is characteristic of herbals, but it can also be found in *materia medica* literature in general (Mäkinen 2002c: 283–4). A similar linguistic co-occurrence pattern in learned medical writing has been identified by Taavitsainen (2001b: 107): the reasons for differences in the presentation of recipes in practical remedybooks and learned treatises lie in the purposes of writing. Recipe collections were a medium for quick reference and were intended for daily use, whereas learned tracts were for the advancement of knowledge and communication between colleagues.[5]

Another reason for the use of the passive voice in herbals is the tradition of *materia medica* literature: in Dioscorides' *De materia medica* the medical substances are arranged according to a polar system, ranging from hot to cold in the humoral theory, and each *materium medicum* is placed on the scale to a place indicated by the degree of its properties (Touwaide 1998: 46–7).[6] In this system each medical substance is usually associated with medicines, cures or remedies in which the instructions are often given in the passive voice. The function of virtual recipes was primarily to provide the reader with the medical knowledge associated with the plant, and secondarily, they were instructions for preparing a medicine (Mäkinen 2002c: 283–4).

According to the material used, in recipe collections the purpose is often given at the beginning of a recipe, whereas in herbals the purpose is often the last element presented in a recipe. This is probably a reflection of the virtues sequences, the recipe paraphrases, and is thus an inherent feature of the recipes in herbals (Mäkinen 2002c: 279). The expected ordering of information in recipes in herbals (both regular and recipe paraphrases) is thus BCDA, or BCDAF, if the additional information is included.

6.3.7 Simples and composita

Simples are recipes for medicines prepared only of one *materium medicum*, and *composita* are recipes with several ingredients. Full recipes (*antidotaria* type) are, by definition, always *composita*, whereas with short recipes (*receptaria* type) one can find both simples and *composita*.

The preliminary survey of my data indicates that the majority of recipes in herbals are simples, and of the *receptaria* type. Simples can also be found in other medical texts, but to observe similarity between herbal and other recipes may be difficult, as many of the simples are of the form *Stampe it* [wormwood] *and ley it to fressh woundes, for it helip hem fere* (*Macer Floridus*, ed. Frisk 1949: 63). Consequently, one cannot say whether the similarity detected is due to intertextuality and transmission of material, or to the 'best use' of the herb, which travels as oral tradition (cf. *experimenta*), or whether it is accepted as common knowledge, and thus does not need be copied from elsewhere. The more complex the detected parallelisms are, the more clearly they indicate intertextuality; consequently the emphasis is on the *composita*.

6.4   Classical, medieval, and vernacular herbals

6.4.1 Greek and Latin herbals

Practically all the classical herbal material that influenced the shaping of Western vernacular herbals was of Greek origin (Singer 1927: 33). Original Latin (and Roman) herbals have not been preserved to our day: their influence on the medieval herbal writing has come down to us through the extant Greek herbals and compiled Latin herbals. The most important extant Latin texts are Pliny the Elder's *Historia naturalis* and Cato the Censor's *De re rustica*, both of which present no original herbal material, but rely heavily on Greek predecessors, especially Theophrastos' work (Pliny also draws on Sextius Niger's lost herbal). *Historia naturalis* is an encyclopaedic text covering a variety of topics within natural philosophy, and *De re rustica* is an instructional text about farming. They both have parts that can be considered as herbals.

The most influential Greek text is Dioscorides' *De materia medica* (first century AD), which also has descriptions of animal and mineral *materia medica*. Dioscorides' text draws on several earlier sources. Most of the borrowed passages originate in the Greek herbals of Krateuas and Sextius Niger (first century BC), and Pamphilos' *Synonyma*, an alphabetical list of plant names in various languages (first century AD) (Singer 1927: 21–4; Collins 2000: 31). Dioscorides writes on over 600 plants, some 35 animal-based subjects, and 90 minerals; the focus is clearly on herbs even though the text is a *materia medica* text. Pliny and Dioscorides were contemporary writers, and they share some of the sources,[7] although they never refer to each other (Collins 2000: 32).

Another Greek text, and the last of the classical era to have authority over medieval compilers and copyists of herbals, is Galen's *De simplicibus*, written in the second century AD. Galen borrowed extensively from Dioscorides, and used Aristotle's and Hippocrates' texts for the theoretical parts of his herbal; his

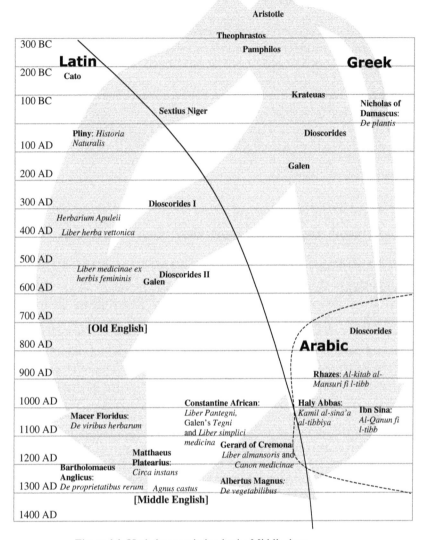

Figure 6.1 Herbal transmission in the Middle Ages

originality was seen in the amalgamation of the medical and herbalistic knowledge (Morton 1981: 72).

6.4.2 Herbal transmission in the Middle Ages

Figure 6.1[8] illustrates the transmission of texts from the Greek originals to Arabic, Latin, and eventually to English manuscripts. Reading Figure 6.1 we can see that medieval herbals derive from only two or three textual nodes: Dioscorides is the most important source of material in Greek, and Pliny can be seen as the lens through which the early Latin lines of transmission travelled. The third node is the one with Theophrastos and Aristotle, but the line leading to the Arabic translations and onward is based partly on Nicholas of Damascus's *De plantis*, which has been considered a corrupt rendering of Aristotle's works. Although the later textual field is broadened by translations and compilations, it is the same material provided by the ancient authorities that is recirculated in new combinations, and as a result the texts remain closely related to each other.

6.4.3 Through Arabic into Latin

The late medieval Latinate herbal tradition would have been weak, had it been based on the early Latin translations of Dioscorides and Galen alone. From the eleventh century onwards, the Latin translations of Arabic masters, such as Rhazes, Haly Abbas and Ibn Sina, revitalised the transmission lines of the somewhat incomplete and corrupt classical medical learning in the West. The interest in classical medicine and science in general within the Muslim learned world had led to the preservation of many texts that would otherwise have been lost. In the ninth and eleventh centuries, Rhazes and Ibn Sina composed *al-Mansuri* and *al-Qanun* respectively, and these works relied directly on the writings of Dioscorides and Galen. Rhazes was the main source for the later Haly Abbas, whose works with Rhazes became the source of the Latinate Galen, *Tegni*, and *Liber Pantegni*. The translation *Liber simplici medicina* was also originally Galen's work.

Galen's and Dioscorides' writings were reintroduced in the West, in Latin, in the eleventh century, when Constantine the African, upon his arrival in Europe, brought with him several Arabic medical texts and translated them into Latin in southern Italy. The influx of 'fresh' texts partly caused increased literary activity in Salerno, an already blooming medical centre near Monte Cassino, where Constantine lived. Dioscorides' works carried over to the West by the writings of Ibn Sina were translated into Latin in Spain, in the twelfth century, by Gerard of Cremona. *Al-Qanun* became *Canon medicinae*, and Rhazes's version translated by Gerard became *Liber almansoris*.

After the translation of the seminal works from Arabic into Latin, Salernitan writings made their way into at least Matthaeus Platearius's *Circa instans* (twelfth century) and Bartholomaeus Anglicus's *De proprietatibus rerum* (turn of the twelfth–thirteenth centuries), and later, in the fourteenth century, into *Agnus castus* as well. *De proprietatibus rerum* was also influenced by Platearius's work, and by the translations made in Spain, especially by *Canon medicinae*. Another author to use Platearius and *Canon medicinae* was Albertus Magnus, in his *De vegetabilibus*. All these Latin works also draw on the earlier Latin tradition, including Pliny. Macer Floridus's *De viribus herbarum* in the eleventh century seems to have been written too early to benefit from the new translations.

6.4.4 English herbals

There are thirteen Old English manuscripts extant which contain herbals or herbalistic cures (*eVK*).[9] Four of these manuscripts contain texts that are regarded as herbals proper.[10] The Old English herbals draw mostly on Pliny, and on the Latinised versions of Galen and Dioscorides, which were translated in the sixth and seventh centuries.[11] Considering the keywords used in this study, some of the Old English recipes using the defined herbal ingredients are very similar to Middle English recipes, at least as far as purpose is concerned (Old English recipes are not included in this study). However, it is unlikely that the influence of Old English manuscripts would have carried over to the period between Old English and Middle English;[12] rather, the intertextuality is based on the same Latin translations recopied and retranslated in the Middle English period.

The late medieval Latin works in Figure 6.1 were all translated into English, and therefore the setting for the intertextuality observed within Middle English herbals is roughly presented there. Dioscorides was not translated into English from Greek before the seventeenth century, accordingly all the Middle English texts reflect the tradition carried over from the Latin translations.

6.5   Intertextual linking of herbals and other medicine

6.5.1 Intertextuality and medieval texts

The manner in which medieval texts, especially practical or theoretical texts were produced stretches slightly the modern concept of intertextuality. The author of a text was usually not creating something new, but keeping to a tradition and reformulating a known text according to the best of his abilities. Kristeva's rendering of the Bakhtinian concept, each text being 'a mosaic of quotations' (Kristeva 1986: 37) is literally true for medieval texts. Medieval intertextuality is insensitive to authorship, but not unconsciously so: the dialogue between texts (textual or structural parallels) is intended, and even demanded of the new reiterations of the existing texts and their traditions (Bergner 1995: 48). The actual textual material may have been worked in a number of ways, thus giving the new translation, copy, compilation, or commentary the individual touch of the author (cf. Plett 1991). Therefore, the textual parallels in medieval practical texts have usually been subject to some kind of editing, if not actual paraphrasing.

MEMT and the herbal corpus provide an opportunity to study recipes in ways that have not previously been possible. As no corpus presents an exhaustive sampling of the material, the parallels observed are reflections of the textual transmission, not way-points on the actual transmission lines. Therefore the links established between the recipes may be seen as indicators of an interrelated system of texts, and markers of intertextuality, rather than succession patterns of the transmission of recipes, or the text lemmata.

The early stages of the analysis strengthened the hypothesis: the herbal recipe material forms a tradition of its own, and is separate from the other medical recipe material, the two being only tangential, only blending in places. Not surprisingly, in other medical writing herbal recipes were most abundant in remedy texts. These texts formed the most closely interrelated textual field of all the material.

6.5.2 Intertextuality in herbals

Simples, as mentioned earlier, are the most common recipe type in herbals. Recipe paraphrases are also numerous in herbals. The first three examples of recipes in herbals, all simples, include one recipe paraphrase, example (3), the rest being recipes proper (the emphases in examples throughout the chapter are mine, indicating the elements shared):

(3)   Also **þe colys of hys stalkys** bownden in a **clene lynene clowt** ȝif þi teth ben well froten þer-wyth **it sleth wormys in þe teth** & kepyth þe teth fro rotyng & fro ake & fro wormys (*Rosemary*, ed. Mäkinen 2002a: 318)

(4)   Of rosmaryni is grene tree,
       Berne a col & bere wyþ þe,
       & lappe hyt **in a lennyn cloþe**,
       Þogt hit grewe, be þou nogt wroþe,
       Rubbe þi teþe þerwyþ at nede,
       & þou schalt haue wel gode spede.
       For **al wormes hyt wol sle**
       & make wenym away to flee. (*Loscombe*, ed. Zettersten 1967: 21)

(5)   Also **take the tymbre therof** & bru∼ne it to coles & make powder therof & tha∼ put it **into a lynen cloth** and **rubbe thy tethe therwith** / & yf there be ony wormes therin it shall slee them & kepe thy tethe from all euyls. (*Herbal*, ed. Larkey and Pyles 1941: H ii)

Despite the differences in syntax the contents are identifiable, and the extracts can all be recognised as renderings of the same recipe. The ailment to be cured is 'worms in the teeth'; the cure is prepared by burning the wood of rosemary branches to make charcoal, and then wrapping the charcoal in a (clean) linen cloth and rubbing this against the teeth.

Table 6.1 compares the different elements and their order in parallel recipes. The letters heading columns stand for the information type, i.e. 'A' stands for purpose, 'B' for ingredients, 'C' for procedure, 'D' for administration, 'E' for justification, and 'F' for additional information. The signs in the respective columns indicate the absence (−) or presence (+, ++, +++, ++++) of an element. The plus and minus signs are comparable to each other in the same column: differences in signs tell of differences between the elements in the recipe extracts, i.e. a + indicates the presence of an element similar to other elements marked by a + in the same column. A ++ in the same column indicates the presence of an element that differs from the first recipe in the table, but is similar to other elements in the same column marked by a ++. The column 'Order' tells the organisation of the elements in the recipe, the letters corresponding to the column names. The expected order of the four essential elements for a recipe in a herbal would be BCDA, and for a recipe in other medical writing ABCD. The column 'Type' indicates whether the example is a recipe proper (rec.) or a recipe paraphrase (par.), *antidota* and *experimenta* count as recipes proper. Under the column label 'S/C' is found the information on the number of ingredients, i.e. 'S' for simples and 'C' for *composita*.

Table 6.1. *Simple recipes in herbals*

Example	Order	Type	S/C	A	B	C	D	E	F
3 *Rosemary*	BCDA	par.	S	+	+	+	+	−	−
4 *Loscombe*	(B)CDFA	rec.	S	+	+	++	+	−	+
5 *Herbal*	BCDA	rec.	S	+	+	++	+	−	−

Legend: A = purpose, B = ingredients, C = procedure, D = administration, E = justification, F = additional information; Type: rec. = recipe proper, par. = recipe paraphrase; S/C: S = simple recipe, C = *composita* recipe; + = element present, − = element absent

Example (3) is formally and linguistically defined as the virtues (the text-type), but functionally it may be perceived as a recipe on account of its explicitness in procedure and ingredients (see section 6.3.6). Examples (4) and (5) are short recipes proper, and essentially the same. The prose version probably allows for a more compact expression as it does not require rhymes; there is looseness in the poem as it carries extra material in order to maintain the rhyme pattern, introducing one new piece of information per couplet. The elements shared by the three recipes can be found in the ingredients (coals, linen cloth), the procedure (burn, rub your teeth), and the purpose indicating components (it will slay the worms in the teeth).[13]

The ordering of components in (3), BCDA (ingredients, *þe colys of hys stalkys*;[14] procedure, *bownden in a clene lynene clowt*; administration, *ʒif þi teth ben well froten þer-myth*; and purpose (cf. note 13), *it sleth wormys in þe teth & kepyth þe teth fro rotyng & fro ake & fro wormys*), is similar to (4) and (5), although the latter two are recipes proper. Example (4) differs from the others due to the absence of ingredients and the interrupting additional information sequence (*And þou schalt haue wel gode spede*). The extract is part of a poem on rosemary, thus the one ingredient in this simple is known and not repeated. The element of additional information (F) does not fit the expected pattern, but it may be used in the poem in order to maintain the rhyme scheme. The reason for the uniform ordering of information in all the three extracts may be the established recipe paraphrase structure, in which the purpose is often indicated towards the end (Mäkinen 2002c: 278–9).

Composita recipes are not uncommon in herbals, although they are distinctly rarer than simples. A herbal entry, or a herbal treatise on one plant only, deals with the description and properties of a singular *materium medicum*, thus simples are the kinds of recipes one would expect to find in herbals. The herbal recipes including multiple ingredients are, in a way, transgressing the boundary between herbals and recipe collections, and are therefore also potential places for textual parallels. Examples (6) and (7) illustrate *composita* recipes:

(6)   Also take **an hundred peper greynes** & þer wyth þe jows of his flourys & his lewys & wyth a **lytyll hony** make **ij pelotes** & **ete þe ton at morwyn & þe toþer at ewen** and mythtely it delyueryth fro þe cowhe (*Rosemary*, ed. Mäkinen 2002a: 318)

(7)   Also if a man haue a wikked cowhe tak þis herbe and **an hundred pepurcornes** and grynde hym with **tweyn vnces of hony** and make þer-of **peletes** and **3if on of þe peletes in drynk in þe morwenyng** when he aryseth and **anoþer in þe euenyng** when he goth to slepe and he schal be hol in a litel tyme. (*Agnus castus*, ed. Brodin 1950: 201)

Table 6.2. Composita *in herbals I*

Example	Order	Type	S/C	A	B	C	D	E	F
6 *Rosemary*	BCDA	rec.	C	+	+	+	+	−	−
7 *Agnus castus*	ABCBCDF	rec.	C	+	+	+	+	−	+

For the legend, see Table 6.1.

In the two examples given, the similarities in ingredients (*an hundred peper greynes, an hundred pepur-cornes; a lytyll hony, tweyn vnces of hony*) and in the administration of the medicine (*ete þe ton at morwyn & þe toþer at ewen, 3if on of þe peletes in drynk in þe morwenyng . . . and anoþer in þe euenyng*) justify these as textual parallels. The differences can be found in the ordering of elements: in example (6) the purpose is indicated at the end of the recipe, whereas example (7) gives the purpose at the beginning of the recipe. The repetition of the pattern 'BC' (ingredients–procedure) in example (7) is characteristic of recipes with several ingredients: the introduction of a new ingredient needs a new kind of procedure.

Both examples are recipes proper; the strategy employed in (6) is more expected of a herbal, and (7) resembles more a recipe collection in the choice of the ordering of information. Example (6) is from a treatise on one herb, rosemary, and the text is more theory- than practice-orientated. Example (7) is from an alphabetised herbal with several plants: the text is a reference book with accessible information on each herb, and thus it resembles medical recipe collections in its organisation.[15] The contents of the recipes differ only in the efficacy phrase, which is lacking in (6). Both texts derive from the Salernitan translations and compilations, and the two editions quoted here are even from the same codex (though from different *loci*), thus it is no surprise that they carry similar textual material.[16]

The following extracts are examples of *composita* parallels, in which one or more of the ingredients change from one recipe to another (here wormwood instead of smallage in the last recipe). The possible reasons for the phenomenon may be manifold: a corrupt copy along the transmission line, a 'base recipe template' in which one can add a herb for the desired effect, etc. As recipes in this study have been located by the names of herbs, i.e. by the names of ingredients, the parallels should be most alike within the component of ingredients. However, the parallelisms observed here are confirmed by the uniformity of other components.

(8)   Smalage. Take Smalage sede / **Rewe sede** / **Peper & Salt and grynde them well togyder & tempre them with wyne & drynke it** / for it is good for colde and **wycked humoures in the stomake** & conforteth the stomake / the lyuer / & the longes. (*Herbal*, ed. Larkey and Pyles 1941: H iii)

(9)   Also take smaleche and **rewe the sede and peper and salte and grynde them all to-gedyr and temper them with wyne** and þat **drynke** dothe a-wey colde and **wyckyd humorus yn þe stomake** and comfortat þe stomake and þe lyver and longges. (*Vertues*, ed. Grymonprez 1981: 99)

(10)   For þe stomak. Take wermode or his rote and **þe seed of rue, salt, and pepir, stampe hem and tempere it with wyn,** sethe hem þan and **drinke hem,** and so shalt þou purge þe **wicked and rawe humourʒ of þe stomak.** (*Macer Floridus*, ed. Frisk 1949: 61–2)

Table 6.3. Composita *in herbals II*

Example	Order	Type	S/C	A	B	C	D	E	F
8 *Herbal*	BCBDEA	rec.	C	+	+	+	+	+	−
9 *Vertues*	BCBDEA	rec.	C	+	+	+	+	+	−
10 *Macer Floridus*	ABCBCDA	rec.	C	+	++	++	+	−	−

For the legend, see Table 6.1.

In addition to the change in ingredients, the recipe in (10) is the only one in this selection that adopts the ordering of information expected of recipe collection recipes, although there the purpose is also restated in the end, in greater detail.

In procedure, (10) has an extra action (*sethe hem þan*) compared to the other recipes, and the purpose lacks a sequence the other recipes have (*and comfortat þe stomake and þe lyver and longges*). The purpose and administration sequences are identical, and so are the ingredients, save for the one herb mentioned earlier. Example (8) from *Herbal*, which is a sixteenth-century compilation (cf. note 2) of several medieval herbals, follows the organisation pattern set in *Vertues*, or in similar texts. *Vertues*, which is exemplified in example (9), is an unorganised collection of herb entries, i.e. it is not organised according to the humoral theory, or the initials of Middle English herb names. Recipes proper are more frequent in *Macer Floridus* than in *Vertues*. *Macer Floridus* has more sequences that could pass as extracts from a recipe collection within other medical writing (cf. example 10). There seems to be a continuum within herbals from more theoretical texts to practical texts and reference works: the texts discussed so far seem to have *Rosemary* and *Vertues* closer to the theoretical end of the continuum, and *Macer Floridus* closer to the practical end, *Agnus castus* being placed somewhere in the middle. *Herbal* is, as already mentioned, a compilation of earlier works, and thus its place in the continuum changes from extract to extract.

The final examples of intertextuality within herbals further illustrate the relation between *composita* recipes proper and recipe paraphrases: here also the main difference is the ordering of information, the elements themselves being essentially the same, save for slight variation in procedure and administration:

(11)   Also **watir þat his** [rosemary's] **lewys arn sothyn in** to þe myddys or to þe thredde del and þanne clense it & medele it wyth **wyn** & dronkyn: **first mad soppys þer inne** and it astoryth **apetyt lost** (*Rosemary*, ed. Mäkinen 2002a: 318)

(12)   Also yf thou be feble with vnkydly swette / take and **boyle the leues** [of rosemary] **in clene water** / & whan þ~ water is colde do therto as moche of whyte **wyne** / & than **make therin soppes** & ete thou well therof / & thou shal **recouer appetyte**. (*Herbal*, ed. Larkey and Pyles 1941: H ii)[17]

Table 6.4. Composita *in herbals III*

Example	Order	Type	S/C	A	B	C	D	E	F
11 *Rosemary*	BCBDA	par.	C	+	+	+	+	−	−
12 *Herbal*	ACBCBDA	rec.	C	+	+	++	++	−	−

For the legend, see Table 6.1.

As we have seen, recipe and recipe paraphrase parallels in herbals are prone to variation, but variation seems to prefer some elements to others. Most often fluctuation may be observed within procedure, sometimes in administration. Additional data may vary greatly from one recipe to its copy, and it may even be left out as it is unnecessary information for the function of a recipe. Ingredients are the means to locate the parallels in this study, therefore the similarity between recipes within the ingredients is expected. The variation within the ingredients is also chosen at the selection of recipes for this study. As a result, the uniformity or variation of ingredients is not always directly comparable to other recipe components.

6.5.3 Recipe intertextuality in other medical writing

In the course of this chapter, I have noted that practical remedybooks seem to be the most tightly knit textual 'population' in the Middle English period, that is, according to the material at my disposal, and the search parameters I have chosen. It is obvious that most parallels should be found within texts containing recipes for all purposes, and not within treatises and tracts focusing on a distinct ailment, cure, or skill (surgeries and specialised treatises), nor within the genre of herbals of which the readily accessible data are scarce. In this section the first extracts from (13) to (17) are all from remedy texts or recipe collections, and they are *composita* recipes. Surgical texts and treatises on special subjects (e.g. gynaecology or ophthalmology) did yield hits within recipes, but only a few, and with only one or two parallels in other texts. Simples are rarer than *composita* in recipe collections, but there will be examples of simples as well in section 6.5.4.

(13)   For a stynkyng brethe at þe nose. Take þe juce off **mynte** and off **rew** and put yt to-gyddyr and **do yt in-to þe nose-thyrlys**. (*Burgundy*, ed. Schöffler 1919: 196)

(14)   another medecyne for the same Take **rede mynte** and **rewe** of either like moche and stamp hem and wring out the juse and **put therof in his nostrel** when he gothe to bed and it schal a mende him (*Naples*, ed. Vallese 1940: 19)

(15)   For stoppede nos terlis þat comiþ of feble brayn. Tak þe ius of þe **mynte**. and þe ius of þe **rewe** y temprid to gedere. and **do hit to his nosterlis ofte**. hit is goud (*Leechbook I*, ed. Edmar 1967: 81)

(16)   Pro fetore alitus per nasum. tak **rede myntes** &~ **rewe** ana, &~ **wrynge þe jus in to seke nese þrelles**, at even, when he gooþ to bedde. (*Mediz-inbuch*, ed. Heinrich 1896: 70)

(17)   ffor stinkinge breth through the nose. Take **red myntes** and **rue** of either like quantytie & **wringe the juyce in to the pacyent his nostrelles** at night upon he goeth to bed. (*Leechbook III*, ed. Dawson 1934b: 333)

These *composita* recipes are governed by the same ingredients and a common ailment: they all deal with a malady affecting the nose, except (14), which is for a 'cold in the head', but there also the ingredients and administration are similar to the other recipes. The differences that are found are related to the definition of

Table 6.5. Composita *in other medical writing*

Example	Order	Type	S/C	A	B	C	D	E	F
13 *Burgundy*	ABCD	rec.	C	+	+	+	+	−	−
14 *Naples*	ABCDF	rec.	C	++	+	++	+	−	+
15 *Leechbook I*	ABCDF	rec.	C	+	+	++	+	−	++
16 *Medizinbuch*	ABCD	rec.	C	+	+	++	+	−	−
17 *Leechbook III*	ABCD	rec.	C	+	+	++	+	−	−

For the legend, see Table 6.1.

the disease, to the time of administration of the medicine (including frequency), and to the efficacy phrases in additional data. All the examples conform to the pattern of a recipe collection recipe, starting with the purpose, followed by the ingredients, procedure and administration, and rounded off by an efficacy phrase in half of them. These texts probably draw on the same few source texts, and on each other. The intertextuality in these recipes is likely to reflect the transmission lines of the recipes, the construction of which, however, would require an accurate timeline of the manuscripts, and information from the unedited texts of the stemmata.

Earlier in this chapter I noted that recipe parallels are easier to detect in complex recipes. The following are examples of complex *composita* recipes which have changed very little during the copying processes. Complexity in itself does not explain the small degree of variation, but the length of a recipe may correlate with the greater prestige value of a complex *composita* recipe, and the motivation to copy it correctly may have been higher than with 'regular' recipes.

(18)   For þe hefd-ache. Take and seþe **verueyn** and **betany** and **wormod**; and þere-with wasche þe seke-ys hefd; and þan make a playstere a-boue on þe molde on þes manere; tak þe same herbys wan þey bene sodyn, and wryng hem and grynd hem smale in a morter; and tempre hem with þe same licoure a-ȝen; and do þere-to wete-bren for to holdyn in þe lycour; and **mak a garlond of a kerche**, and bynde þe sek hefd and ley þe playster on þe molde with þe garlond, as hoot as þe sek may sufre it; and bynd þe hefd with a voliper, and set a kap a-boue and do þes but þre tymys, and þe seke schal bene hool; on warantyse. (*Medical works*, ed. Henslow 1899: 135)

(19)   Pro dolore capitis. take and seþe **verueyne**, and **betonye**, and **wermod** and þer wyþ wasche þe seke heued, &~ þanne make a plasture aboue on þe moolde on þis manere Take þe same erbys, when þey beon sodyn, and wrynge hem and grynde hem smale in a morter, and tempre hem wyþ þe same licour a ȝeyne, &~ do þer to wheton branne, to holde in þe licour, and **make a garlande of akerchef**, and bynde þe seke heued, and ley þe plasture on þe molde wyþ ynne þe garlaunde, as hoot as þe seke may

suffre, and bynde þe hed wyþ a volyper, and sette a kappe aboue, and þys do bote þre dayes, and þe seke shal be hool on warantyse. (*Medizinbuch*, ed. Heinrich 1896: 65–6)

(20)   For hed-ake. Take and sethe **verueyne, betonye,** and **wormode,** and þer-with wasch þe seke hed, and make a playstre abowe on þe molde on þis maner; take þe same erbys, qhwanne he ben sothen, wrynge hem, and grynde hem smale in a morter, and tempere hem with þe same erbis, and do þer-to qwete-bryn for to holde in þe lycour; and **make a garlond of a kerchefe** and bynde þe seke hed, and ley þe playster on þe molde with-inne þe garlond as hoot as he may suffre it, and bynd þe hed with a wolypere and sette a cappe abowe; and do þus III tymes, and þe seke schal ben hole a warantyse. (*Stockholm*, ed. Müller 1929b: 50–1)

Table 6.6. *Complex* composita *in other medical writing*

Example	Order	Type	S/C	A	B	C	D	E	F
18 *Medical works*	ACBDBCBDF	rec.	C	+	+	+	+	−	+
19 *Medizinbuch*	ACBDBCBDF	rec.	C	+	+	+	+	−	+
20 *Stockholm*	ACBDBCBDF	rec.	C	+	+	+	+	−	+

For the legend, see Table 6.1.

In complex *composita*, as in examples (18–20), the parallel material is fairly easy to detect, providing that the recipe has not grown in length during the compilation process, and received additional, possibly prestige ingredients. These three extracts are primarily chosen for the curiosity confirming the parallels, *a garlond of a kerchefe*; otherwise the recipes echo each other almost verbatim, only differing over an odd *and*.

The extracts contain two sub-sequences, i.e. the same ingredients are used for the same purpose by different procedures. The sub-recipes (CBD and BCBD) are both introduced by the same purpose element and as they are not joined by an interrupting 'for the same' or 'another', they can be regarded as parts of a longer recipe.

Examples (19) and (20) belong to the Stockholm and British Library Additional 33996 groups of manuscripts which are related to Norfolk and Lincolnshire (see Jones in this volume).[18] The texts related to these groups in this chapter will be further discussed with Figure 6.2.

Examples (21) to (23) counterbalance the coherent recipes of the preceding examples. Here, small differences can be observed both in ingredients and in procedure. Not even the identifying sequence (*5 cornys of peper*) is without variation; yet these recipes are parallels:

(21) An oþ~ [for the head-ache] Take **bitayne verveyn** celidony **wormod**
weybred Rubb wal wort sawge **fyue cornys of pep**~ and **hony** and seith
all in wat~ and **Drynke hitt fastynge** (*Leechbook II*, ed. Dawson 1934a:
18)

(22) a drinke to distroy the hed ache Take **betanye** and **vervayne warmot**
and celidon and **6 cornys of pepir** and **hony** and sethe ham al in watir
and kepe the watir in a viol of glas and **drinke therof fasting** and use it
and it schal save the from al evil in the hed (*Naples*, ed. Vallese 1940: 23)

(23) Anoþer for þe hevede: Tak **betayne** & **vervayne**, **wormet**, celidoine,
waybred, rew, walworth, sange, & **v cornys of pepyr**, & stamp þam & seth
þam togidder in water, & **drynk þam fastande**. (*Daniel*, ed. Jasin 1983:
43)

Table 6.7. *Variation in* composita *in other medical writing*

Example	Order	Type	S/C	A	B	C	D	E	F
21 *Leechbook II*	ABCD	rec.	C	+	+	+	+	−	−
22 *Naples*	ABCD	rec.	C	+	++	++	+	−	−
23 *Daniel*	ABCBD	rec.	C	+	+++	+++	+	−	−

For the legend, see Table 6.1.

All the recipes in Table 6.7 belong to the *receptaria* type, and are from recipe
collections. The ordering of information is the same in all of the examples, and
the organisation pattern here is the default of recipe collection recipes.

Very few hits have been retrieved from among specialised treatises and surgical
texts; in the following, a rare occurrence of an encyclopaedic recipe (25) with
parallels from remedybooks, (24) and (26), has been found in Gilbertus Anglicus's
work:

(24) Ach off hede. make þ~ for **lye of verveyne** or ellys of **betenye** ether of
wormod and þ~ with **wasshe thyne hede thrise in þe weke** (*Leechbook
II*, ed. Dawson 1934a: 18)

(25) But if þe hede-ache be of flevme, þat is to sei, of cooldenes and of moystnes,
let him wasshe his fete with warme salt watir euery ny3te. And let him often
kembe his hede with an yvery combe. And of þe asshis of heyne-houe and of
elern bowes in grete quantite, and of þe asshis of egrimoyn and of **betayn**,
make **lye** and **wasshe þerwith his hede**, for þis is gode boþe for falling
awey of heris and to do awey þe ache (*Gilbertus*, ed. Getz 1991: 2)

(26) For hedwark: Mak **lee of verveyne** & of **betayne** or of **wormede**, &
þarewith **wasch þi hevede twys or thrys in a weyk** (*Daniel*, ed. Jasin
1983: 43)[19]

Table 6.8. Composita *from remedybooks and an encyclopaedia*

Example	Order	Type	S/C	A	B	C	D	E	F
24 *Leechbook II*	ACBD	rec.	C	+	+	+	+	–	–
25 *Gilbertus*	(AEDBD)BCDA	rec.	C	+	++	+	++	+	–
26 *Daniel*	ACBD	rec.	C	+	+	+	+	–	–

For the legend, see Table 6.1.

The ordering of information is more complex in (25) than in the other two: the encyclopaedic extract here presents an initial (DBD) sequence after the purpose, describing an alternative treatment for the ailment. The sequence following is the actual parallel to (24) and (26), but it is also introduced with the purpose element at the beginning of the extract. The differences in contents are slight: in (25) extra ingredients have been introduced, and the difference in administration is merely an omission of the frequency of treatment.

Recipes may change involuntarily as well, as may be seen in the next selection of recipes. Examples (27) and (28) are commonsense recipes that one does not stop to decipher, whereas (29) is probably an edition of a corrupt copy:

(27)   for ache in a man is hyndis Take **an egge shil ful** of the **juce of betany** a nothir of wyne **a sponeful of hony 9 cornys of pepir** and stamp ham to gadir and lete him drink therof 3 daies and he schal a mendy (*Naples*, ed. Vallese 1940: 41)

(28)   For werkynge of lendys: Tak **a nege schelfull** of **jus of betane** & menge with **a sponfull of hony**, & grynd **ix pepir cornys**, & do þareto, & menge it with wyne. (*Daniel*, ed. Jasin 1983: 48)

(29)   ffor ach of lendis or of reynes Take **betayn** and stamp it and take **an ey shell** ther with and **a sponfull off hony** and grynd **ix pep~ cornes** and menge al thies in wyne & geue þe seke (*Leechbook II*, ed. Dawson 1934a: 36)

Table 6.9. Composita *with one corrupt copy*

Example	Order	Type	S/C	A	B	C	D	E	F
27 *Naples*	ABCDF	rec.	C	+	+	+	+	–	+
28 *Daniel*	ABCBCBC	rec.	C	+	++	+	–	–	–
29 *Leechbook II*	ABCBCBCBD	rec.	C	+	+++	+	+	–	–

For the legend, see Table 6.1.

The basic ordering of information is similar from recipe to recipe, save for the repetition of the pattern ingredients-procedure in (28) and (29). All the recipes are of the *receptaria* type, although in (28) the administration has been dropped (this is not uncommon, cf. section 6.3.4). The diagnostic sequence is *9 cornys of pepir*, and it confirms the parallelisms, as the rest are fairly common ingredients. Example (29) is the only recipe to have dropped ingredients (*an eggshellful of betony juice* has become *an eggshell*), but it is still recognisable as a member of the stemma. The dropped ingredients do not render (29) unintelligible; however, it does make the recipe sound rather strange. A possible reason for the change may be a scribal error; here, as the study is based on an edited text, it is the best assumption we can make.

The recipes which were sampled from other medical writing have shown us some characteristics of the medicine of the period, especially the extent to which remedybooks and *materia medica* texts are interrelated. Figure 6.2 illustrates the field of Middle English medical recipes in the light shed by the *MEMT* corpus, and the cues used in this study. Continuous lines indicate a closer relationship, i.e. identical or near identical recipes shared by the joined texts. Dashed lines indicate that the texts in question share only some elements in the parallel recipes, often it is an indication of a recipe/recipe paraphrase connection. The dash–dot lines are the only temporal indication in Figure 6.2: they mark a later text, Dawson 1934b, which is the only post-1475 recipe collection quoted in this study. Texts plotted in Figure 6.2 are almost exclusively *materia medica* texts, or recipe collections; the few treatises focusing on a special topic or of encyclopaedic character are the surgical treatises *Cyrurgie* (ed. Ogden 1971) and *Morstede* (ed. Beck 1974) (*The Cyrurgie of Guy de Chauliac* and *A Fair Book of Surgery* by Thomas Morstede), and *Epilepsy* (ed. Keiser 1994) and *Gilbertus* (ed. Getz 1991) (actually both extracts of Gilbertus Anglicus's pharmaceutical writings in a Middle English translation, and presented here for their link to the recipe collection *Liber de diversis medicinis*).[20] The surgical treatises link only to each other, at least with respect to recipes containing the cues chosen for this study; Morstede was probably familiar with Chauliac's writings. The network depicted here confirms the observations in the course of this chapter: in the Middle English period, *materia medica* texts and recipe collections formed an interrelated system of texts with close affiliations to each other. The network is not a rendering of the transmission lines, but intertextual evidence of the transmission that has taken place in the communities which used and produced the texts. The figure is based on the three keywords used in this study, therefore it is only a glimpse of the intertextual relations of the texts studied; a more concise picture could be attained with a larger keyword database.

A similar field of intertextuality has been noticed in Michael Benskin's study on an Irish manuscript (Dublin, Trinity Colleges MS 158). His list of parallel texts is (Benskin lists only published texts): *Medizinbuch* (ed. Heinrich 1896), *Medical works* (ed. Henslow 1899), *Burgundy* (ed. Schöffler 1919), *Leechbook II* (ed. Dawson 1934a), *Stockholm* (ed. Müller 1929), *Diversis medicinis* (ed. Ogden 1938), and *Macer Floridus* (ed. Frisk 1949) (Benskin 1997: 139–40). All the texts Benskin mentions are included in my study, and in Figure 6.2 (except *Macer Floridus*, as it is a herbal).

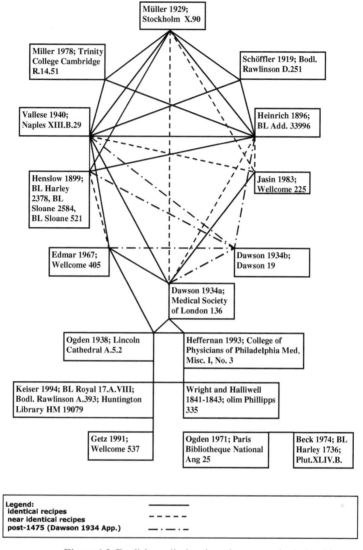

Figure 6.2 English medical recipes: intertextual relationships

6.5.4 Intertextuality – herbal recipes and recipes in herbals

Recipes that other medical writing shares with herbals are almost exclusively of the *receptaria* type, or pairs of *receptaria* recipes/recipe paraphrases. As was noted earlier in this chapter, simples are rarer in recipe collections, whereas they are very common in herbals. Examples (30–2) are from *MEMT*, and (33–4) from herbals, both of which are recipe paraphrases:

(30)　A gude drynke for **bane of þe hede broken**, secundum R. de O. Stamp **betoyne** wele & drynk þe jus þer-of & lay þe drafe appon þe wounde & it **sall brynge a-way þe broken banes & hele þe wond** (*Diversis medicinis*, ed. Ogden 1938: 76)

(31)　For **bonis þat buþ brokin in þe heued**. Nim **betayne** and drinke of þe jus and **þe bonis willun gon out and þe wounde wele hele** (*Leechbook I*, ed. Edmar 1967: 93)

(32)　Ether drynke **betayn** and **it will kest vp the bones** and hele the wounde (*Leechbook II*, ed. Dawson 1934a: 40)

(33)　If **it** [betony] be stamped and tha~ layde to a wounde in the heed that is smyten with a stroke / **it shall hele the wounde fayre** / and **drawe out the broken bones** yf there be ony as the leches do say. (*Herbal*, ed. Larkey and Pyles 1941: B i)

(34)　Also **it** [betony] **wyll drawe out brokyn bonys in a wounde** as summe auȝtoures seyn. (*Agnus castus*, ed. Brodin 1950: 133)

Table 6.10. *Simple recipes shared by herbals and other medical writing*

Example	Order	Type	S/C	A	B	C	D	E	F
30 *Diversis medicinis*	AFCBCDF	rec.	S	+	+	+	+	−	+
31 *Leechbook I*	ABDF	rec.	S	+	+	−	+	−	+
32 *Leechbook II*	ADBAF	rec.	S	+	+	−	+	−	+
33 *Herbal*	BCDAF	par.	S	+	+	+	++	−	+
34 *Agnus castus*	BAF	par.	S	+	+	−	−	−	+

For the legend, see Table 6.1.

The variation in the contents of these recipes concentrates on procedure, administration, and justification. As the examples are all simples, the places for variation have been narrowed down. The interesting feature is the ordering of information: almost all of the examples have a pattern of their own, and only one, (33), is an example expected of its genre, although even that pattern carries the rare justification in the end. Recipe collections and herbals do abide by their conventions: in recipe collection recipes the purpose comes at the beginning of the recipe (examples 30 to 32), whereas the recipes in herbals leave the purpose as the last or second to last element. The great variation in patterns may be due to the fact that the recipes are simples: including one ingredient in a recipe is syntactically more flexible than including multiple ingredients.

Composita are the prevalent type of the shared recipes. Examples (35) to (38) exemplify shared recipes in which the text is similar (but not identical), and the recipes both in herbals and other medical writing are for a similar (but not the same) purpose:

(35)   Also take the leues [of **rosemary**] and boyle them in **stronge Aysell** &
       bynde them in a clothe to thy **stomake** / & it shall delyuer þ~ of all euylles.
       (*Herbal*, ed. Larkey and Pyles 1941: H ii)

(36)   For swellyng of þe stomake. [. . .] Or ellis take **rosemary** and sede yt in
       strong esyll and ley it to þe **stomake**. (*Burgundy*, ed. Schöffler 1919:
       207–8)

(37)   Also his [**rosemary's**] lewys sothyn in **strong eysyl** or **vinegre** and bown-
       den in a lynene clout to þe **wombe** and to þe nowele it helyth þe wombe
       flyx (*Rosemary*, ed. Mäkinen 2002a: 317)

(38)   Also yf thou haue the flux boyle þ~ leues [of **rosemary**] in **stronge Aysell**
       & than bynde them in a lyne~ lothe and bynde it to thy **wombe** & anone
       the flux shal withdrawe. (*Herbal*, ed. Larkey and Pyles 1941: H ii)

Table 6.11. Composita *shared by herbals and other medical writing I*[21]

Example	Order	Type	S/C	A	B	C	D	E	F
35 *Herbal*	ABCBDA	rec.	C	+	+	+	+	−	−
36 *Burgundy*	ABCBD	rec.	C	+	+	+	+	−	−
37 *Rosemary*	BCBDA	par.	C	++	+	+	+	−	−
38 *Herbal*	ACBDAF	rec.	C	++	+	+	+	−	+

For the legend, see Table 6.1.

Despite the variation in the purpose column, all the recipes treat a stomach ailment. The differences can be seen in purpose and in additional data. Interestingly,
both examples from *Herbal*, (35) and (38) (paraphrases of the same recipe within
the same herbal entry), conform to the recipe collection pattern of organising the
information; only (37), an example from a herbal treatise, presents the default
pattern of a recipe in herbals.

There are also identical or almost identical shared *composita* recipes where the
purposes do not match (i.e. the ingredients and procedures are the same, but the
rubric/label/title/name is different):

(39)   whoso hathe the pose Take **rewe** and **comyn** and sethe them bothe in a
       panne with **hony** and **pepir** and ete a sponeful at morowe a nother at none
       and a nother at night (*Naples*, ed. Vallese 1940: 19)

(40)   Contra periculosam tussim. Take **sawge**, and **rewe**, &~ **comyn**, &~
       pouder of pepur, and medle hem to gedir in **hony**, &~ **make aletewa**
       rie, &~ vse þer of a sponful at euen, &~ anoþer at morowe. (*Medizinbuch*,
       ed. Heinrich 1896: 72)

(41) ffor the prlouse coughe a good medycyne. Take sawge, **rue** & **comyn** & **pouder pepper** beate them together & put them in **honey** & make a lettuarye & use a sponefull at even & an other in the morninge. (*Leechbook III*, ed. Dawson 1934b: 334)

(42) Also take **rewe** / **comyn** / and **Peper** / of yche lyke moche by weyght / & grynde them small togyder and medle them with **hony** and **vyneger**. And it it is good for the ache in the brest and in the reynes. (*Herbal*, ed. Larkey and Pyles 1941: H ii)

(43) Also take **rewe comyn** and **peper** off eyþer y-lyche moche and grynde them well to-gedyr. And medell with **hony** and **vynegar** and thys ys a presyous oyntment for ache yn þe breste and yn þe bowell and off þe raynes. (*Vertues*, ed. Grymonprez 1981: 73)

Table 6.12. Composita *shared by herbals and other medical writing II*

Example	Order	Type	S/C	A	B	C	D	E	F
39 *Naples*	ABCBD	rec.	C	+	+	+	+	–	–
40 *Medizinbuch*	ABCBCD	rec.	C	++	++	++	+	–	–
41 *Leechbook III*	ABCD	rec.	C	++	++	++	+	–	–
42 *Herbal*	BCBA	rec.	C	+++	+++	++	–	–	+
43 *Vertues*	BCBAD	rec.	C	+++	+++	++	++	–	+

For the legend, see Table 6.1.

Although the B column indicates differences in the ingredients, it is only a question of sage and vinegar added or omitted; the rest of the ingredients are the same. The information patterns correspond to the defaults at least concerning the position of the purpose sequence. It is noteworthy that the herbal text extracts are also recipes proper, and not recipe paraphrases.

The final group is a mixed bag of recipes or recipe paraphrases which share some elements, mainly ingredients, but differ from each other in many ways:

(44) Also **yf a man may not holde his meet** within hym / take þ~ same medycyne [**powder of betony and honey**] and gyue hym .iii. spo~full therof with a sponefull of water. (*Herbal*, ed. Larkey and Pyles 1941: B ii)

(45) Item **pulvis** [of betony] potatus post cenam juvat stomacum et **facit digestionem**. (*Vertues*, ed. Grymonprez 1981: 87)

(46) **Powdre of betayne** j dronke wiþ water is goud for **digestun** of blod and hit is goud for þe **cow3e** and **comfortiþ þe stommak** (*Leechbook I*, ed. Edmar 1967: 58)

(47)   Also ʒef a man may noʒt kepe hys mete with hym tak iiij dragmos of
poudre of betonye and medle it with hony and lat ben sothen a lytyl in
water and þanne make pelotys as grete as walnotis and ʒyf hym iij days
iche day on and do hym drynke ij sponfwl of lewk water and so he schal
ben holpyn (*Agnus castus*, ed. Brodin 1950: 134)

(48)   To make a man holde mete and drynk þat he takeþe. Take VII plantes
of Betoigne and boyle hem wele in hony til hit be somewhat thyk, and þan
make yt on smal pellettes, and drynke hit often in wyne, and þou schalte
be alle hole. (*Hoote somere*, ed. Miller 1978: 22)

(49)   Also for Coughe take þ~ ioyce or powder of Betyne and medle it with
hony / and make therof a lectuary / & vse it .ix. dayes and thou shalbe
hole. (*Herbal*, ed. Larkey and Pyles 1941: B ii)

(50)   Also ʒef þou hawe þe cowʒwe tak ij vnces of þe poudre of þis betonye
with a lytyl hony and sethe it in water and þanne vse it ix dayes and be þat
tyme þou schalt be hol (*Agnus castus*, ed. Brodin 1950: 134)

(51)   Betayne ysode wiþ honi is goud for þe dropeseye (*Leechbook I*, ed. Edmar
1967: 58)

(52)   ffor blode in yen this ys a poruede medecyne.
Jus of betoigne with hony ys gode,
To dryue away euell blode.
There with anoynte hem at morowe and eue,
It schall doo gode, hit may not greue,
ffor it ys trewe and prouebe ys
And cleres wele þe yen ywys. (*Hoote somere*, ed. Miller 1978: 2)

Table 6.13. *Partial recipe parallels in herbals and other medical writing*

Example	Order	Type	S/C	A	B	C	D	E	F
44 *Herbal*	AB[C]D	rec.	C	+	+	[+]	+	−	−
45 *Vertues*	C[B]CDA	par.	S	+	[++]	++	+	−	−
46 *Leechbook I*	CBDA	par.	S	+	++	+	+	−	−
47 *Agnus castus*	ABCBCDF	rec.	C	+	+	+++	++	−	+
48 *Hoote somere*	ABCBCDF	rec.	C	+	+	+++	++	−	+
49 *Herbal*	ACBCBCDF	rec.	C	++	+	++++	+++	−	+
50 *Agnus castus*	ABCBCDF	rec.	C	++	+	++++	+++	−	+
51 *Leechbook I*	BCBA	par.	C	+++	+	++++	−	−	−
52 *Hoote somere*	AFCBEDF	par.	C	++++	+	++++	++++	+	+

For the legend, see Table 6.1.

As already noted, these recipes are governed by the ingredients, with the variation of adding or omitting 'honey'. As a result, this selection of recipes has both simples and *composita*. The sources of the extracts are herbals or recipe collections only, and the type of recipes is *receptaria*, or recipe paraphrases. The purposes vary from 'digestion' to 'cough', 'eyes' and 'dropsy', but although the recipes are here presented as separate entities, some of them are parts of longer entries. Thus (44), for digestion, is the latter part of an entry for betony started by (49), for cough. Also in *Agnus castus*, (47) and (50) are recipes for digestion and cough respectively, from the same entry. In *Leechbook I*, (46) and (51), recipes for digestion and dropsy, are also from the same entry. Consequently, we may note that again most variation takes place in procedure and administration.

The ordering of information is mostly that of recipe collection recipes, even in recipes in herbals. Only (45) from *Vertues* presents the default position of purpose for recipes in herbals. This phenomenon seems to be a pattern in the intertextual links between herbals and recipe collections: the recipes in herbals with recipe collection parallels are more often ordered according to the recipe collection pattern than according to the recipe paraphrase pattern. *Leechbook I* in London, Wellcome Library (MS 405, see Plate 5a (p. 192) for the manuscript page; example 51 starts on line 1, and example 46 on line 7) stands out as an anomaly by using the herbal order of information, but then the extracts are very much like a herbal entry: the medical properties of the plant are listed using participial adjectives, recipes proper starting first in the second folio of the opening. In example (52) the verse form may be the cause of the extraordinary information pattern. In examples (45) and (46), we find the regular herbal pattern preceded by procedure: this is due to the word 'powder', which requires some kind of processing of the ingredient, thus it may be read as an indication of a procedure. Again, many of the recipes present a pattern in which ingredients alternate with procedure; cf. the discussion of Table 6.2 earlier in this chapter.

6.6   Conclusion

The medical recipes of the Middle English period have a common source, the *materia medica* literature of antiquity. The few original texts and the nature of medieval book production brought about a closely interrelated textual field in the Middle Ages. For this reason the intertextuality of recipes may be studied by the aid of computerised material which is based on the edited medical texts.

With regard to the scope of the corpora and cues used in this study, both the herbal recipes in Middle English medical texts and the recipes in Middle English herbals seem to have several interconnecting links, but still embody traditions of their own and meet only tangentially here and there. The intertextual links are almost solely between herbals and remedybooks or recipe collections, keeping specialised treatises and surgical texts separate. The reason is clear: the *materia medica* literature in the Middle Ages was dominated by the works of Dioscorides and Pliny, who drew on the same sources, whereas treatises on surgery or on focused topics seldom presented the material of all-purpose recipe reference books. As a result, most of the data gathered are *receptaria* recipes, and therefore also *composita*, due to the recipe collections which form the main body of the remedybooks and the *materia medica* part of *MEMT*.

The recipes in common with the two textual traditions of herbals and other medical writing often conform to the remedybook pattern of organising information. Recipe paraphrases in herbals do occur as intertextual pairs to the recipe collection recipes, but they are in the minority. The conceivable reasons for this are two: firstly, it is the herbal end of an intertextual link which adapts to the recipe collections, or the direction of borrowing recipes is usually from recipe collections to herbals.[22] Secondly, the recipe paraphrase type is so much more difficult to detect from among the material that it affects the outcome of the study. There are also cases where it seems that textual material has been borrowed from herbals to recipe collections, but they are rare. Therefore it can be assumed (acknowledging the restrictions of this study) that the customary direction of borrowing recipe material was from other medical writing to herbals, and material was borrowed almost solely from recipe collections and *materia medica* literature.[23]

Notes

1. For example, Dioscorides' *De materia medica* has been reorganised and recompiled many times over: the original organisation of animal, herbal, and mineral ingredients according to the humoral theory has often been rearranged, even to the extent of producing separate bestiaries, herbals, and lapidaries based on the information in *De materia medica*.

2. The current size of the herbal corpus is 100,000 words. At the moment the Middle English part consists of six texts (*c*. 60,000 words): I have chosen previously edited Middle English texts as the material of the corpus, and the six texts included form a representative sample of the accessible material. In addition to these texts, I have included in this study an Early Modern English text, Bancke's *Herbal* printed in 1525 (ed. Larkey and Pyles 1941), as it is mainly a compilation of the antecedent medieval manuscript herbals, and thus a valuable piece of evidence for the transmission of the medieval herbal texts beyond the period of my study. Texts still to be added to the Middle English part of the corpus include *synonyma* (lists of plant names in various languages) and herbalistic sections of medical treatises. For *MEMT*, see Pahta and Taavitsainen, p. 7 in this volume. In addition to the texts in *MEMT*, I have included three medical texts in this study, edited by Müller (1929b), Vallese (1940), Miller (1978) and Dawson (1934b). Müller, Vallese and Miller are fifteenth-century recipe collections, and Dawson is a sixteenth-century commonplace book of remedies.

3. *Corpus Presenter* is a Windows compatible application suite designed and written by Prof. Raymond Hickey for various kinds of text, corpus and database processing that a corpus user might need. A description of the earlier version of *Corpus Presenter* can be found in Hickey (2000). See also Hickey (2003).

4. By covert instruction I mean the use of the passive voice in order to convey instruction for procedures, etc., thus covert instruction may not formally be distinguished as instruction.

5. The vernacular language of the learned texts would suggest another kind of audience, but already the topics seem to presuppose a learned audience.

6. The kind of *materia medica* text that Dioscorides wrote and compiled was intended for a medical practitioner who knew the classification system based on the humoral theory by heart. The indexing system led one to the knowledge of a medical substance by its properties, not by its initial. Thus, knowing the cause of the illness, it was possible to find effective substances to treat it just by knowing the required properties of the substance; the name of the substance may well have been unknown to the medical practitioner. Herbals, which are renderings of *materia medica* focused on plants, were often transformed from the humoral order to the alphabetical order. This was also common for full copies or compilations of *materia medica*. Recipe paraphrases in herbals grew to quite extensive lists of remedies and medicines, their purpose being still the same; it must be noted here that recipes proper still occur in herbals, i.e. their primary purpose is not annulled by recipe paraphrases. Thus herbals reflect the blending of genres, using the instructive mode familiar to us from learned tracts, as well as practical handbook devices, such as alphabetised ordering of plants, in order to facilitate the everyday use of the text.

7. Pliny and Dioscorides have both borrowed 106 almost identical passages from Sextius Niger (Arber 1986: xxv–vi).

8. Figure 6.1 and sections 6.4.2–6.4.4 are based on Singer (1927), Brodin (1950), Morton (1981), de Vriend (1984), Arber (1986), Cameron (1993), Burnett and Jacquart (1994), Collins (2000), and Pollington (2000).

9. The manuscripts are London, British Library, Harley MS 55; British Library, Harley MS 585; British Library, Harley MS 6258B; British Library, Royal MS 12.D.17; British Library, Additional MS 43703; British Library, Cotton Faustina MS A.X; British Library, Cotton Domitian MS A.I; British Library, Cotton Vitellius MS C.III; British Library, Cotton Galba MS A.XIV; British Library, Cotton Otho MS B.XI; Oxford, Bodleian Library, Hatton MS 76; Cambridge, Corpus Christi College MS 41, and Louvain, Bibliothèque Centrale de l'Université, Fragmenta H. Omont 3 (*eVK*).

10. There are three Old English texts that can be regarded as herbals proper: *Liber de herba vettonica* (often falsely attributed to Antonius Musa, Pliny the Elder's contemporary), *Herbarium Apuleii*, and Pseudo-Dioscorides' *Liber medicinae ex herbis femininis*. These three texts are extant in four manuscripts (London, British Library, Harley MS 585; British Library, Harley MS 6258B; British Library, Royal MS 12.D.17; Oxford, Bodleian Library, Hatton MS 76), and together they form a text which is called the *Old English Herbarium* (de Vriend 1984: lv–lx). Although the *Nine Herbs Charm* in *Lacnunga* and the *Healing Powers of Mulberry* in *Medicina de quadrupedibus* both relate to the medicinal properties of plants, they are not herbal entries as such, but

more like incomplete parts of herbal entries or lists of recipes (cf. de Vriend 1984: 238–41; Pollington 2000: 214–15).

11. Despite the ascription of *Liber de herba vettonica* and *Herbarium Apuleii* to Antonius Musa and Lucius Apuleius of Madaura respectively, the Latin originals seem to be somewhat later in origin, from the fourth century AD (Singer presents a differing view on the origin of *Herbarium Apuleii* (1927: 37)). They are both closely related to Pliny's *Historia naturalis. Liber medicinae ex herbis femininis*, the third herbal translated into Old English (probably composed before the sixth century AD), draws on Dioscorides' and Galen's works, although it has some original textual material (de Vriend 1984: lvi–lx). The textual material in the Old English herbal lore may also partly be of native origin (Rohde 1922/1971: 12; Frisk 1949: 13; Pollington 2000: 74).

12. I have not commented on the text of *Peri didaxeon* in London, British Library Harley MS 6258B (from *c.* 1200), partly because it does not include a herbal or parts of one, and partly because its language divides scholars: it has been identified both as an Old English and a Middle English text (cf. Löweneck 1896; Cameron 1993: 64).

13. In recipes in herbals, the purpose indicating element may also function as an efficacy phrase (additional data), especially when a promise of the effect is included in the element (cf. example 5, *yf there be ony wormes therin it shall slee them*). I have often analysed the elements with a possible dual function as 'purpose' alone, as according to Stannard (1982: 70–3) the element including efficacy phrases is incidental or additional data, and therefore a recipe is complete without it, whereas an element with the functions of both 'purpose' and 'additional data' cannot be left out.

14. Here *colys* is also an indicator of the procedure.

15. Medieval recipe collections are usually not alphabetised, but organised according to some other principle, such as the kinds of medicine, body parts, or maladies.

16. Both texts are from Stockholm, Royal Library X.90 (*Rosemary* pp. 80–86; *Agnus castus* pp. 156–216), and they are written in the same hand (Mäkinen 2002a: 309; *LALME* 3: 361).

17. I have found yet another parallel for this recipe, in John Lelamour's Macer (London, British Library Sloane MS 5) (as quoted in the electronic *MED*, s.v. *soppe*): 'Take þe levis of that erbe wiþ wyne and water and make þere in soppis of brede and ete þe soppis and þou shalt haue gode appetide to þi mete'.

18. I have found a fourth, probable parallel for this recipe, an incipit in *eVK* (the modern English version by the authors): 'Take and make him a bath of vervain or of betony or of wormwood and therewith wash the head' (San Marino, Huntington HM 64, ff. 114–20). This manuscript has also been discussed in this volume by Jones.

19. Example (26) is connected with Henry Daniel's *Liber uricrisiarum*, and is a list of recipes for ailments. The recipes have been included in the remedybook category in *MEMT*, although the rest of the text is a treatise on a specialised subject.

20. Gilbertus has features of both an encyclopaedia, and a recipe collection. The part of the text in *MEMT* is mostly recipes.

21. *Also* in the beginning of a recipe or a recipe paraphrase may be used as an indicator of a new item in a list, as here in example (35). However, this is not

always the case, and for this reason not all the cases of *Also* have been analysed as indicators of purpose.

22. Recipes in herbals often exemplify the medical properties of the plant in question, and therefore they are only secondarily meant for preparing medicines, and thus often presented as recipe paraphrases (Mäkinen 2002c: 283).

23. This study will be pursued further in my forthcoming dissertation.

7   Middle English recipes: Vernacularisation of a text-type[1]

RUTH CARROLL

7.1   Introduction

The process of vernacularisation involves several tasks. Language variation gains a new dimension (see Taavitsainen 'House-styles' in this volume) and the vocabulary stock is increased (see Norri in this volume). In addition, vernacular text-types are established: norms are developed for the creation and reception of texts. This chapter addresses the formulation of the recipe text-type in Middle English after the Anglo-Saxon scientific prose tradition had been severed by the Norman Conquest.

As will be illustrated below, the recipe text-type can be seen to have varied from one medieval European vernacular to another. It is also the case that the Middle English recipe differs noticeably from its Modern English counterpart. Clearly, the process of vernacularisation of English recipes involved the gradual evolution of norms for recipe writing. Over time, conventions were established with regard to the linguistic characteristics of recipes, the range of functions they served, and their contextualisation within manuscripts or even within other texts. However, these conventions, like most discoursal norms, represented prototypicality, and were not always strictly adhered to.

In order to demonstrate different ways in which recipes were vernacularised, this chapter focuses in particular on two texts containing recipes, *Diuersa cibaria* (ed. Hieatt and Butler 1985) and *Horse Leechynge* (ed. Svinhufvud 1978), both of which were translated or adapted into English. The chapter also draws on evidence from other roughly contemporary recipe collections, in order to convey the range of variation found within what might now be called the Middle English recipe genre or text-type. Rather than limiting the study to recipes for human medicine, this chapter tests the borders of the genre by including in its consideration a wide range of recipes. The two texts studied here in most detail, however, both belong to the broad field of medicine. *Horse Leechynge* is a veterinary text and *Diuersa cibaria* a collection of culinary recipes (food and drink comprised one of the six categories of non-naturals in the humoral understanding of factors influencing health and sickness).[2]

7.2 The Old English background

As noted by Pahta and Taavitsainen (p. 9 above), the process of vernacularisation began in England earlier than in other European nations, and this was true of medical recipes and other scientific writing as well as of religious texts and poetry, for example. Non-vernacular medicinal recipes and other texts were available in England before the mid-eighth century (Cameron 1983b). The earliest extant manuscripts containing vernacular recipes date from the early tenth century, but some of these show evidence of much earlier composition.

Commonly referred to by the name of the man who is said to have commissioned the work, *Bald's Leechbook* (ed. Wright 1955) claims to have been written by Cild and has been dated to the early tenth century.[3] Although much of the text has been shown to draw on classical sources, no sources have been identified for most of the recipes. Some are ascribed by the text itself to natives Oxa and Dun. The recipes comprising the third book are now considered a separate text, being 'quite different from the other two books in tone and intent' (Cameron 1983b: 147).[4]

The *Lacnunga* (ed. Grattan and Singer 1952; ed. Pettit 2001) includes two hundred recipes and charms, and is extant in a manuscript which has been dated to 1050. Grattan and Singer's title, *Anglo-Saxon Magic . . . Illustrated Specially from the Semi-pagan Text* Lacnunga, indicates the extent to which modern readers find this text superstitious and non-scientific; we must heed Liuzza's warning against anachronistic distinctions between ' "popular" ways of thinking, writing and acting and the ways of "high" or "élite" culture' (2001: 182–3, 211).

The Old English *Medicina de quadrupedibus* (ed. de Vriend 1984), as extant, is a tenth-century text, but appears to be based on an earlier, perhaps eighth-century, Anglian exemplar. The Old English *Herbarium*, perhaps translated (or adapted) from Latin as early as the eighth century, is extant in four manuscripts with the *Medicina de quadrupedibus*. Although it is understood to be based on classical sources, not all have been identified (de Vriend 1984: xli–xliii). As with later herbals, the *Herbarium* is organised by herb, listing treatments which use each herb. Both texts contain some passages serving a recipe-like function, some in the imperative, some using the past participle (the use of verb forms in Middle English is discussed below):

(1) *Wið eagena sár genim þære ylcan wyrte wyrttruman, seoð on wætere to þriddan dæle; 7 of þam wætere beþa þa [eagan];* . . .
[For pain in the eyes, take the same plant root. Boil in water, reducing to a third, and bathe the eyes . . .] (*Herbarium*, ed. de Vriend, 1984: 30)

(2) *Wið scurfum rammes smeoru, 7 meng ðærto sot 7 sealt 7 sand, 7 hyt wulla onweg; 7 æfter smyre, hyt byðeft liðre. IX. 1. Wið ælc sar bares brægen gesoden 7 to drence [geworht] on wine, ealle sár hyt geliðegaþ.*
[For scurf [a scaly skin condition], ram's fat; mix therewith soot, salt and sand. Use wool to wipe it away, and then rub. Afterwards it will be smooth.

IX. 1. For every sore, boar's brain, boiled and prepared in wine to drink. It relieves all sores.] (*Medicina de quadrupedibus*, ed. de Vriend, 1984: 260)

The Anglo-Saxon development of scientific prose in the vernacular, in Voigts's words, 'came to naught, however, with the Norman Conquest of 1066' (1995b: 184). When recipes again began to be written in the vernacular in England following the Conquest, it was initially in the Anglo-Norman vernacular. There are over 80 twelfth-century Anglo-Norman medicinal recipes extant, 40 in London, British Library, Royal MS 8.D.v, and some 33 others in British Library, Royal MS 5.E.vi, in addition to more isolated examples of marginal recipes (Hunt 1990: 64–6). The earliest extant culinary recipes from England are found in two Anglo-Norman collections, both of 'which can be assumed to include recipes of thirteenth-century origin' (Hieatt and Butler 1985: 7), described below.

7.3   Middle English recipes

7.3.1   The breadth of the tradition

Anglo-Norman recipes are found translated into Middle English from the early fourteenth century (see below). At least three other fourteenth-century Middle English culinary recipe collections (presumed to have been primarily composed in English) survive, the earliest extant manuscript dated to *c.* 1381 (Oxford, Bodleian Library, Douce MS 257; Keiser 1998: 3888). However, culinary recipes in English were still considered a novelty in the fourteenth century (Hieatt and Butler 1985: 18). Middle English medicinal recipes also appear from the fourteenth century: Voigts and Kurtz's index (*eVK*) contains no recipes from the thirteenth century, but 85 collections from the fourteenth century.

Recipes fall into at least two categories or traditions: those found in remedybooks and those found in scientific treatises (Taavitsainen 2001c; Voigts 1984; they may also be found outside collections, for example in manuscript margins). Remedybooks are not always considered to be science proper. Voigts, for example, appears inclined to dismiss remedybooks when she notes that 'no codices containing science or medicine in Middle English *other than remedy-books* appear to have been written before 1375' (1989b: 352, emphasis added) and therefore restricts her study to the period after that date. Yet remedybooks are important for the study of vernacularisation, since they appear in English earlier than scientific treatises do (cf. Taavitsainen and Pahta 1997: 212). Also, as Taavitsainen (2001c) has noted, remedybook recipes are more standardised as a text-type than those appearing in academic texts.

The present discussion focuses in particular on two texts, neither composed originally in English, and each representing one tradition. *Diuersa cibaria* contains translations from both the collections of Anglo-Norman culinary recipes mentioned above, as well as of other Anglo-Norman recipes no longer extant in the original. The collection is found in London, British Library, Additional

MS 46919, dated to the first quarter of the fourteenth century, and the fifteenth-century London, British Library, Cotton Julius MS D.viii. A few of the recipes are also found in other manuscripts (see Hieatt and Butler 1985: 43–4). As this is a straightforward collection of short-recipe texts, with no intervening prose and not attributed to any authoritative source, it may be considered representative of the remedybook tradition. The recipes are primarily culinary rather than exclusively medicinal, but as I pointed out earlier, this distinction is not as strict for medieval collections (see also Carroll 1999: 37–8). *Diuersa cibaria* is a fascinating collection of translated recipes because so many of the source texts have been identified.

Horse Leechynge, a veterinary text rather than a treatise on human medicine, represents the scholarly tradition. The text relies on authoritative sources (*olde wise clerckus*, p. 85), although they are not named (*sum men*, p. 143), and it was adapted from the *Practica equorum* of Theodoric, Bishop of Cervia (1206–98; pp. 13–15). The bulk of the text is made up of instruction in caring for a horse, describing ailments a horse may suffer, and explaining how they may be prevented or cured. Recipes are found embedded within the paragraphs detailing cures for the various diseases. The text is found in London, British Library, Sloane MS 2584; no other manuscript exemplars were discovered by Svinhufvud, or listed in *eVK*. Doyle said of the hand that he was 'inclined to think that it must be of the first half of the fifteenth century, although it could be late in the fourteenth' (quoted by Svinhufvud 1978: 26); the *MED* dates the text *c.*1450.

Using veterinary and culinary recipes calls attention to the breadth of subject matter covered by medieval recipes. Their use extends beyond the register of human medicine to other fields of practical instruction. For example, another of the relatively early Middle English recipe collections (London, British Library, Harley MS 2253, dated by the *MED* to *c.*1325) contains recipes for dyes (Keller 1971). Extant Middle English instructional texts also include recipes for laces,[5] alchemical recipes (Grund 2000), and recipes for gunpowder (Braswell 1984: 345); Voigts and Kurtz list 28 subcategories of recipe in their subject index, including recipes for soap, artificial jewels, and glue (*eVK*). That these texts may all be called 'recipes' by Modern English researchers calls attention to their similarities in form and function:

(3)   Culinary recipe from the *Forme of Cury*:[6]
      For to make drawen benes. Take benes and seeþ hem, and grynde hem in
      a morter, and drawe hem vp with gode broth; & do oynouns in the broth
      grete mynced, & do þerto; and colour it with safroun, and serue it forth.
      (ed. Hieatt and Butler 1985: 98)

(4)   Medicinal recipe:
      Pro male videntibus uel oculos rubeos habentibus. [t]ake white gyngire,
      and robbe hit on a whestoon in a fayre bacin of metal, and take as mykel
      salt, as þow hast pouder, and grynd hem wel to gedur in þe bacin, and
      tempre hem wyþ white wyn, and let hit stonde a day and a ny3t, & þenne

take þe þynne, þat stondes aboue, & do hit in to a viol of glas, and when þe
seke goos to bedde, take a feþer, and wete þer ynne, & anoynt wel þe sore
eyen þer wyþ, & he shal be hool. (ed. Heinrich 1896: 68)

(5)   Recipe for dye:
Vor te make Cynople. Tac brasyl ant seoþ in dichwatur to þe halfendel
oþer to þe þridde partie. and seþþe tac a ston of chalk ant mak an hole i
þe chalk. as deop ant as much. as þu wenest þat þi watur wol gon in. ant
held it þer-in. ant seþþe anon riht quic-liche. tak a bord oþer a ston. ant
keouer hit þat non eyr ne passe out. ant let hit stonde vor te hit beo colt.
(ed. Keller 1971: 96)

(6)   Veterinary recipe (for the care of hawks):
For the dry Frounce. Take the rote of Polypody that groweth on okis and
seth hem a grete while; then take it fro the fire and lete cole in to mylke
warme, then wash your flesch ther in and feede your hauke iij tymes, and
withoute doute he schalle be hole. (ed. Swaen 1943: 10)

(7)   Recipe for lace:
FOR to make a lace endented: Take iij bowys of o colour and set on A [first
finger] and C [third finger] of þe lyft h(ond) and also B [second finger] of
þe ryȝt hond, and ij bowys of anoþer colour, and set on B of þe lyfte hond
& C of þe ryȝth hond, and wirke in þe maner of þe round lace of v bowes.
(ed. Stanley 1974: 96)

However, given that text-types vary geographically and historically, care must be
taken not to over-impose a researcher's own cultural or linguistic expectations on
historical texts. It is helpful to use Diller's (2001) distinction between producers'
genres/text-types and those perceived by the recipient, and extend it so as to
distinguish between medieval English genres/text-types and those perceived by
scholars or other readers of medieval texts today.

7.3.2 Characteristics

7.3.2.1 Form. The formal characteristics of a recipe are what define it as a 'text-
type', while a recipe's function (analysed below) determines its 'genre'.[7] Analyses
of text-types drawn with very broad brush-strokes, such as that of Werlich for
English, identify linguistic characteristics common to many different kinds of
instruction, including the use of commands or requests, first- or second-person
point of view, topical coherence, topic-giving introductions, and the text being
structured either analytically or like a list (Werlich 1976: 122–5). It is in this
regard that Görlach (1992) is able to sketch out a diachronic study of the English
recipe, considering texts from the Old English period as variants of the same text-
type as is found in present-day English. A finer-grained study, however, such as
that of Sánchez-Roura (2001), shows the Middle English recipe text-type to be
significantly different from that of Modern English.

The Middle English recipe could be comprised of four parts: the heading, ingredients, procedure, and application. Of these, only the procedure was obligatory (Stannard 1982). The Middle English recipe in example (8) below is vague with regard to which herbs were required as ingredients (as well as what quantity was to be used (see Carroll 1999: 32–3; Taavitsainen 2001c: 103)). Like many Middle English recipes, it does not separate the ingredients section from the procedure. It is the procedure which comprises the largest part of the text:

(8)   Frytour of erbes. Take gode erbys; grynde hem and medle hem with flour and water, & a lytel ȝest, and salt, and frye hem in oyle. And ete hem with clere hony. (ed. Hieatt and Butler 1985: 132)

Hunt's analysis of Anglo-Norman recipes (1990) identifies six components, all optional. His *rubric* and *indication* together correspond to Stannard's *heading*, and he adds the *efficacy statement*. His survey thus encompasses recipes varying in length from three words to 'whole pages of manuscript' (1990: 17). The Anglo-Norman recipes of London, British Library, Royal MS 12.C.xii consist largely of lists of ingredients (example 9). Their Middle English translations (example 10) follow the originals so closely that some omit the procedure component, thus failing to adhere to the expected Middle English pattern.

(9)   Dragonee. Let d'alemaunz, flur de rys, braon de chapoun, sucre, canel; colour, vermail de sang dragon. (ed. Hieatt and Jones 1986: 867)

(10)   Dragone. Milke of alemauns, flour of rys, braun of chapoun, sucre & kanele; þe colour red of sanc dragoun. (ed. Hieatt and Butler 1985: 47)

This might be analysed in one of three ways: either as an overly slavish translation, an indication that the Middle English recipe text-type norms had not yet been established by the early fourteenth century, or that the Middle English recipe text-type shows prototypicality effects. The translator is not so slavish as to always translate word for word. He feels free to add words in his translation of *Diacre*, translating *losenges plaunté desuis; colour, vermail* (ed. Hieatt and Jones 1986: 867) into Middle English *losenges ystreyed abouen; þe colour red ase blod* (ed. Hieatt and Butler 1985: 47). The striking similarities found when comparing the linguistic characteristics of various medieval English texts for practical instruction (as in examples 3–7 above) illustrate the diffusion and acceptance of norms for recipes.

This leaves the third possibility, that of prototype effects, as the most likely explanation for the divergent recipe form. All text-types, including recipes, can be somewhat inconsistent in terms of linguistic characteristics, and it is indeed helpful to think in terms of prototypes and fuzzy boundaries. Linguistic characteristics of text-types can be said to be tendencies; in the words of Eggins and Martin (1997), they are 'probabilistic' rather than 'deterministic'.

Prototypically, then, Middle English recipes were based upon short, paratactic, imperative clauses (Carroll 1999). To the English reader this may seem obvious, since Modern English recipes are also based upon imperative clauses. However, recipes, like all text-types, may vary from one speech community to another, geographically and across time, and with regard to its heavy use of the imperative the Middle English text-type differs from other medieval vernacular recipe text-types, such as the Catalan and the Spanish. Medieval Catalan recipes include future tense (example 11) and indicative mood (12) in addition to imperatives (13–14).

(11)   E aprés doneràs piment
        [And afterwards you will add pepper] (ed. Grewe 1979: 198)

(12)   Primerament posats lo pex al ffoch
        [First you put the fish to the fire] (ed. Grewe 1979: 211)

(13)   e suffrigex-ho un poc per la seba
        [and sauté it a little for the onion] (ed. Grewe 1979: 119)

(14)   leva-lla del ffoc
        [carry it from the fire] (ed. Grewe 1979: 137)

In comparison, Middle English recipes do not make use of the second-person indicative or the future in this way. Alonso Almeida (2002) has demonstrated in a comparative study of medieval English and Spanish medicinal recipes that Spanish uses the infinitive form (with an imperative function), while English is more reliant on imperative forms.

Although the recipes translated from MS Royal 12.C.xii rely heavily upon past participial forms, as in example (15), the more prototypical Middle English recipes are overwhelmingly imperative.

(15)   þin angeylles ifried & þe lyuere iholden, & þe gobouns ipoudred in poudre
        of kanele (ed. Hieatt and Butler 1985: 47)

In another Anglo-Norman recipe group, that translated from London, British Library, Additional MS 32085, the imperative is used almost seven times as often as any other verb form (116 tokens as compared with sixteen instances of the indicative present):

(16)   Nym clanlyche frissiaus & soþþen grind in an morter, & soþþen nim
        milke . . . & tempre wyþ ius of frissiaus; & soþþen do a lute bred of wastel,
        & lye wel . . . (ed. Hieatt and Butler 1985: 50)

The use of imperatives rather than modal verbs has been shown to be one distinguishing characteristic of recipes as opposed to herbals (Carroll 1999; Mäkinen 2002c; see also Mäkinen's chapter in this volume). Herbals are also distinguishable from recipe collections by their discourse organisation, and this distinction represents one of the boundaries of the recipe text-type.

By the fifteenth century, the prototypical short imperative phrases of the recipe text-type were well known enough to be evoked in the song of the fiends of hell in Mirk's *Festial*:

(17) Sle, sle, sle, sle, sle, sle, open þe broche, rost hote, cast ynto þe cawdren, sethe fast yn pyche, and cood, and brymston, and hot leed! (ed. Erbe 1905: 5)[8]

The Middle English use of the imperative is particularly visible in what Taavitsainen has called the 'conventional formula' of using the imperative *take* to begin instruction (2001c: 95), as evidenced from examples (3–7) cited above. To open a recipe with *take*, however, is not a requirement.

Recipes can begin with synonyms such as *accipe, nim* or *recipe* (examples 18–19) or with something quite different (20–2):

(18) Mortrellus blanc. **Nym** pyggus and hennys & oþer maner fresch flesch . . . (ed. Hieatt and Butler 1985: 71)

(19) For an hors yat has a sore bak. **Recipe** honbolok, and stampe hem . . . (ed. Braekman 1986d: 101)

(20) For to make blomanger, **do** ris in water . . . (ed. Hieatt and Butler 1985: 68)

(21) A tenche in syuee. **Scalde** þy tenche . . . (ed. Hieatt and Butler 1985: 84)

(22) For ye malaunder. **Rost** paryngges of chese . . . (ed. Braekman 1986d: 103)

The *Diuersa cibaria* translations of MS Additional 32085 consistently use *nim*, translating *pernez*. Each recipe begins with imperative *nim* except the last, which begins with *make* (*festes* in the original), having *nim* as the second imperative verb in the text (ed. Hieatt and Butler 1985: 53).

Examples (18–22) also serve to show the range of forms available for the Middle English recipe's heading. Most commonly, the heading consists either of a noun phrase or a *to*-infinitive, with or without *for*. It was unprototypical for a recipe to lack a heading, but this does occur in the academic treatise, where the surrounding text serves the function of introducing the recipe and indicating what it is for:

(23) And when it is drie þen schalt þou grece it with an oynement þat is ymade on þis manere. (ed. Svinhufvud 1978: 105)

The headings, particularly those naming the final product, are the one component of the text-type frequently left untranslated. This is one notable distinction between recipes and charms, which are more lexically fixed. Since the power of a charm is in its words, the words should remain as they are given; thus charms may be seen to feature code-switching as an 'essential feature' (Taavitsainen 2001c: 92; see also Pahta pp. 88–9 above). The distinction between charms and recipes defines another of the boundaries of the recipe text-type. Although Hunt, for example, includes charms within his first category of 'therapeutic' receipts, he is nonetheless able to distinguish them from recipes, as evidenced by his separate treatment of them (1990: 78–99).

Of Werlich's list of general characteristics of instruction, the use of commands has been shown to be effected in the Middle English recipes prototypically by the use of the imperative, and topic-giving introductions in the form of the headings beginning most recipes. The headings also serve to emphasise topical coherence, something easily achieved in texts so short. The longest recipe in Hieatt and Butler's collection is 462 words long (*To mak anneys in counfyte*, from Harley 2378), but such length is very unusual except perhaps in alchemical texts; Grund (personal communication) has noted that alchemical recipes may be extremely long, even embedded one within another. Much more common are recipes ranging in length from 40 to 120 words, and some are even shorter.

Other linguistic characteristics include the use of possessive pronouns, which illustrate the first- or second-person point of view expected of instruction, and the structuring of the texts by means of temporally ordered clauses, sometimes lexically reinforced. The latter is seen clearly both in the recipes translated from MS Additional 32085 and their sources (24–25) as well as in *Horse Leechynge* (26):

(24)   e pus metez ses mosseus en cel bro; e pus le dressez e metez des bons especes
[and then put these pieces in that broth; and then serve it and add good spices] (ed. Hieatt and Jones 1986: 865)

(25)   & soþþen do mossels in þilke broþ, & soþþen dresse & do god poudre of speces (ed. Hieatt and Butler 1985: 52)

(26)   And þen aftur þou make a plaster of auence & of þe rote of radische of boþe I-liche muche. & a litel swope. & as muche hony. & grynde hem al to-geder & þen þou schalte schaue þe heere . . . (ed. Svinhufvud 1978: 93–5).

By highlighting the addressee, Staczek has argued, possessive pronouns make the recipe more personalised, creating social involvement (1996: 246). Although noun phrase determiners in the recipes are articles even more commonly than possessive pronouns (Carroll 1999, Grund 2000, and Taavitsainen 2001c provide more detail), it is noteworthy that they tend not to be elided as they are in modern English written recipes. The relatively conservative *Diuersa cibaria* translation of the Anglo-Norman recipe *Soree* follows the emerging Middle English tendency to allow possessive pronouns, adding *þin* to the text (27) which is not found in the Anglo-Norman original of this recipe (28),[9] although possessive pronouns are found elsewhere in Anglo-Norman recipes; for example *vostre past* (ed. Hieatt and Jones 1986: 865) is translated *þi past* (ed. Hieatt and Butler 1985: 53).

(27)   & oþur maner vihs; þin angeylles ifried (ed. Hieatt and Butler 1985: 47)

(28) e autre manere de pesshoun; anguilles fris
      [and other kinds of fish; fresh eels] (ed. Hieatt and Jones 1986: 867)

This feature was less common in medical recipes from the academic tradition than in remedybooks (Taavitsainen 2001c: 100–1). *Horse Leechynge*, as expected, contains possessive pronouns more rarely than definite or indefinite articles, but when they do appear they may occur side by side with the articles:

(29) And mylte þi pylk & do þe poudur of þe oþer forsaide þer-to (ed. Svinhufvud 1978: 131)

(30) when þe capytel is made ... ȝif it synk not þi capytel is good (ed. Svinhufvud 1978: 106)

7.3.2.2 Discourse location. The layout of the text, the placement of recipes within a larger context, is also an important feature of the form of the text-type. Görlach has also noted that recipes can join with other texts (including other recipes) to form larger 'conglomerate' or 'composite' texts (1991: 202). Note, however, that recipes need not be inserted into a larger text in any cohesive way, or indeed in such a way as to be treated as part of the whole. Marginal, or in other ways isolated, recipes abound. Oxford, Bodleian Library, Digby MS 29, for example, contains a single recipe for glue on folio 113v, followed by a uroscopy text (*eVK*). The most common composite text-types containing recipes, as said above, fall into two categories: the remedybook and the learned academic medicinal treatise. In the academic tradition, Taavitsainen notes that recipes may be 'inserted in the middle of the running text, without any indication of the switch' (2001c: 95).

Horse Leechynge, like other more academic scientific treatises, includes instructive passages amongst expository ones (cf. Taavitsainen and Pahta 1995: 522):

(31) Swellynge of þe side aftur prykynge of þe spore wol come when þat cold watur is entred with-ynne þe prikynge of þe spore. & it is with-ynne þe skyn. And nameliche if þe hors stonde too daius with-oute trauaile. or swetynge. ȝif it so bi-falle þen schalt þou take walwort & louache & calamynte & wermod or ellus sum of þese if þou myȝt not come to all. & seþe hem riȝt wel . . . (ed. Svinhufvud 1978: 129)

The writer of *Horse Leechynge* was inconsistent in his use of the formal features of recipes and did not use the text-type to structure his text. In this, his recipes are in sharp contrast to charms, which he did name and set apart. His recipes were not isolated in paragraphs in the way charms were, unlike charms were not named, and were not standardised in their relationship of form to function. Rather, what we today might call 'recipes' (a recipients' genre, in the terminology of Diller (2001)) are contained within the producer's genre of 'cures':

(32) I wol schewe ȝou as j haue jlerned sum curus for hors (ed. Svinhufvud 1978: 85)

(33)   Cure þerfore now wol I schewe (ed. Svinhufvud 1978: 93)

(34)   þerfore in þis cure þus schalt þou don (ed. Svinhufvud 1978: 115)

The cure includes not just the instructions for preparation of medicines, written in short paratactic imperative clauses, but a complete account of veterinary care, incorporating subordinate clauses and varying approaches to treatment:

(35)   But loke þou do not þe last cure of lettynge of blod but if þe þynke be good syngnes þat it be nede. þat is to say. þat blod be enchesoun. (ed. Svinhufvud 1978: 117)

Remedybook recipes are not only more consistent in their linguistic formal structure, but in their discourse placement and identity. Remedybooks are a medieval example of 'discourse colonies',[10] texts composed of components which 'do not derive their meaning from the sequence in which they are placed', and which usually all have the same function (Hoey 2001: 72–92). Simply put, remedybooks, culinary collections, and other such discourse colonies consist largely of a collection of recipes, one following after another.

Although some compilers strive towards following broad organisational principles (medicinal collections, for example, may be structured *de capite ad pedem*), the fact that recipes may be read in any order or indeed individually, means that organisational ideals are rarely met. The medical recipe collection found in London, British Library, Additional MS 33996 (ed. Heinrich 1896) scatters recipes for the eyes from folio 81r to folio 144v, with recipes for the stomach presented as early as folio 82v. Although recipes for the eyes are grouped so that several fall together, these groupings may be found alongside recipes for headache (f.86r), the teeth (f.91r), or the nose (f.125v) (see Rand Schmidt 1994 for more exceptions to the 'rule' of *de capite ad pedem* ordering). The extent to which a text follows organisational principles is a point of contrast between remedybooks and academic treatises. *Horse Leechynge* is a text which is ordered by disease, consistently presenting all cures for farcy in one section and all cures for abscesses in another.

Diuersa cibaria is a token of a medieval discourse colony, a cookbook organised like a remedybook. It begins without an incipit (at least in the MS Additional 46919 version, something which is perhaps unusual for medieval discourse colonies), with 32 recipes which we now know to be translations from MS Royal 12.C.xii. With no textual indication of any break, the *Diuersa cibaria* collection continues with thirteen recipes translated from MS Additional 32085, and then sixteen from an unknown source or sources. A heading follows the eleventh of these (the 56th recipe in the entire collection); a Latin explicit, the only Latin in *Diuersa cibaria*, ends the collection:[11]

(36)   Explicit doctrina faciendi diuersa cibaria (ed. Hieatt and Butler 1985: 58)

With the exception of the 38 words comprising the heading and explicit, *Diuersa cibaria* is made up entirely of recipes. There is little cohesion to the text as a whole, with a recipe for white plum pottage followed by a recipe for salmon, followed by one for galentine.

When a reader comes across a discourse colony, a collection of similar components, or 'sister-texts', they are perceived as all being tokens of the same text-type, despite relatively minor differences between them. Thus, it is not just the linguistic form within a text which affects its text-type classification, but also the context in which it is found. A text such as the following:

(37)   Þe heyroun schal be diȝht as is þe swan and it come quyk to kechen. Þe sauce schal be mad of hym as a chaudoun of gynger & of galyngale, & þat it be coloured with þe blood or with brende crustes þat arn tosted. (ed. Hieatt and Butler 1985: 86)

is classifiable as a recipe despite its lack of imperative verbs, heading, and other typical features, largely because of its placement in a collection of culinary recipes, *Utilis coquinario*. Followed by two similar texts, it appears immediately following two recipes for swan (one of which is referred to in its first line).

Already, an example has been given of a text which evokes a recipe but is found in a sermon (17). The following text, out of context, appears to be unambiguously a recipe:

(38)   Take new chese & pyke hit full of smale holes & cast wyne or vinegur vp-on hit & ley hit in þe son.

However, its larger context is not a recipe for cheese or anything else to eat; it is in fact the recommended way of collecting maggots for use as fishing bait. The context for this sentence is given here:

(39)   In Jule take for þe cheveyn & dub þi hoke with þe tayle of a rede worme & þen take þe codworme, & þou may fynde hyt, or ellys take þe magod þat is mad of shepes fete or ellys þat is made of new chese. Take new chese & pyke hit full of smale holes & cast wyne or vinegur vp-on hit & ley hit in þe son. Also take þe gresshop or þe whit bee . . . (ed. Bitterling 1981, lines 45–8)

The larger text itself can only be considered functionally a recipe by using the wider definition of the function of a recipe which will be discussed below. It is in fact catalogued as being part of 'a collection of medical and other receipts' (Bitterling 1981: 110, citing the *Catalogue of Additional Manuscripts: Sloane 1599–1777*), but here again, the distinction between the recipients' text-type and that of the producer must be borne in mind.

Most discourse-analytical studies of medieval recipes to date have focused on the recipes themselves rather than the larger contexts in which they are found. Although the reasons for this are understandable (as discussed in Carroll forthcoming) care must be taken in lifting recipes out of their surrounding context.

In addition to a recipe's immediate context, the medievalist should also consider the larger context, other manuscript *matere*. Both *Diuersa cibaria* and the treatise on hunting preceding it in the manuscript (*Till all those that will of venery lere I shall them teach as I have learned*) are included in *eVK* (nos. 3602.00, 3811.00 (hunting prologue), and 7573.00), although there is no further information on the manuscript contents available in the database. The manuscript was compiled by William Herebert, of Hereford (*d.* 1333), and is described by Reimer (1998) as containing 'materials which might be useful for an itinerant preacher, from theological works and sermon aids to recipes gastronomic and medicinal'. The theological works include an Anglo-Norman poem relating a debate between Mary and the Cross, English translations of Latin hymns, and six Latin sermons. The manuscript also includes proverbs, and an Anglo-Norman poem of motherly advice on choosing a husband (Hieatt and Butler 1985: 7).

The recipes are likely to have been drawn from at least four sources. Recipes 1–32 represent a very close translation of a collection of Anglo-Norman recipes found in MS Royal 12.C.xii, dated *c.* 1320–40. Recipes 33–45 translate a selection of Anglo-Norman recipes found in MS Additional 32085 (both Anglo-Norman collections were edited by Hieatt and Jones in 1986). MS Additional 32085 has been dated to the late thirteenth century, so is perhaps unlikely to be the actual source for the translation, but the manuscript shares the scribal errors which explain oddities in the English text (Hieatt and Butler 1985: 7; Hieatt and Jones 1986: 860). The 'original' contains 29 recipes, of which numbers 13–25 were translated for MS Additional 46919.

MS Additional 46919's recipes 46–56 and 57–63 may represent two source collections, as there is a heading between recipes 56 and 57. The heading is so broad, mentioning *diuers potages & metes*, that it seems unlikely to have been intended to separate one section of a recipe collection from another, but rather to introduce a recipe collection as distinct from another text in a manuscript. In contrast, the collection found in Oxford, Bodleian Library, Douce MS 257 contains a Latin heading distinguishing the section of recipes containing meat dishes from the section containing fish dishes (see Hieatt and Butler 1985: 74; cf. Pahta, pp. 89–90 above). However, the suggestion that MS Additional 46919's recipes 46–63 might have come from two sources remains speculative, as no sources for any of these recipes have yet been identified.

Diuersa cibaria is also extant in London, British Library, Cotton Julius MS D.viii, along with texts on the winds, estate management, horticulture, medical, veterinary and codicological recipes, a herbal, and the 'Manner of bleaching linen cloth' (*eVK*).

Horse Leechynge is also found among the practical and instructional texts of a commonplace book. London, British Library, Sloane MS 2584 contains many other medicinal and recipe texts (see *eVK* for a complete listing), lists of lucky and unlucky days, metallurgical recipes, and arithmetical texts.

7.3.2.3 Function. As noted above, to define recipes by function rather than form would be to consider them as a genre. However, to consider the functions handled by the textual units having the form of a recipe is to continue in the analysis of the text-type. The function of a recipe as commonly accepted for both Middle and Modern English is to give instructions on how to prepare something. Instruction, in Werlich's analysis for example, is that communication in which someone is told what to do (1976: 40). Görlach's functional definition of a recipe is restricted to culinary recipes, 'the instruction on however to prepare a meal' (1992: 745). Taavitsainen's (for Middle English medical recipes) is broader: 'instructions on how to prepare medicine, a dish, or some household utility like ink' (2001c: 86). The verb *create* might be inserted alongside *prepare*, since some recipes adapt something which already exists (*noumbles* or *funges* (ed. Hieatt and Butler 1985: 100)), while others create a new entity from other ingredients (*makerouns* or *cold brewet* (ed. Hieatt and Butler 1985: 119, 128)). Grund's (2000) study of alchemical texts includes recipes for powder of silver (*calce of lune*) and water of mercury (*aqua mercurij*), expanding the scope of recipes beyond the household utilities mentioned by Taavitsainen (2001c).

The broad range of products which recipes may give instructions for, and hence the broad range of topics they cover, is one reason for discounting vocabulary as an important linguistic feature defining recipes. Within a given field it is possible to make a preliminary analysis of lexis; for example Taavitsainen points out that there is a narrow 'semantic range of transitive verbs' found in medicinal recipes. Her list of core verbs includes the Cooking Verbs *boyle*, *fry*, and *seethe*, Verbs of Combining like *meddle*, *mix*, *temper*, and other active verbs like *beat*, *strain*, and *cut* (2001c: 100). In a volume on vernacularisation, it is worth noting that her list contains by far more words which were drawn from the Old English word-stock than Middle English Romance borrowings.

An analysis of the *Diuersa cibaria* translations of the 32 Anglo-Norman recipes of MS Royal 12.C.xii shows that more recipe verbs are drawn from Anglo-Saxon lexis (58 tokens of eighteen lexemes) than new Romance loans (35 tokens of twelve lexemes, the most common being *trien*, *abaten*, and *boillen*). Anglo-Norman *mettre* is always translated as *don*. Of sixteen tokens of Anglo-Norman *planter*, twelve are translated *strien*, and only one *plaunten*, although *plantian* had already been present in Old English as a Latin loan (*MED* s.v. *plaunten*).

For nouns denoting food-stuffs and ingredients the opposite is true. Only 109 of the translations of 301 tokens of words denoting food are drawn from the wordstock of Old English (28 lexemes), while 190 tokens (47 lexemes) are borrowings new to Middle English. Almost every student of the history of English is taught that English kept its native terminology to describe farmyard animals, but borrowed Norman terms to denote their meat. *Diuersa cibaria* contains two fewer tokens of words denoting food than the Anglo-Norman original, because twice it was unnecessary to translate the word *char* 'flesh':

(40)   char de veel moudree, char de veel chiselé a manere de dees
        [flesh of calf, ground; flesh of calf cut in the manner of dice] (ed. Hieatt and Jones 1986: 866)

(41)   veel ipolled, veel icoruen ase deez (ed. Hieatt and Butler 1985: 45)

Note also that Anglo-Norman recipes included Germanic and Middle English lexis (*bro* 'broth' and *curnel* 'kernel').

However, when considering the range of Middle English recipes as a whole, it is preferable to link vocabulary not with text-type but with subject matter. Eggins and Martin (1997), operating within the framework of functional linguistics, call this 'field', a part of the larger 'register' within which the text-type is situated. There clearly are texts which do contain recipe vocabulary yet are not recipes, such as the proclamation (42) and the description of the cook in the *Canterbury Tales* (43):

(42)   wyne of Spayne, Rochell & oþer remenauntz of brokyn, **sodyn, reboyllid**, and vnthrifty wynes of oþer Contrees . . . ('Proclamacioun of Romeny . . .' *A Book of London English* 1384–1425, Helsinki Corpus)

(43)   He koude rooste, and sethe, and broille, and frye, Maken mortreux, and wel bake a pye. (ed. Benson, I.383–4)

More importantly, there are texts which share the form of recipes but which contain very little of this core vocabulary. Consider the following instructions for salvaging meat which has gone bad:

(44)   For to do awey restyng of venisoun, tak þe venisoun þat ys rest & do yt in cold water & after mak an hole in þe herþe & lat yt be þereyn þre dayes & þre ny3t; & after tak yt vp & frot yt wel wyþ gret salt of poite þere were þe restyng ys. & after lat yt hange in reyn water al ny3t or more. (ed. Hieatt and Butler 1985: 73)

The only verbs from Taavitsainen's list found in the above text are *do*, here meaning 'put', and *mak*, 'make', both of which are so general as to be unhelpful, and the first word after the title, *tak* 'take'. The latter is the most compelling, since it often serves as the opening for a recipe, as mentioned above.

Example (44) not only illustrates that recipes need not necessarily contain vocabulary generally typical of recipes, but also illustrates that the definition of a medieval English recipe given above (a text giving instructions on how to make or prepare medicine, a culinary dish, or other product) is still too narrow. In addition to telling how to make things, recipes may tell how to do things. In some cases it is easy to paraphrase: example (19) may be a recipe which tells how to do something (cure a horse with a sore back) or make something (a cure for a horse with a sore back).

But other examples of clear 'how to do' recipes may also be found:

(45)   For to make two pecys of flessh to fasten togyder (ed. Hieatt and Butler 1985: 143)

(46)   Ad purgandum caput. Take peletur of spayne, and chewe þe rote þre dayes a good quantite, and hit shal purge þe heued . . . (ed. Heinrich 1896: 66)

Stannard, whose study includes recipes in many medieval European languages, including Dutch, German, Icelandic, Italian, Latin, and English, notes that '[t]here are many different kinds of recipes in the Middle Ages and they occur in many different literary genres'. He restricts his study to '*only* . . . three kinds' (1982: 59, emphasis my own): medicinal, culinary, and secreta, the latter being 'those whose aim was the production of some object for purposes not specifically medicinal or culinary'. He does not explicitly say what has then been omitted from his study, but as it cannot be recipes for how to make anything (since the secreta are recipes for making everything other than food and medicine), it must be recipes for how to do things.

Hargreaves, on the other hand, does include 'how to do' recipes in his brief survey of the wide range of medieval recipes (1981: 91). He notes that in addition to extant medical, culinary, and veterinary recipes in Middle English, there are also what he calls 'general recipes' (such as 'how to make all apples fall from a tree') and 'magical recipes' ('how to make fire go out of a vessel full of water'). Hunt, too, considers such texts as instructions for curling hair and getting rid of flies to be 'receipts' (1990: 17, 146).

7.4   Conclusion

The Middle English recipe was vernacularised, according to the extant evidence, in the fourteenth century. The vernacularisation of recipes began with the remedybook tradition, and the recipe text-type was standardised more quickly in that tradition. The early Middle English recipe writers may well have followed models provided by Anglo-Norman; a closer study will make clearer the extent to which this is true. What is certain is that the Middle English recipe differed in form from other European vernacular recipes, such as those from Iberia.

Middle English recipes, medicinal, veterinary, even culinary and others, shared a common resemblance to a prototype consisting of short imperative clauses, temporally ordered according to the procedure to be followed. Prototypical recipes prefaced this procedural component with a heading, included specification of ingredients to be used, and ended with an application component. Noun determiners were not elided, and could be either articles or possessive pronouns.

Recipes may be found on their own, or in very small groupings, but also form discourse colonies such as remedybooks and culinary collections. Although the recipes in a discourse colony are usually very consistent with regard to form and function, an aberrant member may be recognised as a recipe by virtue of its discourse context, amongst its sister-texts. Academic treatises are a composite text-type into which recipes are inserted in a cohesive way, and within which recipes tend to display greater formal variation. A common manuscript context for text containing recipes is within a commonplace book, as is the case with both *Diuersa cibaria* and *Horse Leechynge*.

The function of a recipe has been shown to be broader than it has previously been defined, texts enabling the reader to create new items, prepare existing ingredients, or do things such as salvaging rancid meat. The subject matter (*field*) of recipes may extend far beyond the present-day recipients' genre of science or medicine, and the varied vocabulary of recipes reflects this. However, some boundaries of the genre/text-type have been sketched out, with recipes shown to be distinguishable from charms (both producers and present-day recipients treat them differently), and herbals as distinct from discourse colonies of remedybook recipes.

Diller's distinction (2001) between producers' genres and recipients' genres has been shown to be salient not only for synchronic studies, but also for attempting to distinguish medieval producers' or recipients' genres from contemporary perceptions thereof (present-day recipients' genres). As a final note, it is instructive to remind ourselves that the earliest *Middle English Dictionary* citation for the use of *receipt* as the name of a text-type is 1395 (s.v. *receite*; also *recepte*), later than the earliest extant texts containing text-types we would now call recipes. Neither *Diuersa cibaria* nor *Horse Leechynge* contains the word *recipe*, indicating that this was not yet a text-type regularly named by its producers.

Notes

1. Part of this research was carried out while I was a visiting scholar at the University of Helsinki. Earlier versions of portions of this chapter were presented at the SHEL (Los Angeles, 2000) and Cardiff (Santiago de Compostela, 2001) conferences. I am grateful to CIMO for funding my accommodation and travel expenses in Helsinki, and to Turun Yliopistosäätiö for funding my trip to Los Angeles. The chapter has benefited from comments by an anonymous reviewer.
2. For concise explanations of the interrelationship of culinary and medical concerns, see Sass (1981) and Scully (1995).
3. A new edition of the *Leechbook* is in preparation by Sally Crawford and Tony Randall.
4. See also, for example, the bibliography of The Anglo-Saxon Plant-Name Survey (University of Glasgow), which credits Bald with compiling books I and II, but not III.
5. My study of the *Directions for Laces* text (ed. Stanley 1974) was presented at the NAES conference (Gothenburg, 2001); the written version is forthcoming.
6. I have not reproduced editorial indications of expansion of abbreviations.
7. The distinction of 'text-type' from 'genre' is often but not always made, and the terminology and definitions vary from one researcher to the next. For some uses of 'text-type' similar to that used here, see Biber (1988), Diller (2001), Taavitsainen (2001c), as well as papers in *EJES* 5/2 (2001) and Uhlig and Zimmermann (1991).
8. I am grateful to Dr Matti Peikola for drawing my attention to this passage.
9. Hieatt and Jones's edition includes some discussion of translation errors such as this 'fried' for 'fresh'. Although I presented some evaluation of medieval culinary

translations at the Cardiff conference talk upon which this section of the chapter is based, it falls outside the scope of the present volume.

10. I presented a fuller treatment of the medieval culinary recipe as discourse colony at the ICEHL12 conference (Glasgow, 2002). A written version of that paper is now in preparation; see also Carroll forthcoming.

11. For the use of Latin as a text-organising device, see Pahta in this volume.

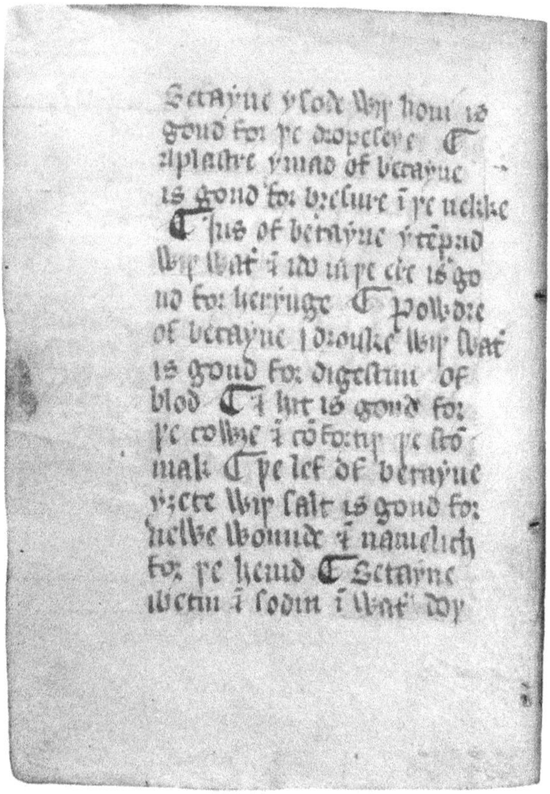

Setayne yſod wiþ hony is
goud for þe dropesye   ¶
A plaſtre ymad of verayne
is goud for vlecſure i þe uelike
¶ Ius of verayne ytepad
wiþ wat i lad iu þe ere is go
ud for werruge   ¶ Powdre
of verayne i dronke wiþ wat
is goud for digeſtiu of
blod   ¶ i lut is goud for
þe colwe i coforty þe ſto
mak   ¶ þe lef of verayne
yꝛete wiþ ſalt is goud for
helwe wounde i nauielich
for þe heud   ¶ Setayne
wetin i ſodin i wat doy

Plate 5a

Plate 5b Plates 5a and 5b Two pages from a Middle English leechbook, early fifteenth century. Wellcome MS 405, f. 17r.

117

Plate 6 A manuscript page from a surgical text from 1392 in Wellcome MS 564, f. 117r.

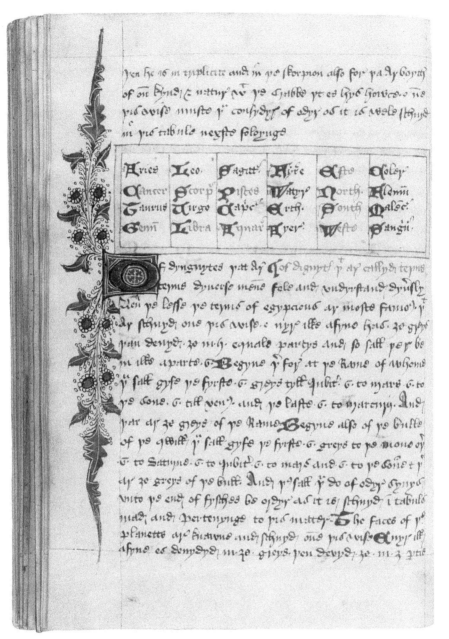

Plate 7 Middle English version W of the *Declaracions* of Richard of Wallingford. Wellcome MS 8004, f. 33v, with table of correspondences.

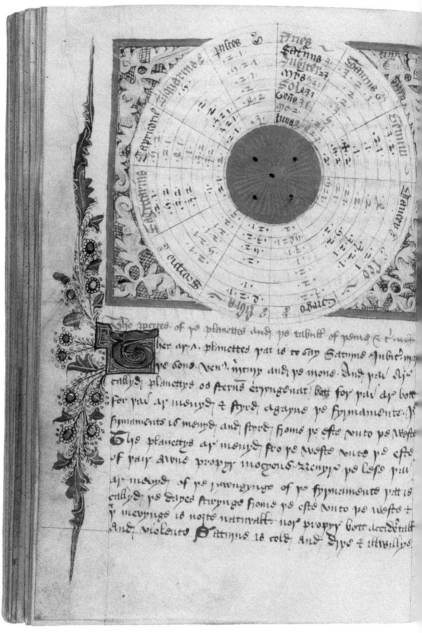

Plate 8 Middle English version W of the *Declaracions* of Richard of Wallingford. Wellcome MS 8004, f. 34v, diagram following the text showing relationships of signs of the zodiac to planets.

8   The *Declaracions* of Richard of Wallingford: A case study of a Middle English astrological treatise

LINDA EHRSAM VOIGTS

Middle English scientific and medical texts often survive in multiple versions, sometimes with dialectal variations within a single textual tradition. A case study that forcefully illustrates the challenges inherent in making such a text accessible to the modern reader is that of the Middle English versions of a fourteenth-century Latin treatise by the learned Abbot of St Albans, Richard of Wallingford.

Any consideration of Richard's *Declaraciones abbatis Sancti Albani* in Middle English requires some discussion of the author and of the Latin treatise with its own vexed tradition. Richard of Wallingford was born the son of a blacksmith *c*. 1292 and served as Abbot of St Albans 1327–36. He was afflicted with leprosy at least by 1328, suffered impairment of speech from the disease from the early 1330s and died of it in 1336. In his short life, of which at least fifteen years were spent studying and teaching in the faculties of arts and theology at Oxford, he wrote treatises on mathematics, astronomy, horology, and the Benedictine statutes. He invented astronomical and geometrical instruments and was responsible for the first and perhaps most elaborate astronomical clock in England, one with an astrolabe face 10 feet across. He also for nine years administered with rigor the royal abbey of St Albans, restoring it to solvency and addressing conflicts between the abbey and townspeople and within the house itself.[1]

While at Oxford (1308–15 and 1318–27) this remarkable Benedictine began his career of scientific writing. His treatises include canons for John Maudith's astronomical tables that rectified the Toledan or Alfonsine tables for the latitude of Oxford, and he was responsible for the first comprehensive discussion of trigonometry written in Christian Europe, the *Quadripartitum*. His surviving works include treatises on the astronomical instruments he invented, the Albion (a pun on all-by-one), the rectangulus, and his St Albans astronomical clock. He was also responsible for the *Exafrenon pronosticacionum temporis* on astrological meteorology, which until recently was thought to be the only work by Richard translated into English in the medieval period.[2]

It is, however, another Latin treatise, attributed to Richard and edited by John North in his three-volume edition of Richard's writings, not hitherto known to have been translated into Middle English, that is the subject of study here.[3] This text on astronomical-astrological terminology is part of the vast medieval written tradition on the impact of the celestial upon the terrestrial, the 'natural law' underlying much medieval science.[4] John North concluded that this work was based on texts by Grosseteste or Roger Bacon, along with another treatise containing much of the *Liber introductorius* of Alcabitius (al-Qabisi). Richard's text does indeed bear a strong resemblance to the Alcabitius text, also known as the *Isagoge*, an introduction to the principles of astrology that was widely disseminated in medieval Europe.[5]

This Latin text survives in widely varying versions in four fifteenth-century manuscripts, and bits of it in a fourteenth-century codex.[6] The rubrics in two of those manuscripts, London, British Library, MSS Harley 1612 and Harley 321, provide the two variant titles by which the treatise is known:

Canon supra kalendarum abbatis Sancti Albani

Declaraciones abbatis Sancti Albani super Kalendarium regine[7]

The *Canon* or *Declaraciones* begins with a discussion of kinds of degrees which can be assigned to planets (e.g., masculine and feminine, light and dark), and then addresses one by one, in descending order of strength, the five 'dignities', that is, the five ways a planet can be related to the zodiac. It begins with 'houses', emphasising the principal house which accords with a planet in two qualities, for example Leo, the principal house of the sun. It also takes up accidental and secondary houses, which accord in only one quality, before discussing the second dignity, the 'exaltation', identifying the location of a planet in a sign in terms of numbers of degrees. The third dignity, the 'triplicity', when a planet is in the sign of the same complexion, is explained discursively and the reader is referred to a table.

The fourth dignity, the 'term', is acknowledged to be a subject of controversy, and the division of the thirty degrees allotted to each sign is further broken down into five equal units of six degrees, each assigned to a planet. The reader is also referred to a table at this point.[8] The fifth and last dignity, the 'face', divides the thirty degrees of each sign into three units, each assigned to a planet. The shorter version of the text ends here, where the fuller version goes on to describe a circular diagram on which the five kinds of dignities or strengths can be plotted for each planet (Plate 8). No Middle English text extends beyond this point, but North's edition of the Latin treatise contains a continuation not found in the English-language texts.[9]

Of the two Latin titles the second most closely resembles that found in two of the six Middle English manuscripts: *Declaracions of þe Abbot of saynt Alban Vpon þe kalender of the queen*.[10] No calendar linked with an English queen from the first half of the fourteenth century has been identified, but North and Carey suggest two candidates for this dedication: Phillipa of Hainault, queen of Edward III, who came to London in 1327 and died in 1369; and her mother-in-law, the dowager queen Isabella, who lived until 1358. Although the dowager Isabella possessed a library that included calendars, she may be a less likely candidate than her daughter-in-law Phillipa, both because at least one of Phillipa's twelve children was baptised at St Albans, and because Richard carried on a protracted lawsuit against the dowager Isabella, from whom he successfully collected (North 1976, 2: 372–3; Carey 1992: 80). On the other hand, it is not impossible that the treatise was a reconciliation offering to Isabella.

In his three-volume edition and study of the writings of Richard of Wallingford, John North edited from three manuscripts the Latin text that I shall refer to as the *Declaraciones*. I have also transcribed the Latin text from another manuscript, Oxford, Bodleian Library, MS Digby Roll 3, which North did not use, but which in some instances seems to be relevant to the three English versions.[11]

Although North had identified among Richard's writings only the *Exafrenon* as surviving in a translation in the English vernacular,[12] computer searching of Voigts and Kurtz, *Scientific and Medical Writings in Old and Middle English: An Electronic Reference (eVK)* makes it possible to identify several texts of the *Declaraciones* in Middle English. Patricia Kurtz and I had identified, in the course of data entry, the text in Cambridge, Gonville and Caius MS 84/166 as Richard's, on the basis of the title which sent us to the Latin version in the North edition. However, we found in the database no identical texts in terms of either title or incipit. Knowing that many Middle English scientific texts survive in widely varying versions, we looked in that preliminary version of *eVK* for other instances of the text using a simple keyword search. Because Latin versions begin 'Si fiat questio de nativitate viri' we searched for the word 'question' and turned up four additional manuscripts containing this text. In none of the four was the text identified by author or title. The appearance of a sixth witness to this text occurred late in *eVK* data collection with the appearance in 1999 at the Christie's sale of what is now Wellcome Library MS 8004.[13] For the incipits for the six versions see Figure 8.1.

Discussion of the six manuscripts will use the following sigils.

R: London, British Library, Royal MS 17.A.iii, ff. 74–75v
G: Cambridge, Gonville and Caius College MS 336/725, ff. 43–44
S: London, British Library, Sloane MS 965, ff. 3–6
T: Cambridge, Trinity College MS R.14.52, ff. 259–260
C: Cambridge, Gonville and Caius College MS 84/166, pp. 196–197
   Rubric: *Declaracions of þe Abbot of saynt Alban Vpon þe kalender of the queen*
W: London, Wellcome MS 8004, ff. 31v–34
   Rubric: *Declaracyons of þe Abbott of Sanct Albans Apoun þe calender of þe queene*

In three of the six manuscripts, the Middle English texts are closely related, almost certainly copies of the same translation. One might call R, G, and S the triplets.[14] All are found in mixed Latin–English scientific and medical miscellanies dating from the late fourteenth century to the late fifteenth century. These compendia can be found in the Royal and Sloane Collections in the British Library

R ¶ If þere be maad a questyoun of þe natiuite of
G Iff þer be maad a questioun of þe nativite of
S Yef there be made a questioun of the natiuite of
T If questioun be made of the nativite of
C If þer be a question made of the byrth of
W If þer be a questyone mad of þe byrth of

———

R a man & þe planetis ben in þe grees of þe signe
G a man & þe planetis be in þe degrees of þe signe
S man and the planetis ben in the grees of the signe
T man and the planetis bien in grees
C mon and the planetys bee in the
W manne and þe planetts be in þe

———

R of masculyn þt schal be to hem a strengþe ¶ And
G masculyne. þat schal be to hem a strenkþe ¶ And
S of masculyn that shall be to hem a strengthe ¶ And
T males this shal be to hem strong And
C masculyne grece þat is to say in grece of mon þat shall
    be to hym a stronge natiuite. And
W masculyne grece þat is to say in þe grece of mane þat sall
    be to þeme a stronge mayntynyte. And

———

R if a questioun be maad of þe natiuyte of a womman
G if a questioun be maad of þe natiuite of a womman
S yef a questioun be made of the natiuite of woman
T if the questioun be of the nativite of womman
C ther be a question made of the byrth of a womon
W if þer be a questyone mad of þe byrth of womane

Figure 8.1 *Declaracions*: incipits

and at Gonville and Caius College, Cambridge.[15] As the examples in Figures
8.1–8.4 illustrate, R and S appear to be more closely related to one another than
to G, and it is possible that the version in S was copied from R.

The dialects of R and G are not distinctive, and both manuscripts have London
associations. R is a large codex from the end of the fourteenth century containing
40 Middle English texts on science and medicine as identified in *eVK*. There
are in addition Latin scientific and medical texts. It also contains an English
translation of the 1365 Charter of the London Weavers' Guild (f. 126). G is an
illuminated manuscript written nearly a century later. It contains 26 texts on
science and medicine in Middle English (*eVK*) as well as Latin texts. It includes
a core of texts transmitted together that is associated with manuscripts produced

R deefnes & blyndnes lesinge & fallinge of lymes
G deefnesse blyndnes lesynge & faylynge of lymes
S defnes blyndenesse lesynge and fallyng of lymes
T def blynd losse of membres
C defenes blendynes losyng of membrus or lyms
W defnesse blyndnesse losynge of members or lymys

R & siche oþere whiche a man haþ is his liif
G & siche oþere. Whiche a man haþ in þis lyf
S and suiche other Whiche a man hathe in his lyff
T and like thynges whiche a man hath in this lif.
C and such maner thyngus os mon hath in þis lyfe.
W and schuch manere of þinges as mane hath is þis lyfe.

R ¶ Whanne þe mone is in ony of þese grees in þe
G ¶ Whanne þe moone is in ony of þese grees in þe
S ¶ Whanne the mone is in any of these grees in the
T ¶ Therfor whan the moone is in any of thiese grees in the
C Therfore when þe mone schall be in any of þise grece in the
W Therfore qwene þe mone sall be in any of þies greys in þe

R natiuite of man or of a womman sum sich defaute schal falle to hem
G natiuite of ony man or womman sum sich defaute schal falle to hem
S natiuite of man or woman sum seche defaute shal fall to hem
T nativite of any ther fallith to hem sum of thiese defautis
C byrth of any mon or womon sum of thoo foresayde maymes
    schall fall tyll þem.
W byrth of any mane or womane sume of þo forsayd mames sall fall vnto þem

Figure 8.2 *Declaracions*: on the effects of azamena

in London in the mid-fifteenth century (Voigts 1990: 26–57; especially pp. 27, 33, 53).

The small manuscript S appears at first glance to be the anomaly in the group of triplets in terms of dialect. It contains some Latin, but most texts are Middle English (33 texts in *eVK*). The presence of epact tables beginning 1449 suggests a mid-fifteenth-century date, and London saints are named in the calendar. While the listing of local saints is by no means unequivocal evidence of a London origin for the manuscript, it should not be ignored. The dialect of this manuscript has been identified in *A Linguistic Atlas of Late Mediaeval English* (*LALME*) as north-east Leicestershire or Rutland, but such an identification need not rule out book production in London. Taavitsainen argues in this volume that the so-called '*Rosarium* type' dialect associated with Eastern Midlands,

R to þt planete in qualitees ¶ The hous of þe sunne
G to þat planete in qualitees ¶ The hous of þe sunne
S to that planete in qualitees The hous of the sunne
T to that planete in qualitees ¶ Therfor is leo the
C tyll þe selfe planet in qualite The lyon is þe
W tyll þe selfe planete is qualitys. The lyon is þe

R is leo of þe mone cancer þe principal hous of
G is leo Of þe moone Cancer The principal hous of
S is Leo of the mone cancer the principal hous of
T house of the sonne Cancer of the moone
C howce of þe son. The crab is þe howce of þe mone.
W howce of þe sonne. þe crabe is þ [sic, no e] howce of þe mone
---

R mercurye is virgo of venus libra of mars Aries
G mercurie. virgo libra of venus Aries of maris
S mercurie is virgo of venus libra of Mars Aries
T Virgo the principal house of mercurii libra the principal house of Venus Aries
    the principal house of mars
C The virgin is þe principall howce of mercury. The balance is þe principall
    howce of Venus. The ram is þe principall howce of mars.
W The virgyne is þe principall howce of marcury. The belauns is þe principall
    howce of venus. The rame is þe principall howce of marse.

Figure 8.3 *Declaracions*: on planetary houses

including Leicestershire and Rutland, may well have been the language of some metropolitan scientific and medical manuscripts.[16]

   The text passages in Figures 8.1–8.4 are presented as diplomatic transcriptions of the manuscripts with abbreviations expanded. However, spelling has been normalised in the subsequent discussion of lexical variations in the six versions, using modern orthography so as to more clearly demarcate the patterns of relationship. To compare variations within the triplets RGS, consider in Figure 8.2 RS 'falling' against G 'failing', and RS 'his' against G 'this'. Note, however, the relatively minor three-way divergence in the last collated line.

   In Figure 8.3, in the third group of collated lines, G retains the Latin inflected form 'maris' against RS 'Mars'. Although RGS are very close, accidental variations, of course occur. Note in Figure 8.4, in the third group of collated lines dittography ('that that') in R not found in GS.

   In addition to the triplets, there are two other versions of this Middle English text, T, and the twins C and W.[17] See Figure 8.1. These three manuscripts are also scientific and medical miscellanies from the second half of the fifteenth century, perhaps representing a later tradition than RGS. T is a compendious

R ¶ The triplicite of planetis is seid whanne he
G ¶ The triplicite of a planete is seid whanne he
S ¶ The triplicite of planetis is said whan he
T fforsoth triplicitees of planetis so shewen and bien saide
C The triplicites of planetis are knowyn and schewyd on þis wyse and þai are
    sayde to be
W þe triplicites of planettis ar knawne & schuyd oun þis wyse and
    þai ar sayd to be

R is in a signe of þe same complexioun þt þe signe
G is in a signe of þe same complexioun þat þe signe
S is in a signe of the same complexioun that the signe
[*expanded material in TCW*]
T of the same nature wt the propre signe of hem as if the zodiac
C of the same nature wt þe propyr syne of hem. As if þe gre þat is
    callid Zodiake
W of þe same nature wyth þe propyre syne of þem. As if þe gree þat is
    callyd zodiake
T be divided in iiii partis ther shal be in everiche iii signes. Therfor
C be dividit into iiii parteys iii synes schall be in euer ylke parte of hem
    Therfore
W be deuydyd into 4 partys 3 synes sall be in euer ilke a parte of þem.
    Therfore
T theese iii signes whiche bien of oon nature nat as thei folowen nombred
C lett þer be chosen iii synes þat are of on nature nat as þai are
    numeryd consequenli
W latt þer be closen [sic] 3 synes þt ar of a nature nott as þai ar nowmbyrd
    consequently
T in the Zodiac and bien saide ¶ But tho signes to make a triplicite in so
C in Zodiak and þe synes are sayde to make triplicite in alls
W in zodiake and þo syns ar sayd to make triplicite in al so

R is of þat þat he was maad ynne ¶ As whanne þe
G is of þt he was maad ynne As whanne þe
S is of that he was made Inne ¶ As whanne the
T moche that thei bien convenient in oon nature As if the
C mycull as þai acorde in on nature and kynde. As yf þe
W mykyll as þai acord in oun nature and kynd. Os if þe

Figure 8.4 *Declaracions*: on triplicities

manuscript of some 111 texts, almost entirely in English. There are many reasons to associate this manuscript with London towards the end of the fifteenth century; these include scribal hands and the presence of personal names in the codex.[18] C, providing one of the two titled instances of the text, contains considerably fewer English texts; most of the medical treatises in the codex are Latin. It belonged at the end of the fifteenth century to the Padua-trained physician and provost of King's College, Cambridge, John Argentine (Talbot and Hammond 1965: 112–15). C is unusual among surviving Middle English manuscripts in that all three hands in the codex wrote in a Derbyshire dialect (*LALME*, 1: 63, 186). W, also containing the title, can be dated to 1454 and is written in a single hand. It is almost entirely Middle English, containing 58 calendrical, mathematical, and medical texts, along with what is apparently a unique pilgrimage account from London to Jerusalem.[19] The dialect of W is, like that of C, from the Danelaw. Margaret Laing places it in central west Lincolnshire or east Nottinghamshire.[20] Unlike RGST, C and W contain a table and a diagram that explains and amplifies the text. See Plates 7 and 8.

T and CW differ significantly from RGS as translations of the *Declaraciones* and may be based on a fuller Latin version than RGS. Only this fuller version contains the final section with the circle diagram. A comparison of the incipits in the six versions in Figure 8.1 establishes the general pattern of variation between RGS on one hand and TCW on the other. As is illustrated in Figure 8.3, we find consistently in RGS the construction 'the house of the [planet] is the [sign of the zodiac]'. In contrast TC and W consistently use the construction 'the [sign of the zodiac] is the house of the [planet]'. In any consideration of the differences between T on one hand and CW on the other, these parallels must not be overlooked, nor should the fact that the text is often much fuller in CW and T than in RGS. See Figure 8.4.

What bears further examination and is most problematic in understanding the relationships among the six manuscript witnesses is the relationship between T and CW, because both CW and T contain material not found in RGS, and English syntax in the two is often similar, although by no means always. On the other hand, there are striking differences in lexicon when T is compared to CW, and in CW we find a pattern of doublets not occurring in T.

T, like RG, also uses a relatively Latinate vocabulary, whereas C, in a Derbyshire dialect, resolutely Englishes almost every Latin word, preferring, for example, 'birth' to 'nativity' (*LALME*, 1: 63, 186). That is also the case with W, in a dialect that has also been identified with the Danelaw, in Lincolnshire or east Nottinghamshire (see note 20). Equally important in any consideration of the lexicons of T and CW is that often in CW, when a Latin-derived word is used, it is paired in a doublet with a native English synonym, as for example, 'triplicity or a threefoldness'.

The translator responsible for CW follows an anomalous English practice of preferring English terms even for the names of most of the signs of the zodiac, whereas T, like RGS, uses the traditional names found in Latin texts. CW use 'the ram', 'the bull', and 'the twinlings' for Aries, Taurus, and Gemini; 'the crab', 'the lion' and 'the virgin' for Cancer, Leo, and Virgo; 'the balance', 'the scorpion', and 'the shooter' for Libra, Scorpio, and Sagittarius; and 'the fishes' for Pisces, but 'Capricorn' and 'Aquary' for Capricorn and Aquarius.[21]

I am not aware of any other texts with such resolute anglicisation of the zodiacal names as is found in the Danelaw versions CW, although similar lexical choices occur in medieval German astrological texts. In one of two mid-fifteenth-century German-language texts in Munich manuscripts we find 'der Wider, der Stier, der Czwilig, der Chrews, der Lebe, die Junckfraw, die Wag, der Scorp, der Schuscz, der Stainpock, der Wasserman, die Vische'. In the other the names used are 'der Wider, der Ochs, die Zwilein, der Chrebs, der Lewe, die Junchfraw, die Wag, der Schorp, der Schiezzer, der Stainpokch, der Giezzer, der Fisch'.[22]

If T and CW derive from the same translation, the differences between the two must be explained. Whether T represents an urban redactor attempting to improve upon CW by paring out doublets and restoring Latin names to the signs of the zodiac or whether CW represents a modification of the text towards more complete anglicisation of the text as found in T may not be possible to say, although the case for the latter explanation is traditionally considered the stronger one in textual study.

Consider that in the first group of collated lines in Figure 8.2 T has 'deaf blind loss of members' against CW 'deafness blindness losing of members or limbs'. T mixes adjectives and nouns, where C and W use a series of nouns, concluding with the doublet pairing the Latinate 'members' with the Old English-derived 'limbs'. In the second group of lines we find T 'like things which' against CW 'such manner things as' and in the third group T 'is in' against CW 'shall be in'. In the fourth group T has 'nativity of any' against CW 'birth of any man or woman' and T 'there falleth to them some of these defaults' against CW 'some of those foresaid maims shall fall till/unto them'.

Figure 8.3 illustrates the anglicised names of the signs of the zodiac in CW but not in T. In addition T has the RGS reading 'to that' against CW 'till the self' and T plural 'qualities' against the singular in C, but not W. T also includes a 'therefore' not found in the other five manuscripts. In the second group T differs from CW in 'the moon' against 'the house of the moon'.

In the first group of lines in Figure 8.4, T has 'forsooth' not found elsewhere, but C and W use a longer construction that includes a doublet. In the second group T has 'not as they follow numbered' against CW 'not as they are numbered consequently'. The Latin text reads 'non ut consequenter numerantur in zodiaco', suggesting that CW, which sounds 'more English', may actually be closer to the Latin. In the last group, in addition to dialectal differences, we find T 'been convenient' against CW 'accord', and T lacks the CW doublet where the native English 'kynde' is paired with the Latinate 'nature'.

As is apparent from this comparison of these six witnesses to the Middle English *Declaracions* of Richard of Wallingford, the differences do not lend themselves to easy explanation, and the relationship between T and CW is particularly intractable. In comparing some passages, it appears that T and CW are discrete translations of the same Latin version, one fuller than the text translated by RGS. A consideration of other passages, however, where T resembles CW against RGS, suggests either that T is a modification of CW or that CW expands and anglicises T.

What is significant in a case study of these three versions of the Middle English *Declaracions* in six manuscripts is that they are representative of the variations found among the different surviving manuscript witnesses to many vernacular English medieval writings on science and medicine. It can also be argued that, even if it were possible to produce a critical Lachmannian edition based on the RGS triplets, such an edition would misleadingly prioritise one version simply because more witnesses of it survive. Furthermore, it would not be possible to produce anything other than a bizarre hybrid in any edition based on T and CW with their widely differing vocabularies. The most we can hope to do, if we are to represent accurately the Middle English *Declaracions*, is to reduce six manuscript witnesses to three vernacular versions of the Richard of Wallingford text, and even then it remains unclear whether we have three translations or two, one of which survives in both a 'more' and a 'less' English version.

In a relatively brief text such as this one, the presentation of three versions is not an unrealistic possibility in an edition, and the opportunity to see three versions in parallel has much to commend it.[23] The three versions taken together tellingly illustrate different translation strategies. They reveal varying resolutions of syntactic differences between source and target language, and they provide convincing evidence of the fluid state of the lexicon for scientific and medical writing in the late medieval English vernacular (cf. Norri in this volume). The six Middle English witnesses to Richard of Wallingford's *Declaracions* illustrate above all the plethora of lexical and syntactic possibilities that characterised Middle English translation of science and medicine, a variety of choices that ceased to remain available in Modern English.

Notes

1. Biographical summaries can be found in North (1990) and Emden (1957–59, 3). For editions of Richard's works and further biographical information, see North (1976).
2. For an edition of both Latin and Middle English versions of Richard's *Exafrenon*, see North (1976, 1: 181–7). On the importance of astrology for meteorology in fourteenth-century England, see Carey (1992), especially Chapters 4 and 5, and on this text, p. 80.
3. *eVK*, nos. 2621, 2685, 2686 (two manuscripts), 2691, 2692.
4. Because educated people today understand astrology as a superstition, it is important to recall its pre-modern role as the cosmological model on which most medieval

science was based. As the eminent historian of science Lynn Thorndike observed, the underlying 'law' of medieval science was that natural phenomena are controlled by the celestial, as can be observed in seasons, weather, tides, and the growth and death of plant and animal life, in short that 'all operations of the inferior world of nature spring from and are controlled by the eternal movement of the incorruptible celestial bodies' (Thorndike 1955/2000). See also Plate 1.

5. North (1976, 1: 558–63; 2: 371–8). *TK*, entry 1148F. The relationship of many medieval texts to the treatise of Alcabitius will be clearer with the appearance of Al-Qabisi, *Introduction to Astrology: The Arabic and Latin Texts, and Greek Fragments, with an English Translation*, edited and translated by Charles Burnett, Keiji Yamamoto and Michio Yano, Warburg Institute Studies and Texts, London, 2003.

6. London, British Library, Harley MS 321, ff. 18–19; Harley MS 1612, ff. 13–13v; Oxford, Bodleian Library, Ashmole MS 191, ff. 7–10v; Bodleian Library, MS Digby Roll 3; Cambridge University Library, MS Gg.VI.3, f. 284 (14th century).

7. Harley 321, f. 18; Harley 1612, f. 13.

8. The first two tables mentioned in the text are wanting in the Middle English versions, although the final, circular diagram is found in CW (Plate 8). CW also contain a basic table of correspondences not mentioned in the text (Plate 7). Medieval astrology was firmly grounded in mathematics. Tables went to fractions of seconds, and the tools of geometry and trigonometry were essential (Thorndike 1955/2000: 243). Richard of Wallingford's treatise on trigonometry was related to his larger concern with astronomy and astrology.

9. The five additional sections found in some, but not all, of the Latin manuscripts deal with the eighth sphere; the influence of signs of the zodiac on parts of the body; four kinds of triplicity; fixed, movable, and common signs; and five aspects of planets (North 1976, 1: 561–3).

10. Cambridge, Gonville and Caius College MS 84/166 and London, Wellcome Library MS 8004; Figure 8.1.

11. North's edition is based on the two Harley manuscripts and the Ashmole codex. See above, note 6.

12. See above, note 2. The Latin text is *TK*, entry 56J, and the Middle English versions are *eVK*, nos. 6701 and 7750.

13. Christie's Catalogue, sale, 29 November 1999, No. 9, 'Physician's Handbook', pp. 28–31. Digital images can be viewed on the Wellcome Library web site.

14. *eVK*, nos. 2685, 2691, 2692.

15. On Royal 17.A.iii, see Warner and Gilson (1921, 2: 214–15). On Gonville and Caius 336/725, see James (1907–08, 1: 378–80). On Sloane 965, see Sloane Catalogue, pp. 187–8.

16. *LALME*, 1: 115, 210, 233; and Taavitsainen 'House-styles' in this volume.

17. *eVK*, nos. 2621 (T) and 2686 (C and W). On Trinity College R.14.52, see James (1900–04, 2: 338–9). On Gonville and Caius 84/166, see James (1907–08, 1: 79–82). On W, see Christie's sale catalogue, cited in note 13.

18. Many studies have addressed this important manuscript. A full bibliography is to be found in Tavormina (forthcoming b). See also Pahta (1998).

19. See above, note 13. Fifty-two texts are cited in *eVK* as 'Physician's Handbook' on the basis of information provided by Christie's. Revised *eVK* will contain citations to 58 texts.

20. Private communication, 2 September 2002.
21. Note, however, that 'Aquarius' has been anglicised to 'Aquary'.
22. The manuscripts are Munich, Hofbibliothek cod. lat. 700 (dated 1458) and Hofbib-liothek cod. germ. 32 (both ed. Sudhoff 1914).
23. The question of determining a single version when length of text proscribes a multiple-version edition is beyond the scope of this study.

9 Scriptorial 'house-styles' and discourse communities

IRMA TAAVITSAINEN

> . . . someone writes the materials of others, adding or changing nothing, and this person is said to be merely the scribe.
>
> (Bonaventura, translated by Minnis 1984: 84)[1]

9.1 Introduction

The vernacularisation of scientific writing began towards the end of the fourteenth century at the time when the English language consisted of local dialects, and no language variety was yet recognised over larger areas of the country. Manuscripts with local features continue to be written beyond the Middle English period, but there is a clear change after the first quarter of the fifteenth century. The compilers of *A Linguistic Atlas of Late Mediaeval English* (*LALME*) report an increasing number of manuscripts that escape localisation. They may be cases of *Mischsprachen* (see the *LALME* Introduction), or fifteenth-century texts which represent the 'colourless' use of language, i.e. they are written in a language in which the local elements are muted and replaced by items with a wider currency. The growth of centres of education, especially grammar-schools, was instrumental in changing the patterns: regional spellings which had hitherto varied from parish to parish became less specific to given places and appear in combination in the spelling systems of individual writers (*LALME*, 1: 47, 22). Temporal variation is important for the present study and needs to be considered in connection with the present assessment of regional features, 'house-styles' of scriptoria, and metropolitan language use. Most of the manuscripts containing scientific texts in the vernacular were written after the *LALME* period, but regional features can be identified and they are prominent, for example in surgical texts. Social variation and facts about the audiences of early medical texts are scarce, but the possibility of incipient register variation and social variation within scientific writing according to the discourse communities cannot be ruled out.[2]

9.2 The aim of this study

The aim of this chapter is to consider the provenance of vernacular medical, especially surgical manuscripts, and discuss their language patterns from the angle

209

of regionality, discourse community, and metropolitan language use in the mid-fifteenth century. These texts have special characteristics. They contain combinations of features some of which are localisable with considerable precision, but others are found in a larger but still distinctly regional area. In an earlier article I argued that features of a language type connected with the 'Central Midland Standard' were fairly widespread in the new register of scientific writing. By an empirical study I was able to prove that spelling forms of Central Midlands were more widely disseminated in the texts included in the *Corpus of Early English Medical Writing* (*CEEM*) than noted earlier in the literature.[3] It seems that different language types can be discerned in the scientific/medical register: one is a variety of Central Midlands, related to the language of the Wycliffite writings, yet it is not identical to the repertoire of forms in their religious language (see Samuels 1989; Taavitsainen 2000b). Another type of language is more eastern and this language has been localised fairly precisely to East Midlands (see below).[4] Location and time of writing defined by extralinguistic facts would be of primary significance, but facts are scarce. As pointed out above, variation in Late Middle English has traditionally been associated with regional variation over larger geographical areas, and the language patterns of late medieval London with immigrants from various dialect areas as well as specialised book production have not been considered in connection with the types of language in medical texts. The core question is the position of the Central and East Midland dialects in medical writing, and the currency of Midland features in London English in the fifteenth century. It is possible to go even further and ask the question whether there is anything that definitely rules out London as the location of the scriptoria from where the vernacular versions of certain types of medical, especially surgical, texts were disseminated. The amount of variation found in some of the medical texts seems to be very high, and the co-occurring features are unexpected. It is possible that the new metropolis has something to do with this. In the light of the new trends of sociolinguistics and sociohistorical contextualisation (see below), the variant forms are also likely to reflect the changing patterns of 'social network' ties in the fifteenth century (see Jones in this volume), and the new developments in book trade with the rise of communities that would act as customers in specialised book production. The evidence is elusive and difficult to interpret because of the lack of sociohistorical facts.

9.3   Changing language patterns in medieval England: London English manuscripts

9.3.1 *Manuscripts and copying practices*

Current research interests in the study of late medieval vernacular manuscripts have increasingly been directed to codices as artefacts in the communication between the author, the text producer, and the audience(s), and the importance of sociohistorical context has been emphasised (see e.g. Pearsall 1989). The present assessment outlines some core types of language in fifteenth-century medical texts. What we have in the manuscripts as objects is their external features such as layout, size and format, handwriting, perhaps watermarks and ascriptions, even notes that tell us about provenance and use. Language-internal features encoded into the text provide another major category of evidence. The copying practices of manuscripts in scriptoria need to be taken into account. The well-known classification divides scribal practices into three main types: *litteratim* copying, and partial or full translation into the scribes' own dialect (*LALME*, 1: 13). These considerations are relevant to the present assessment as it deals with copies of surgical texts that seem to be connected with specialised book production that answer the need of a discourse community. The three types of copying have become an axiom in the field, and if a text shows a great deal of variation, it can usually be explained by layers of copying and relict forms from earlier texts. The time factor, however, complicates the issue as new patterns emerge with changing sociohistorical conditions. In the fifteenth century, variation with some incompatible forms can sometimes plausibly be explained by the scribes' personal histories, the place of birth, schooling, and working location (Samuels and Smith 1981; Smith 1988). London is the most likely place for specialised book trade, and metropolitan language use may provide an explanation for unexpected forms.

9.3.2 Urban dialectology

The assessment of urban cities as spaces provides a perspective worth pursuing: various standards and types of language within the London area may have been associated with different types of work, and with particular scribes and scriptoria (Samuels 1989; cf. Keene 2000). This remark needs further study on the linguistic repertoire of manuscripts produced in London. Urban dialectology has focused on phonological variation and patterns of pronunciation, though interest in historical aspects as manifested in written materials has also increased (see below). It seems feasible to assume that abundant variation is a characteristic of metropolitan centres especially in a period before generally accepted standards of writing. Another characteristic would be the occurrence of some widely spread features co-occurring with those limited to a different region. The levelling phase of the model of urban evolution in modern dialectology does not show as such in the present material, but what we have here is dialect mixing, typical of frequent contact situations perhaps as an outcome of increased mobility.[5]

The estimates of London's population keep its size at a fairly steady level from the thirteenth to the fifteenth century, with a peak in growth in the sixteenth (see the figures in Keene 2000). Compared to the cities next in importance, London's population was manifold, for example an estimate gives 70,000 for London in the 1470s, whereas the other cities remain in the range of 10,000–12,000. In the period of rapid growth, a more integrated system of communication was established, as London interacted directly with many provincial districts. The capital needed provincial resources and skills, and regional identities are said to have become more pronounced (Keene 2000: 93). The focus of historians is increasingly on centrality and dominance of the city, the increasing force of metropolitan culture, and immigration patterns with a flow of people to and from the city. The distances are measured in time and cost according to modern methods; for example there were several important harbours and a ready sea route along the coast from the East Midlands to London (see the maps in Keene 2000). New explanatory models of distance and space can be applied to linguistic modelling of changing language patterns as well. For example, we know that the direction of change in London English in Late Middle English was from the Essex type to more Central Midland, and on the whole the Midland component became more prominent, which correlates with immigration patterns into the metropolis and good transport and communication connections (see Ekwall 1956; Samuels 1989: 74; Keene 2000). The hinterland shaped London and was itself shaped by the impact of the city (Keene 2000: 94). This interaction is one of the challenges to both historical and linguistic studies.

The changes that were taking place in London English in the early fifteenth century (1400–1420) have been attributed to immigrants from various parts of the country, particularly from Central Midlands, but also from the North, north West Midlands and south West Midlands; Coventry, Leicester, and Northampton appear as parts of a region with relatively high interaction associated with London (Keene 2000: 102). Scribes came from all these parts, and Samuels talks about tiers of scribes who would start from different thresholds and therefore achieve different repertoires (Samuels 1988: 40–1). Immigrant scribes might continue to use their own regional spellings in London, thus contributing to the confusion by exotic forms, or they might attempt to adapt their own regional spelling systems to what they conceived to be more acceptable in London, thus contributing more subtly to the confusion (Samuels 1988: 40–1). Evidence of conflicting spellings in manuscripts copied in London in the early decades is abundant. In particular, the lack of common currency at which immigrant scribes might aim led to some extraordinary shifts and vacillations. Unusual combinations of linguistic features have been interpreted as evidence, for example some curious relict northern strata tell of northerners at work in London *c*. 1400. Such forms are found, for example, in London, British Library, Additional MS 27944 of Trevisa's translation of *De proprietatibus rerum*, copied by Scribe D of London (see Samuels 1988: 41, and below). It has also been pointed out that cities usually show a higher rate of innovation than surrounding areas; peripheral areas are usually conservative (Samuels 1972: 93). Furthermore, ongoing linguistic changes do not follow the shifting isoglosses neatly, but many forms appear first in London as isolated enclaves before they reach the surrounding areas (Samuels 1972: 168–9).

The patterns of Central Midland features penetrating London dialect emerge through written texts, and there may be differences according to the registers of writing. According to Ian Doyle (1983: 169) the multiplication of Lollard manuscripts could have got going in the metropolis in the 1390s and after 1408, the time when the production in the vernacular was expanding and beginning to concentrate in London; the majority of Lollard books produced in the late fourteenth and early fifteenth centuries were London work (Doyle 1983: 169). Knowledge of scientific texts circulating in the capital and the extent to which Central Midland features are present in them would be important.[6]

9.3.3 Types of London language

London is by far the most important area for the development of writing standards in the Late Middle English period, but the history of London English leaves a great deal unanswered. We know that London English changed in type several times, and different layers are found in it. The dialects of the capital during the later fourteenth and fifteenth centuries are notably heterogeneous (Benskin 1981: 9). The most important account of the characteristics of London English and an overview of the phases and types 1340–1420 are found in Samuels's article from 1963 (revised in 1989). It has been taken as a basis for several new studies and the issues raised in it are very topical (Smith 1996; Stenroos forthcoming). The following main types have been discerned: Type I, 'Central Midland Standard' was the most homogeneous language form; Type II and Type III consist of heterogeneous London texts in which each scribe had idiosyncratic features; and Type IV is the 'Chancery Standard'. The linguistic profiles from London in *LALME* represent Types II and III (LPs 6380 (*The Scale of Perfection*), 6390 (Guild Hall Letter Books I), 6400 (*olim* Hengwrt), 6420 (Hoccleve), 6430 (*Mirror of Simple Souls*), 6500 (*olim* Auchinlech)). According to *LALME*, earlier London texts are placed east and north-east of the city centre, the later ones centrally or north and north-west of the centre (1: 12), but on the whole there is very little about London English.

Of the types of language connected with London, Type I, the Central Midland Standard, is important in connection with scientific writing. It has been described as an 'incipient standard' because it showed wider currency than the original geographical location(s) of its features. It also continued to be copied over a long period, from before 1430 till the later fifteenth century, the time when the dialects of the capital converged markedly on the Central Midland type (Samuels 1989: 68; Benskin 1992: 92; Blake 1996: 170, 173; cf. below). This language type has been described as a distinct, well-defined language form based on the dialects of Northamptonshire, Huntingdonshire, and Bedfordshire (Samuels 1989; *LALME*, 1: 40), but on the whole it has proved difficult or impossible to localise texts written in it or other Central Midland dialects (see below). It has been generally accepted that the Central Midland Standard has the best claim to be the first literary standard after the period of French and Latin dominion (Blake 1996: 169). The main bulk of writing known in this language type is Wycliffite tracts, and other religious and devotional treatises. The connections to special scriptoria are still to be shown, but it is possible that the use of this language type is connected with scriptorial 'house-styles'.

Medical texts are found in this type of language as well. Samuels lists three medical manuscripts written in Central Midland Standard in a footnote of his seminal article (1989: 79, footnote 5, item vii). He mentions Oxford, Bodleian Library, Ashmole MS 1396 with Lanfranc's *Cirurgerie* (base text of Fleischhacker's edition from 1894), London, British Library, Royal MS 17.A.III (an astrological miscellany, R in Voigts's study),[7] and London, British Library, Sloane MS 73 (a mainly alchemical manuscript). In subsequent studies in the British Library on recipe materials (Taavitsainen 2001a), I discovered a fourth manuscript written in a very similar language variety. It is a recipe collection in British Library, Sloane MS 2948, ff. 72–79; the codex also contains pages of a London Sloane Group manuscript (see below). The medical manuscripts written in the Central Midland Standard have not been localised on external evidence as produced in London, but Samuels associates the Central Midland Standard with London (Samuels 1988: 34; and Samuels 1989: 67) in passages like the following: 'There was no standardisation in London . . . until the emergence, ca 1430, of what I have termed Chancery Standard or Type IV. Before that time there are three other types that may be considered, but of these only Type I (Central Midland Standard) comes anywhere near the kind of homogeneity . . .'. During the whole period, apart from Type I, the spelling of each scribe is idiosyncratic (1988: 38–9). In the light of the present assessment, 'house-styles' of scriptoria should be considered in this connection, as they seem to have had an influence on the scribes' writing habits, making them converge more or less in their spelling; even syntactic patterns seem to be affected (see below).

9.4   A hypothetical East Midland scriptorium of mainly surgical texts

A centre of scribal activity producing manuscripts written in the East Midland type of language has been pointed out by McIntosh in 1983. The output of this scriptorium focuses on surgical and anatomical writings, especially by Chauliac and Arderne, but not exclusively. A theological text in the Wycliffite tradition, the *Rosarium*,[8] is firmly associated with it and shows close affinities with some of the medical texts. The history of the identification of this language type is of interest and direct relevance to the present concerns: at first the language of Tokyo, Takamiya MS 59 was considered an unlocalisable *Mischsprache*, with forms of apparently southern origin, like *-eth* in the present indicative plural, co-occurring with northerly features like *-thoff (all)* 'although', and certain other features like *nez* '-ness' and *-ez* in the noun plural, recalling the language of *Sir Gawain and the Green Knight* (see *LALME* LP 26, Cheshire). The facts indicated a 'very circumscribed area of origin with which most of the other features could not possibly be reconciled' (Benskin 1981: 10). In subsequent studies, however, the manuscript was compared with the forms of the *Rosarium* manuscript, localised by Margaret Laing along the Rutland–Lincolnshire–Soke borders. This led to a larger complex of manuscripts with similar features among so far unlocalised texts which in one way or another had been thought dialectally suspect.[9] The result was unexpected: texts by about 50 scribes had similar combinations (Benskin 1981: 10–11). The conclusions are reported in Angus McIntosh's article (1983). The above discovery poses new questions as the connections between the manuscripts are complex, and no conventional explanatory model seems to apply. According to McIntosh's inventory, London, British Library, Sloane MS 1 with Guy de Chauliac's texts is very like Tokyo, Takamiya MS 59, which is another Chauliac manuscript; Sloane 563 (hand C, Arderne), Sloane 3666 (Chauliac), and New York Academy of Medicine, MS 12 (Chauliac) have affinities with both (1983: 243). Two copies of Arderne's texts, British Library manuscripts Sloane 6 (base text of the edition; contains several other learned medical texts as well) and Sloane 277 (Arderne, William of Saliceto, and recipes) are quite similar in language to the *Rosarium*. McIntosh concludes that wherever in the area they originated, they share so many characteristics that they must have been produced in a single scriptorium. Furthermore, McIntosh implies that the manuscripts in the list above are only a few of the whole complex of texts (1983: 243; cf. Benskin 1981), and notes that further studies are needed. This statement is specified in a note where he lists medical manuscripts that merit closer examination in relation to the above-mentioned groups. Sloane 610 (miscellany of medical texts) is indicated as dialectally mixed; Sloane 374 (urinaries and recipes), Sloane 505,[10] Sloane 965 (miscellany, S in Voigts's study), Sloane 1721 (Henry Daniel, *Liber uricrisiarum*), Sloane 2187 (John of Bordeaux, Trevisa, recipes), Sloane 2464 (*Secreta secretum*), Sloane 3466 (recipes, herbals), Sloane 3486 (miscellaneous items, e.g. Gilbertus, Chauliac, and recipes), Paris Bibliothèque Nationale MS Anglais 25 (Chauliac), and London, British Library Additional MS 60577 (herbal lore) 'deserve a mention here' (McIntosh 1983: 243). The meaning of this implication remains unspecified, and to my knowledge it has not been taken up in any subsequent study. What we have here is obviously a widespread and complex pattern of linguistic variation in multiple copies of learned texts. I shall call this type of language the 'Chauliac/*Rosarium* type' to distinguish it from the Central Midland type described by Samuels. All evidence for this complex of scribes comes from linguistic features. There is no knowledge of a medical school in the geographical dialect area of Eastern Midlands that would have promoted the vernacularisation of Guy de Chauliac, Arderne, and other important works. As most of the books in this type of language are medical 'one naturally wonders about the circumstances in which such a large body of materia medica is associated with so small an area' (Benskin 1981: 11).

9.5   External evidence of medical book production in London

The most comprehensive assessment of the conditions of scientific book production in the late medieval period has been made by Linda Voigts (1989b). She outlines the field of scientific writing and its special characteristics. An important observation is that the beginnings of professional book production in scriptoria can be traced to the earlier part of the fifteenth century. Traditionally such practices are associated with the advent of printing, but she suggests antedating Caxton by 50 years (Voigts 1989b: 348). Other studies have also proved that the mode of book trade and manufacture in fifteenth-century London was quite different from that practised earlier in monastic scriptoria (Christianson 1989b: 96). Secular copying flourished and several scribes were active and produced a great number of manuscripts, for example John Shirley is a well-known figure of fifteenth-century literary London.[11] Some scribes focused on the scientific register. There is factual evidence of at least 67 manuscripts and books that can be associated with London book artisans. The works of three textwriters are listed in detail by Christianson (1989b: 107, note 43), but only one of them seems to be relevant in the present connection (Voigts 1989b: 379, 382, 385; Voigts 1995b; Getz 1990b: 259–60). A large number of texts are associated with this scribe, but only one scientific manuscript, consisting of medical texts, Cambridge, Trinity College MS R.14.52, has been ascribed to him (the issue is discussed in Gross 1996: 116–17; Pahta 1998: 123–6; Tavormina forthcoming b).[12]

9.5.1 The Delta Scribe

The above scribes produced some medical manuscripts and texts, but there is even more sociohistorical evidence of a specialised production of medico-scientific codices on a larger scale in London. The Delta Scribe produced scientific or medical manuscripts in prose in the early fifteenth century (Doyle and Parkes 1978; Voigts 1989: 384; Waldron 1991 and 2004). He is perhaps best known for his copies of the *Polychronicon* in three manuscripts, Cambridge, St John's College MS H.1 (204), London, British Library Additional MS 24194 and Princeton, MS Garrett 151. Another very important text by him is Guy de Chauliac's *Cyrurgie*, now in Paris, Bibliothèque Nationale MS Anglais 25 (base text of Ogden's edition). This manuscript was mentioned as deserving special attention by McIntosh (1983). It is the only extant manuscript of version two (Keiser 1998: 251), and a different translation from the other versions (Ogden 1971: vi).

The Delta Scribe is important for the present assessment for several reasons: his language provides evidence for London use in academic scientific texts in the vernacular, and there seems to be a London network of scribal connections. The hand of Scribe Delta is very similar to that of Scribe D who copied the text of *Of the Properties of Things* in London, British Library, Additional MS 27944 (the base text of the edition). This manuscript contains a medical section included in *The Corpus of Middle English Medical Texts* (*MEMT*), and it proved to contain Central Midland features (see above, and Taavitsainen 2000b). The relation of the two scribes has caused some speculation. The most likely explanation for the similarities is perhaps that they were independent practitioners in the same neighbourhood, as evidence for a stronger statement is lacking; this statement would be that the two scribes worked in the same scriptorium or had a master–apprentice relationship (Doyle and Parkes 1978: 206–7; Voigts 1989b: 384). Both scribes seem to have belonged to a group that was copying English works in the

London area during the first quarter of the fifteenth century. This way of thinking is in accordance with the approach to urban environments in terms of spaces (see above), especially as the network can be extended to other scribes who worked in London in Paternoster Row in *c.* 1404 (Waldron 1991: 82; Christianson 1987: 50 and 1989b: 96).[13] In his recent study Waldron (2004) discusses the language of the Delta Scribe and related manuscripts further, paying attention to 'some kind of control exercised over the practice of individual scribes and overriding their own local habits, whether through the establishment of a workshop norm . . . or simply through a policy of reproducing an authoritative exemplar more or less exactly' (Waldron 1991: 86). He also points out a layer of Central Midland features underlying the Central Southern Midland picture emerging from the *Polychronicon* manuscripts. This layer includes features like the P-paradigm (see below), and has led Waldron to suggest another translation, besides Trevisa's, originating in the Central Midland area (Waldron forthcoming).

9.5.2 The Sloane Group

Another very important group of manuscripts from the present viewpoint is the so-called Sloane Group produced in London or Westminster in the mid-fifteenth century (for a discussion on the discourse community, see Jones in this volume). This group comprises a number of medical, alchemical, and astrological manuscripts. Evidence for grouping these manuscripts together and ascribing them to London comes mainly from the physical appearance of the manuscripts. They are so similar that it appears that an individual or a group co-ordinated and controlled their contents and presentation (Voigts 1989b: 384–5; 1990: 37).[14]

The language of the Sloane Group manuscripts is mostly Latin, but some texts are written in English. This vernacular material is not very comprehensive, and the scope of texts varies, nevertheless the linguistic forms in it are important for my study as they provide an anchorage point. The date of several of these manuscripts is known and their provenance has been established. Such socio-historical facts are invaluable, and, for example, the Boston manuscript provides an exceptional case among medical manuscripts as the factors of production are known. The scribe was William Ebesham of London (before 1468), a freelance scribe, working on and off at Westminster, moving backwards and forwards to Norfolk like his employer Sir John Paston (Doyle 1983: 178). Thus in spite of the very professional contents of the manuscript, it was written for a lay person; the links with the East Anglian discourse community show how medical knowledge disseminated from the capital to other parts of the country (see Jones in this volume). The Middle English part in the Boston manuscript has been edited (Harley 1982), and the language of the Boston manuscript has been described by the editor as East Midland.[15] The features in these manuscripts deserve detailed scrutiny as they give first-hand evidence and provide potentially very important information about mid-fifteenth-century London and Westminster English in the scientific register.

9.6   Types of language within medical writing: 'House-styles' of scriptoria?

The above connections with London were made on external evidence, and both the Delta scribe and the D Scribe as well as the Sloane Group provide evidence of specialised book production. More evidence for medical scriptoria has been presented on strictly linguistic grounds. The Central Midland Standard has been defined using linguistic criteria, and McIntosh (1983) assigns a scribal centre focusing on surgical texts to the East Midlands. The occurrence of two different Midland types of language in medical writing seems to point to 'house-styles' of scriptoria with specialised book production. To assess the issue in more depth I shall try to define the features that could potentially reveal the patterns. I compiled a checklist of features containing Samuels's list of Central Midland Standard core forms (Samuels 1989). For the more eastern type of language I studied the linguistic profiles of the scientific texts from the Midlands in *LALME* and compiled a list of possibly diagnostic features. The empirical part of this study is a survey of the linguistic repertoire of features in Guy de Chauliac manuscripts. It would have been futile to make Linguistic Profiles (LPs) of the texts in order to localise them or count the frequencies of various forms. Such an attempt had certainly been made by the *LALME* team at least with some of the manuscripts (see above) and there was no point in trying to repeat it. Instead, a more fruitful way for detecting the possible connections with London was to compare my findings to the English passages in the Sloane Group manuscripts produced in the capital. To complement my assessment, I made electronic searches of some pertinent forms in our electronic database to verify the overall spread of these forms.

9.6.1   Lexical items and spelling variation: Potentially diagnostic features

Samuels (1989) gives the following list of features diagnostic of the Central Midland Standard: SICH 'such', MYCH 'much', ONY 'any', SILF 'self', ȜOUUN 'given', STIDE 'stead', and SIȜ 'saw'. Recent studies (e.g. Smith 1996; Taavitsainen 2000b) have shown that there is some variation in these items, but on the whole, this list serves to characterise the language variety found mainly in Wycliffite writings. The alchemical text of London, British Library, Sloane MS 73 is one of the medical manuscripts written in this language form (LP 4708 in *LALME*).[16] It represents the Bedfordshire variant of the Central Midlands. The other two manuscripts mentioned in Samuels's note (Oxford, Bodleian Library, Ashmole MS 1396 and London, British Library Royal MS 17.A.iii) are not analysed in *LALME* (but see the figures in Voigts's chapter in this volume for some pertinent forms of Royal 17.A.iii). This LP served as the basis of my earlier study of the features that were common in that region, but otherwise limited in their currency. In this study I chose the forms ECH(E, AFTIR, ȜIT, ȜITT, þORUȜ, þOROUȜ, AFTIRWARD, EYR(E, EIR(E 'air', BITWIX, BRENN, BISY, IȜE, YȜE 'eye', FIER, HEED, LYUE, MOUN (pl. 'may'), PUPLE,

Table 9.1. *Variation in Samuels's core list of CMS items in LPs of medical texts from the Midlands*
LP 1 = LP 4708 (Beds): London, British Library, Sloane MS 73, *Book of Quinte Essence.*
LP 2 = LP 432 (Leics): Yale University Medical Library, Foulton MS (Gynecology).
LP 3 = LP 767 (Leics): Tokyo, Takamiya MS 59 (Guy de Chauliac's *Chirurgery*).

LP 1	LP 2	LP 3
siche (sich)	syche, sych ((such))	siche
myche ((miche, mych))	mych (myche)	
	((muche, mykull))	miche (myche)
	ony	any (eny),
	selfe	selfe, silfe ((selffe))
stide, -stede	styd	
ʒoueɳ, ʒeueɳ		giffen (geffen, geven, ʒeuen)
ʒeuen, ʒouen		
siʒen (pt-pl)		sawe

PEPLE, RENN, and TOGIDERE for closer scrutiny. Some of these items proved particularly relevant and seem to characterise the particular Midland varieties in medical texts, and as mentioned above, I could detect a bias towards the Rutland/Leicester area on the basis of this material. This is exactly where McIntosh places the hypothetical East Midland scriptorium. A gynaecological text from Leicestershire has been analysed in full (LP 432) in *LALME*. Another medical manuscript of the Leicestershire area, a translation of Guy de Chauliac's text in Tokyo, Takamiya MS 59 (*olim* Manchester, Chetham's Library 27092) is given as LP 767. Manuscripts with vernacular copies of Chauliac's texts have been mentioned as particularly central in the activities of the hypothetical East Midland scriptorium, and it is also noteworthy that the Delta Scribe of London copied a Chauliac text. LP 767 (Takamiya 59) displays the forms of one of the core manuscripts of Chauliac, which represents the most common version, i.e. version number one. This LP serves as the nearest point of comparison to other surgical manuscripts ascribed to the East Midland scriptorium. Table 9.1 illustrates the scope of variation in the items of Samuels's core list in three LPs of medical manuscripts in *LALME*.

Table 9.2 displays forms that proved especially rewarding in my survey of possibly diagnostic features of the East Midland scriptorium of surgical texts. The list is complementary to the one applied in my previous study (see above). The criteria for the selection of items are the same: the list contains forms that are common in the Midland counties, but otherwise their occurrence is limited. Features that proved most characteristic of the East Midland variety of McIntosh's (1983)

Table 9.2. *Potentially diagnostic features of the Chauliac/Rosarium type of language*
LP 1 = LP 4708 (Beds): London, British Library, Sloane MS 73, *Book of Quinte Essence.*
LP 2 = LP 432 (Leics): Yale University Medical Library, Foulton MS (Gynecology).
LP 3 = LP 767 (Leics): Tokyo, Takamiya MS 59 (Guy de Chauliac's *Chirurgery*).

LP 1	LP 2	LP 3
þo (þose)	þᵒ	þo, tho (þose)
–	though, al-yf	**þof-alle**
		((þof, þoʒ, þoʒ-alle))
þoruʒ	þorogh	þorough
þoruʒt	(þorugh)	
	((þorough))	
bitwene, bitwixe	be-twix	**a-twix**
togidere	to-gedur, to-gedre	to-gider
	(to-gedir, to-gedur)	
((togideres, togedere))		
oon	oon	one (adj. oo, one, o)
oþir	oþer	oþere
	(other, oþur)	(other)
((oþere, oþer, oþire))		
ynowʒ	y-nowe	y-nowe, ynoʒ (Inoʒ)
(y-nowʒ)		
Yʒe	–	eiʒe
yʒen	yeen (yen)	eiʒen ((eyʒen))
((yʒen))		

scriptorium were 'those', 'though', 'through', 'between', 'together', 'one . . . the other', 'enough', and 'eye/eyes'. The pattern emerges from the survey of surgical manuscripts including multiple copies of Chauliac's and Arderne's texts. Table 9.2 shows these core items in the three Midland LPs quoted above. There is considerable variation. The forms that proved most characteristic of the East Midland variety in Chauliac manuscripts in focus in this study are given in bold.

Variation in some other items of the *LALME* questionnaire relevant to this study is shown in Table 9.3. The features of potential interest include 'it', 'they', 'them', 'their', 'are', 'if', 'again', 'since', 'strength', 'air', 'earth', 'enough', 'eye', 'eyes', 'fire', 'flesh', 'give', 'head', high', 'live', 'life', 'neither + nor', 'nigh', 'people', 'fourth', 'sixth', 'two', 'whether', 'why'. I paid special attention to these forms in my empirical survey, but the emerging pattern was not as focused as with the shortlist of items given in Table 9.2. The variation found in LP 3 (the Chauliac MS) seems to describe the present material best.

Table 9.3. *Variation in other pertinent features*
LP 1 = LP 4708 (Beds): London, British Library, Sloane MS 73, *Book of Quinte Essence.*
LP 2 = LP 432 (Leics): Yale University Medical Library, Foulton MS (Gynecology).
LP 3 = LP 767 (Leics): Tokyo, Takamiya MS 59 (Guy de Chauliac's *Chirurgery*).

LP 1	LP 2	LP 3
it	it (yt)	it (hit)
þei	þey ((þei))	þay, þai, thay, thei
		(þei, þaie) ((thai, þaye))
hem ((hem))	þem (hem)	hem (þam)
		((tham, them, hem))
her	hyr	her
((here))	((her, þer, heer))	
ben, beþ	ar, ben	ar ((ben, bene, be, beþ,
(arn, ben)	(be, byn, been)	beþe, beþᵉ))
((ar))		
if	if	if
aȝen	a-ȝeyn, a-ȝeyne	agayne, a-gayne (agayn)
((aȝen))		
siþen	siþe, syþe (syth)	seþ
strengþe	–	strenþe
strenkþe		
eyr	–	aire, ayre
erþe	erthe (ȝerthe)	erþe (erthe)
fier	fyr (fyre)	fire
fleisch	flesche	flesshe (fleshe)
ȝeue	gif (gyfe, gyf)	gif, giff, gif-
heed	hede, hed	heuede (heued, hede)
((heuyd))		
hiȝ	hye (hygh)	hie
lyue	lyu-	liffe
lijf	–	–
neiþer+ne	–	noþer+ne
neiþer +		
nyȝ	ny	ney, nyȝe, nere
–	–	people, peple
fourþe	fourth, fourþe	
–	sixt	sext
two, tueie, tweie	too	two (twayne)
tweye		
((tweyne))		
wheþir	wheþer, wheþer	wheþer
((wheþer))		
–whi	–	whi (why)

Several manuscripts surveyed below have both *it* and *hit* (see Samuels 1972 map 4 for texts with the combined use), several spellings of 'they' and mostly the southern forms of 'them' and 'their'; the present tense indicative, third-person plural of 'be' is manifested in a great variety of forms, especially *ar*, *ben*, and *beþ* in different combinations, *strengþe* seems to be typical, and *-f-* or *-ff-* forms like *life*, *giffe* prevail. Other Midland forms include *als* 'as' in various combinations (*als . . . als*, *als . . . as*, *as . . . als*). Some forms and spellings mentioned in LP 1, for example the *-ij-* spellings, are found in several manuscripts as well, and *-iy-* spellings occur in some (see *LALME* dot maps 1163 and 1164). The characteristics of the *Rosarium* complex also include orthographic variants like *cch* in *mycch*, *ycch*, *-ez* in '-ness', *whilez*, and *-ez* in noun plurals (Benskin 1981: 11). The abbreviations *whᶜ* and *whiᶜ* are also worth attention.

The *Rosarium* contains a large number of variant forms and spellings. The editor points out the great amount of textual variation as a special characteristic (von Nolcken 1979). The following forms were enumerated by the editor of the text as especially characteristic: *War* 'were'; *þof (al)* 'though', *bot* 'but', *hundreþ*, *sex* 'six', *sexte*, *luffe* 'love'; absence of *k* forms in 'which', 'each', 'much'; *-ij-* spellings in words like *lijf*, *cherche* (sporadic), absence of *h* in *it*; absence of *qu-*; unstressed *wiche*, *war*, *wen*, *wy*; *þam* with sporadic *þame*, *þaim(e)*, *hem*; possessive *þar(e)*, *þer*, sporadic *þair*, *her*; *þise (þese)*; endings of verbs in the third-person present indicative *-eþ*, *-iþ*, etc.; *ar* beside *ben(e)*, *be*, *beþ*, *arn*. This list gives the impression of extreme variation. Similar features can be expected of texts ascribed to the same scriptorium.

9.6.2 A morphosyntactic peculiarity of the hypothetical scriptorium: The P-paradigm

The features in the *LALME* questionnaire are mostly concerned with spelling variation and morphological items, but other levels of language may also indicate textual affinities and serve as diagnostic features. A case in point here is the third-person plural ending of the present indicative. The *-eth* ending for the plural can usually be taken as strong evidence of linguistic origin in the southern part of the country, or in the south or central West Midlands. Yet it occurs in a number of Late Middle English texts whose scribes belonged well to the north and east of the main *-eth* area. This morphosyntactic peculiarity was described by McIntosh as the P-paradigm (1983: 238). In this paradigm the present indicative, third-person plural ending is *-eth* when not directly preceded by a personal pronoun, and when preceded by a personal pronoun, either the reduced form or *-en* are found:

(i)   subject not a personal pronoun in contact with the verb
     3rd p. sg. *-eth*
     1, 2, 3 pl. *-eth*
(ii) personal pronouns subject in contact with the verb
     3rd p. sg. *-eth*
     1, 2, 3 pl. *-en* (*-e*, *-ø*)

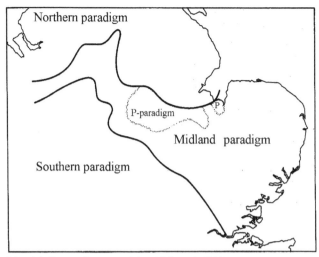

Map 9.1 P-paradigm area (after McIntosh 1983)

The expected paradigm with the repertoire of other linguistic features of these manuscripts would be northern: 3rd p. sg. -*es*; plural not preceded with a personal pronoun -*es*; when preceded -*e*, -*ø* (often -*en* in the south of the northern area). Even the Midland paradigm would be possible: 3rd p. sg. -*eth*; 1, 2, 3 p. pl. -*en* or the reduced forms; -*e* and (though more rarely) -*ø*. The southern -*eth* ending for the plural occurs in the south and west of the Midland area: 3rd p. sg. -*eth*, 1, 2, 3 p. pl. -*eth*; in contrast to the P-paradigm, there are no reduced forms. According to McIntosh's article, the P-paradigm with its 'innovative' -*eth* in the plural is found in a region which includes north-east Leicestershire, Rutland, northern Northamptonshire, the extreme parts of Huntingdonshire, and parts of northern Ely and north-west Norfolk (see map 9.1). In this area, the -*eth* endings do not descend directly from Old English, but they are to be explained as innovations resulting from the influence of a quite different present-tense paradigm, modelled after the northern paradigm immediately to the north of the area in which the P-paradigm was located (McIntosh 1983: 234–8). The combination of northerly features with the -*eth* plural is peculiar, and the extension of -*eth* into the plural has been explained on the basis of equivalence of -*es* and -*eth* in the third-person singular: if -*eth* can be written for -*es* in the singular, then by analogy -*eth* can be extended to place -*es* in the plural (Benskin 1981: 11). This feature is found in the *Rosarium* text, and in the texts of about 50 scribes who combine regular use of -*eth* plural with otherwise northerly-looking features (Benskin 1981). Of these, about a dozen belong to a distinctive sub-set of mostly medical texts, of which the Chauliac manuscripts are screened for this study (see below).

9.7   Vernacular versions of Guy de Chauliac texts

Copies of surgical texts by Guy de Chauliac and John Arderne form the main body of texts using the *Rosarium* type of language. I consulted the most up-to-date reference tools, Keiser (1998) and *eVK* (2000), for information about works by these key authors.[17] My preliminary survey confirmed the affinity, but there was more heterogeneity in the Arderne manuscripts. I shall focus on Chauliac manuscripts in this study. Since 1983 several new copies of his texts have been discovered or identified, and thus my Chauliac material is more comprehensive than that known to McIntosh. I also checked whether the manuscripts were mentioned in the *LALME* list of localised manuscripts. Finally, I surveyed the language of as many of these manuscripts as possible with the aim of detecting similarities or differences between the texts. Guy de Chauliac manuscripts are listed below according to the various versions, as indicated in Keiser (1998); the dates are given according to the information in his list. For practical reasons and limitations of time, it was not possible for me to check all manuscripts in great detail, but I had to confine myself to the passages and to features I considered most pertinent. More comprehensive and detailed accounts remain to be done with studies of individual manuscripts. The survey below is not intended to be comprehensive, but it helps to detect the language type of these surgical texts. I shall comment on the following points:

(1)   Samuels's core forms; Central Midland Standard forms are given in bold. Both *i* and *y* spellings are included as well as forms with or without the final -*e*.

(2)   Features that proved distinctive for the present survey; those that seem most pertinent are given in bold.

(3)   P-paradigm and mixtures, other paradigms.

(4)   Phrases that display the patterns, notes on textual affinities. Other pertinent features noticed while reading passages of the texts.

9.7.1   A London copy of Guy de Chauliac's Chirurgia magna

As the aim of this pilot study is to discuss different language types in medical/surgical texts in relation to scriptoria and metropolitan language use, it seems feasible to start with a manuscript identified on palaeographic evidence as written by a London scribe. It is the copy of Version 2 of Guy de Chauliac's *Chirurgia magna*. This manuscript was said to merit further study in relation to the hypothetical East Midland scriptorium (McIntosh 1983).

1.   **Paris Bibliothèque Nationale, MS Anglais 25**. Copied by Scribe Delta of London; 1425–50.

(1)   *suche, soche; mochil, mochel, moche,* **myche,** *mykel* (see *LALME* dot maps 102, 103, 106 and 109 for this item); *eny, any, self, ʒeuen*

(2)   *tho, þo, þoo, þogh, þoghe, þorgh, bytwene, togedre, togidre, togidres, oon . . . anoþer, oþer, oþir, oþere, inough, inowʒe, eyʒe, eyʒen*

(3) The text shows normal Midland forms:

3rd p. sg.: *þe philosofre scheweth, he saiþ, a corde gooþ*
3rd p. pl. *-n* and reduced forms: *þoo forsoþe þat beeþ written . . . noyen leches forsoþe neden, apostemes þat comen, þai hauen þai ouercome . . . þai trespasse . . .*

Yet there is a passage with mixed forms including *-(e)þ* for 3rd p. pl.:

cordes and ligaments goþ downe and when þai come nygh ioyntes þay beeth made large and þay bynde . . . and þai moven . . . and whan þai passe . . . þoo forsoþe þat beeþ written – such synowes beþ . . . and some forsoþe spryngeþ . . . and passeþ downe . . . but also alle þe synowes forsoþe spryngen . . . þai take felynge

There are reduced forms, but not regularly. The southern paradigm is found in constructions like *when þay passeþ out . . .*

(4) *þoo þinges þat fallen . . . ; euel cokes . . . þai foulen or renten breken or frusshe*

The forms *tho, þo, þoo* are found in the East and Central Midland area, *þogh* shows a wider spread in the same area. The distribution of *þoghe* is more limited, but the form has been recorded from London, too. In contrast, several other forms have not been listed from London. They include *mykel* from list number one, almost all other forms from list two (*tho, þo, þoo, þogh, togedre, inough, inow3e,* and *ey3en*), and some other features like the frequently used *beeþ*. In general, the distribution of the forms confirms a bias towards the East Midland area with regional forms like *eiþer, eyþer* (see *LALME, 4, County Dictionary*). Some spellings like *inough* and *inow3e* have very limited distributions (Northampton and Staffordshire respectively), whereas several forms listed below are common currency.

Some other pertinent features are the co-occurrence of *it* and *hit*, and the preference of *h-* forms in 3rd p. pl. pronouns, except in the nominative: *þei, þai, þay, hem, ham, her, here,* and several forms of 'be': *beþ, beeþ, are, ben* (see *LALME,* 3, dot maps 118, 124, and 128). There is a great deal of variation in all forms, for example *if, 3if, a3eyne, a3en, seþþe, aer, ayre, 3it, from, fro, firste, ferste, werk, chirche, litel, litell, worchyng, wirchynge, worche, wirche, fyry, fleisshe, flesche, 3eue, hede, heed, heued, heuede, hye, hyest, neyþer . . . ne . . . ne, noþer . . . ne, two, tweyne, wheþer, why, whye, ate.* Some of the forms have been mentioned as characteristic of the *Rosarium* type of language, for example *strengþes, lengþe, fourþe,* and *sexte.*

9.7.2 Other copies with no external evidence of their provenance

Version 1:

1. **London, British Library, Harley MS 5915,** fragment 25 (see below New York Academy of Medicine, MS 12)

2. **London, British Library, Sloane MS 1.** Guy de Chauliac, *Chirurgia magna*, ff. 1–7 (*capitulum singulare*, incomplete), ff. 13–312v; 1450–1460. *LALME*: medica, N. Rutland. Wallner version 1.

(1) *siche, suche; miche, myche, moche; silfe, selfe; stede; giffen*
(2) *þo; þof alle, thof alle; atwix, atuix; þorgh; togider; þe tone . . . þe toþer, ynoʒ; eiez, eien*
(3) P-paradigm: 3rd p. sg.: *he seiþ, it goþe, þis same holdeþe*
     3rd p. pl.: *olde men studieþ, lechez forsoþe argueþe*

> . . . *þei come nere . . . þay bynde . . . togider . . . þai moue . . . þei passe . . . þei are . . . þei make . . . thei bene . . . they binde*

But also pl. with -*n*: *þo þingez þat fallen, ligamenteʒ discenden*

(4) *siche is miche, þe toþer two*
> *siche bene like yuel cokez . . . þat kutteþ nozte after þe articulez but brisseþ and crussheþ and ryneþ*

Some other pertinent features:

> There is a great deal of variation in the forms of the 3rd p. pl.: *þay, þaie, þei, þam, her, þaire, þeire, þayre*. Some past participle forms have the prefix *y*-, for example, *yseide; -ff-* spellings are frequent *giffe, giffinge*.

According to McIntosh, this manuscript is close to Tokyo, Takamiya MS 59 (see the LP above).

3. **London, British Library, Sloane MS 965.** Guy de Chauliac, *Chirurgia magna*, ff. 24–106v; *c.* 1450. *LALME*: language of north-east Leicestershire or possibly Rutland. Wallner version 1. (A different kind of manuscript with a calendar and astrological materials.)

(1) *suche, moche, eyen, self*
(2) *tho; though all, though al, thof al; thorugh; atwixte, atwixt, a twixst; togedre, togedir; one, the tone, the thoder, ynoʒ, eye*
(3) P-paradigm: 3rd p. sg.: *he saithe, a muscle gothe, it shewithe*
     3rd p. pl.: *lechez forsothe arguithe . . . , al nerueʒ forsothe springethe. . .*

> *thei go . . . thei with oute for the forsothe strechiþ*
> *thei come nere . . . they bene . . . they bynde . . . togedre . . . thei moue and whanne they passe . . .*

But also pl. with -*n*: *olde men studien, tho thingez that fallen, ligamenteʒ descenden*

(4) *suche is moche*
> *suche ben like euel cokys . . . that cuttithe not after . . . but brosythe crusshithe and ryuithe . . .*

Some other pertinent features:

The forms of the 3rd p. pl. pronouns are *they, thei, them, thaire*; other forms of interest include *flesshe, hede, furst, werking, worchithe, heued, rynnyng water, lyff* (n.), *ageyne, nother* . . . *ne, whedir, ayther, neighing, iche.* Some of them are fairly common, but others have provincial distributions.

Listed by McIntosh among manuscripts meriting further study.

4. **London, British Library, Sloane MS 3666.** Guy de Chauliac, *Chirurgia magna*, ff. 2–7 (*capitulum singulare*), ff. 7–157; 1450–75. Not in *LALME*. Wallner version 1.

    (1) *siche, suych, sich, such; mych, myche; eny, any; silfe, silffe, selfe, selffe; giffen*

    (2) *þo, þose, tho; þof al, thof al, þof alle, þof; þorugh, þorgh; atwix; togider; the tone, þe tone* . . . *the toþere, ynoȝe, eyen, eien, eiez, eiȝen*

    (3) P-paradigm: 3ʳᵈ p. sg.: *he seiþ, he wirkeþ, it goþe*

         3ʳᵈ p. pl.: *olde men studieþ, lechez forsoþe argueþ*

         when þei come nere . . . *þay ben* . . . *þaye bynde* . . . *togider* . . . *þay moue* . . . *and when þei passeþ* . . . *þay ar* . . . *þai make* . . .

But also pl. with *-n*: *crafty men wyrken, and þof al þo þingez þat fallen* . . . , *ligamenteȝ descenden.*

    (4) *sich is mich*
         suche bene like yuel kokez . . . *þat cutteþ nouzt* . . . *but brisseþ or crussheþ and rynethe*

Some other pertinent features:

Both *it* and *hit* are found and the abbreviation *whiᶜ* occurs. Pronoun forms of the 3rd p. pl. include both *th-* and *h-* forms *þei, þai, þay, þam, hem, þaire*; some past participle forms have the prefix *y-*, for example *ytaken, yfounden, -ff-* spellings occur, for example *giffe* (inf.). Other forms of interest include *ȝove, heued, heuede, wyrchingez, whi, oþere, worche, wircheþ, life, aire, agaynez, agayne, rynnyng water, renne, fflessh, flesh, erþe, peple, first, þense, yche, heier, als* . . . *as, þider, hedir and þedir, ȝette, nyȝhing, yche, to ȝove, ychon.*

This manuscript is said to have affinities with London, British Library, Sloane MS 1 and Tokyo Takamiya MS 59 (McIntosh 1983).

5. **New York Academy of Medicine MS 12.** Guy de Chauliac, *Chirurgia Magna*, ff. 8–181v (No. 1, Harley 5915, fragment 25 is the missing leaf from this MS); *c.* 1425. *LALME*: English possibly of north-east Leicestershire or south-west Lincolnshire, but seems to contain an element from further south in Leicestershire or Lincolnshire. Edited by Wallner (included in *MEMT*).

(1) *sich, sych; mich, mych; self*

(2) *þo, tho, þof, þof al, þorgh, atuix, a-tuyx, togider, to-gider, þe tone . . . þe*
     toþer, eye, eyen, yno3

(3) P-paradigm: *he giffeþ*

     in which al men accordeþ, fracturez þat falleþ
     þai say, þai brynge, þai reste . . .

But not regularly: *þai dyen*

(4) Forms of the 3rd p. pl. include both *th-* and *h-* forms: *þai, þei, hem, her, þair;*
     several variants *bene, beþ, ar,* are found. Other forms of interest include
     past participle forms with the prefix *itake, ytake, ysaid,* spellings like *aier,*
     flesh, heued, wirchyng, sithen, siþ, nyz, daiez, strengthez, strengþ, als mych
     as, afore, and the *-f-, -ff-* forms of *life (v.), lyffyn.*

6.   **Tokyo, Takamiya MS 59** (see LP 3 in the above tables); *c.* 1450.
     Version 3:

7.   **Oxford, Bodleian Library, MS 7004, Ashmole MS 1468**; pp. 7–54;
     1400–50. The Chauliac manuscript has not been assessed for *LALME*. Be-
     gins in the middle of Book I, chapter i, and ends in the middle of book VII,
     chapter i. Wallner version 4.

     (1) *suche, moche, ony, eny, any, hymself, hemself, yeven*

     (2) *þoo, tho, all yif, all yf, atwyx, atwix, betwix, thurgh, þurgh, þorugh, togidre,*
          togedre, ynough, eye, ey3e, eyen, ey3en, þe toon . . . þe tother

     (3) The P-paradigm is not found. The ending of the 3rd p. sg. is *-eth: it*
          renneth, renneþe, the 3rd p. pl. has the *-en* ending mostly, but not regularly:

          þei come nygh . . . þey spreden abrode and bynden þe joyntes all aboute . . . w^t
          hem þat couereth þe bones & þe cordes and þe ligamentes mevyn . . . þey make
          some couereth

     (4) Both *it* and *hit* occur (*hit semeth, hit is to witen*); *they, þei, her, their, them,*
          hem; be, ben (summe ben lesse & summe be more), flesshe, toward, lyf(n.), *oon,*
          oo, two, nygh, fourthe, sixt, eyre, hye, seth, sith 'since', *strength, strengthid* pp.,
          heued, neyther . . . neþer, noyther . . . neyþer, for whi, yif, eyther, ayen, litell,
          no3t allonly, natheles, fro, these, þese, theise, hye, heyest, ou3t of þe heued, fro,
          syxe skilles . . . the first . . . the secunde . . . the thirde . . . the fyrthe . . . the
          fyfte . . . the sixte . . .
          n. pl. endings: *-es, -is, -z.*

Some other pertinent features:

     . . . and summe bothe þe ton & þe tother and summe neither þe ton ner þe
     tother . . .
     . . . þei take noon harme nether be not wasted when þey meue to gedir . . .

8.   London, British Library, Sloane MS 3486. Guy de Chauliac, Betrisden, Thomas (attr.), *The Great Surgery, Chirurgia Magna*, ff. 58–80v, incomplete, contains anatomy only. Not in *LALME*; *c.* 1460. Wallner version 4. (A different type of manuscript with several other texts.)

The beginning of the text on f. 58 has distinct regional spellings of the area indicated in map 1, Norfolk and further north (see *LALME* dot map 272) *þe qwych*, and *ffro qwy* but these spellings are soon abandoned in favour of the more common Chauliac variety. The only 3rd p. sg. pres. ind. ending in -*es* is also found at the beginning *Rasys says*. The forms below are from f. 58v on:

(1) *siche, sich, mych, mich, mychel, ony, selfe, yeuen*
(2) *þo, þoo, all if, alle if, þorgh, þur3, atwix, togydre, þe tone . . . þe toþer, ynou3, ye, yen*
(3) P-paradigm is not found. The ending of the 3rd p. sg. is -*eþ: Galien seithe, seiþe, it renneþ* but the 3rd p. pl. follows the normal Midland pattern with -*en* and the reduced forms immediately after the personal pronoun: *phisiciens arguen, veynes þat gone, þei ioyne*. This is, however, not regular: *þei come nye . . . þei spreden . . .*
(4) *neiþer þe tone neiþer þe toþer*

Some other pertinent features:

it, ytt (see *LALME*, 3, dot map 26), *thei, þei, hem, her, ben, bien, 3yf, ferþe* 'fourth', *erþe, rynnyng, it renneþ, flesh, yit, neiþer . . . neiþer, yeve, worcheþ, but, hede, boþe, nye, ayein, þei weren, eyre, seth, hye, hyest.*

Listed by McIntosh as meriting further study in relation to the hypothetical East Midland scriptorium (McIntosh 1983).

9.   Glasgow University Library, Hunter MS 95; *c.* 1425. Not in *LALME*.
(1) *sucche, suche, myche, moche, mochel, eny, enye, self, selfe, stede, 3euen*
(2) *þo, þoo; alle 3if, atwixe, a-twixe, þoru3, þoru3-oute, þurgh, þur3, togider, togidere, þe tone . . . þe toþer*
(3) mixed use: *cordes & ligaments, and whyle þei cumme nei3 . . . þei spreden abrode & bynden . . . wiþ hem þat couereþ þe bones and þo cordes . . . þo ligaments meuen . . .*
(4) *liyf, nei3, nye, 3itte, 3et, lengþe*

10.   New York Academy of Medicine MS 13, ff. 1–51v, falsely attributed to Roger Marshall.[18] Not in *LALME*.
(1) *sich, sucche, mych, myche, moche, enye, selfe, 3euen*
(2) *atuix, a-tuix, atuyx, a-tuyx; y3e*
(3) No P-paradigm, but some mixed use: *cordes & ligaments, and whyle þei cumme neiz . . . þei spreden abrode & bynden . . . with hem þat couereþ þe bones and þo cordes þo ligaments meuen . . . þei waxen rounde . . . þei maken*

(4) *-iy-* spelling *liyf;* other interesting forms *lengþe, fleische* (see dot map 420), *flesche*.

Version 4:

11.   **Cambridge University Library, MS Dd.3.52.** Guy de Chauliac, *Chirurgia magna*, ff. 11–249v; 15 cent. Not in *LALME*.

(1) *sich, siche, suche; eny; mych, mich; self; giffen*

(2) *þo; þof all, þof al; atuix, atwix; þe tone . . . þe toþer; togidre, to gidre, þe tone . . . þe toþer, eiz, eyen, ynoʒ*

(3) P-paradigm: 3rd p. sg.: *he erreþ, it scheweþ*
3rd p. pl.: *lechez forsoþ argueþ, chirurgiens . . . trespasseþ, olde men studieþ*

   þai come ner . . . þai bene . . . þai bynde . . . move . . . þei passe . . . þai ar . . . þai bynde, þai make; thurgh whens þay passe . . . þai go

But also pl. *-n: þof all þo þingez that fallen . . . ligamenteʒ descenden.*

(4) *sich is mych*

   Siche bene lyke evyl cokez . . . þat cutteth noʒt . . . but brusseth and crussheþ and ryneth . . .

Some other pertinent features:

   hit and *it, itte* (see *LALME*, 3, dot map 26); *th-* forms of the 3rd p. pl.: *þai, þam, þair;* and past participle forms with the prefix *ycaste,-ff-* spellings, e.g. *giffe; lyfe* (n.). Other forms of interest include *ar, bene, sith, ʒitte, ayther, fire, fflessh* (see *LALME*, 3, dot map 423), *heved, hiʒe, nowþer, neiʒhyng, tuo* (see *LALME*, 3, dot map 551), *two; whi, yche, fire brent, wheþer, which, wich, rennyng.*

This manuscript is not mentioned by McIntosh (1983). It contains passages of other Guy de Chauliac versions as well, but the treatise studied above forms the main contents of the manuscript (see *eVK* for further information).

12.   **Cambridge, Gonville and Caius College MS 336/725.** Guy de Chauliac, *Chirurgia magna*, ff. 17–42v (incomplete); 15 cent. Not in *LALME*. Wallner version 3.

(1) *sich, siche, miche, myche, ony, silf, ʒolden, ʒouen*

(2) *þo, þouʒ, þouʒ al, þoruʒ, through, bitwixe, togidere, þe oon, þe toon . . . þe toþere, iʒe, iʒen*

(3) P-paradigm forms: 3rd p. sg.: *it springiþ, it goiþ, it byndiþ*
3rd p. pl.: *lechis forsoþe argueþ,*

whanne þei come nere . . . þei binde . . . togidere and þei move . . . þei
passe, ligamentis which descendiþ . . . passiþ

But not regularly:

> *they that touchiþ . . . ȝitt more þei þat touchen . . . owen to be doon . . .*
> *þei ȝeue; alle nerves forsoþe springen*
> (4) *sich is myche, siche ben yuele . . . cokis . . . þat kuttiþ*
> *-ij-* spellings: *sijknes, lijk, sijk, lijknesse, wijn, lijf, arterijs; -iy-* spellings:
> *wiyn.*

Some other pertinent features:

> *þei, hem, her; ben, ȝitt, ȝitte, heed, aftir, strenkþis* (see *LALME*, 3, dot map
> 268), *aȝen, aȝens, neiþir, eiþir, worchinge, axe, axid, rennynge, heed, ffier, eir,*
> *air, heiȝþe, iche, hidirward* (see dot map 442), *þidirward* (see *LALME*, 3,
> dot map 531), *whi* and past participle forms with the prefix *ycast, yseid.*

Not mentioned by McIntosh. The manuscript has some of the items included in
the Sloane Group manuscripts.

13.   **Cambridge, Jesus College MS Q.G.23.** Guy de Chauliac, *Chirurgia*
Magna, ff. 20–408v. 15 cent. Not in *LALME*. Wallner version 3.
(1) *swiche, such; moche, eny, stedis (pl.), silf, ȝouen*
(2) *þo, þoȝ, alþoȝ, þoru oute, bitwene, oþir, togider, togidre, yȝen*
(3) P-paradigm is not found, but the pattern follows the common Midland
   forms:
   3rd p. sg. *-eþ: he seiþ;* 3rd p. pl.: *þo þingis suffisen; þei telle not, þei falle*
(4) *such forsoþe ben lik schrewid cokis . . . þat taken no hede*

Some other pertinent features:

> The paradigm *þei, þem, þeir, here; ben, arn, er* 'before', *ȝif, ȝeueþ, aȝen,*
> *ȝit, ȝut* 'yet', *wich, hundred, þilk* (see dot map 84), *boþe, sith,* and *ech* (see
> *LALME*, 3, dot map 86).

Recently discovered, see Wallner (1991) and Lucas and Lucas (2001). The
manuscript has elaborate ornamentation.

14.   **London, British Library, Sloane MS 2463.** Guy de Chauliac, *Chirurgia*
magna, ff. 2–51v. Not in *LALME*, not mentioned by Keiser (1998). Wallner
version 4 (includes Mondeville).
(1) *suche, moche, silf, self, ony, yeven*
(2) *þo, tho, all yif, alle yif, thurgh, þroughouȝt, þorughouȝt, thorugh, þorulig,*
   togeder, togedir, togedyr, atwix, betwix, betwixt, þe ton . . . þe toþer, þe
   thother, the toþ^{fr}, eye, eyȝe, eyȝen

(3) P-paradigm is not found, but the pattern follows the common Midland paradigm: 3rd p. sg. *-eth, -eþ, -ith: it makiþ . . . wexith, waxith, gothe, goth.* The plural ending is *-en: bothe oolde ffisissiens and yonge studyen; they faylen; þey waxen*

(4) *Galyene lykneth suche surgens to euell cokes . . . they grynden and brosen and wasten . . . neyþer þe ton ner þe toþer.*

Some other pertinent features:

The forms *it, hit,* and *yt* (see *LALME,* 3, dot map 27) co-occur; the pronoun forms of the 3rd p. pl. are *they, þei, hem, them, her, here.* Other forms of interest include *ben, bene, ethir . . . ethyr, ethir . . . ethir, eyther, fourthe, werchyth, yf, yef, yif, ʒif, yet, oon, one, oo, yif* 'give' (see *LALME,* 3, dot map 426), *heued, sixte, renneth, rennen, seth, boþe, bothe, nyhg, fro, eyr, lyf, lif* (n.), *þanne, þen, eche, whether, wheþer, whi, why, flessche, flessch, fleshe, flesh, mowe pl.* 'may', *toward, ayen, sixt, sixte, fourþe, neyther . . . neþer, neþʳ thither.*

Mentioned by McIntosh (1983) as meriting further study.

9.7.3 A related manuscript

In addition to the ones mentioned in the *eVK,* I noticed that the anatomical tract in London, British Library, Harley MS 1736 shows the influence of Chauliac's *Anatomy* very clearly, and some passages derive almost directly from it (anatomy e.g. skin), some other parts show the influence of Arderne's *Fistula in ano* (e.g. the qualities of a surgeon).

London, British Library, Harley MS 1736 Bradmore, John, *Philomena*: London, British Library, Harley MS 1736, ff. 6v-184; ed. Beck 1974 (excerpts) (attributed to Thomas Morstede); Lang 1992 establishes John Bradmore's *Philomena* as Latin original; Lang 1992 ed. London, British Library, Harley MS 1736, ff. 48, 117v. Not in *LALME.*

(1) *swych, syche, sych, mych, selfe, gyffyn*

(2) *ʒif all, throw, betwyx, betwyne, togedyr, all þe tody, othyr, odyr,*

(3) P-paradigm:
3rd p. sg.: *yt semyth, for as galyene sayth*
3rd p. pl.: *The nervys þe wyche . . . takyth the schape*

Sum ligamenttes byndyth; thei shew, thei pase . . . thei make . . . thei bynd . . . and th ei moue yt and thus yt sessys not vnto þe vttyrest partycle, thei wax

But also *-es: þe erbe . . . schewes not* (in the prologue), *yt sessys*

(4) *swych ys mych.*

Some other pertinent features:

The co-occurrence of *yt* and *it*, and *th*-forms of pronouns *thay, them, ther*, and, for example, the following *ar, ben, myrke* (v.), *flesch, fflesch, fleche, flesche, agayne, fyrst, whytyr, wyche, wych, qwyche, syne* 'since' (see *LALME*, 3, dot map 238), *sythe, ychon, hed, hede, agayne, pepull, heyer, eydyr, ner, gyf* 'give', *neydyr . . . nor, aftyr,* and *-f-, -ff-* forms in, for example, *haffe, lufe.*

9.8 Spread of the diagnostic features in the *Corpus of Middle English Medical Texts* (*MEMT*)

Some of the forms indicated as typical of the Central Midland Standard in Samuels's core list (SICH, MYCH, ONY, SILF, 3OUUN, STIDE, SI3) are frequent in *MEMT*, but items vary in their frequency (see Taavitsainen 2000b). The most common are SICH, SYCH. Besides the manuscripts of Lanfranc and *Quinte Essence* (from the manuscripts listed as written in Central Midland Standard by Samuels 1989), several other texts have these forms: Gilbertus Anglicus, the *Phlebotomy*, Arderne, Chauliac, Mondeville, and Chirurgie 1392. MYCH is also fairly frequent, but some other forms of the core list are not found in this material. A more detailed assessment of these features in the corpus remains to be carried out in a future study; my purpose here is to survey the Chauliac manuscripts and to indicate connections between various texts.

Table 9.2 features are rarer in *MEMT* material and focus on certain texts, as could be expected. These forms have limited distributions (*LALME*) so that they can be considered diagnostic of the 'Chauliac/*Rosarium*' type of language in medical writing. The *atwix* type serves best as a distinguishing feature, as it is confined to two relatively compact areas (see *LALME*, 3, dot map 1118). One is on the borders of southern Lincolnshire, eastern Leicestershire and Rutland, the other includes parts of Norfolk, Suffolk, and Cambridgeshire (Benskin 1981: 8). In addition to texts by Chauliac and Arderne, the *atwix* type is found in the *Phlebotomy* in several variant forms: *atuix, atuixe, atwix,* and *atwene*. The type is also found in *Benvenutus Grassus* and Mondeville's surgical treatise. The *between, betwixt* type is more common in general in the present material. Some of the forms are very limited in their geographical spread (see below), partly overlapping with the *atwix*-area, for example the form *bytwyxe*, which was recorded in the survey of manuscripts, but is not found in the corpus at all.

Another feature worth closer scrutiny is 'though' which occurs in a variety of forms: *thof, þof,* and *þof al*. The geographical distributions are limited so that *þof al* is found in Derby and Nottinghamshire only, *thof* in Cheshire, Derby, Leicestershire, Nottinghamshire, East Riding Yorkshire, and West Riding Yorkshire, while *þof* is more widely spread in the same area and a little further north and west. In addition to Chauliac and Arderne, the *Phlebotomy* text has the forms *þof* and *þofe*. Other features are revealing as well. *þoru3* shows a fairly wide spread in *LALME*, including London. In *MEMT*, it is found in Chauliac, *Quinte*

Essence, Lanfranc, Mondeville, Chirurgie 1392. *þorgh* has a similar distribution in *LALME*, and in *MEMT* it occurs in Chauliac, Mondeville, and Chirurgie 1392. *þe tone . . . þe toþer* are very rare forms in *LALME*, and although this item might easily be recorded in different ways by editors and thus be an unreliable feature, a distinct pattern emerges in *MEMT*. The great majority is again found in Chauliac's and Arderne's texts, but they are also found in the gynaecology text from Leicestershire (see LP 2), *Benvenutus Grassus* and in the remedy collection 'In hoote somere' in Cambridge, Trinity College MS R.14.51, ff. 1–45.

The searches of the above features in *MEMT* confirm the pattern of two different Midland types of language: the Central Midland Standard type with the *Quinte Essence* and Lanfranc at the core, and the other more eastern type. The corpus reveals an affinity between Chauliac, Arderne, and the *Phlebotomy* text, which has not been mentioned in this connection before. The *Phlebotomy* contains several diagnostic features of the Chauliac / *Rosarium* type. Further evidence of the affinity can be found in the P-paradigm, which occurs in the *Phlebotomy* as well, for example in the following passages:

> *Also* **sum men** *of custum when þey are flebotomyd* **swoneþ**. . . (ed. Voigts and McVaugh 1984: 39)

> If þis ys hit that **old men** *owth* to be fleobotomyd after mete when **they** have aboue slepp, yong men forsoþ affore mete, for old men are more feble, yong men more strong. Also þer is anothyre resone: for **yong men** sith **þey abovnd** with hote humoris **owth** to be flubotomid in þe ouyr of hote homors – if blode abovnd, afore terce, if colere, atwix terce and none. (ed. Voigts and McVaugh 1984: 39)

Forms in accordance with the Midland paradigm are also found:

> And of fleubotomye þese þynge[s] sufisyn . . . (ed. Voigts and McVaugh 1984: 53)

These features show that the Chauliac / *Rosarium* language type in focus here was not limited to Chauliac and Arderne, but other learned texts contain similar features. I intend to assess this issue in a further study.

9.9 Vernacular texts in the Sloane Group of London and Westminster medical manuscripts

A potentially important group of manuscripts for identifying language patterns in medical manuscripts of London and Westminster scriptoria is the Sloane Group. It provides important evidence of linguistic features in contemporary medical texts in the capital. These manuscripts did not, however, prove very helpful. In the core group, the pertinent folios have texts in Latin, or Latin and French only, for example London, British Library, Sloane MS 2320 (dated 1454), Sloane MS 2948 (dated 1462) and Sloane MS 1313 (dated 1458). Sloane MS 2567 has texts in Latin and English on alchemical processes, but the material is very limited and there is not enough text for real comparison. The following forms are of interest: *thorough, eire* 'air', *eche, after, moche, fyre, fuyr*, and they serve to indicate that this language type is not the same as in the manuscripts discussed above. Two of the Sloane 'half-sister group' manuscripts proved more rewarding (see also Jones in this volume). Boston, Countaway Library of Medicine, MS 19, is valuable for the knowledge of its provenance, but it does not yield much material for dialectal analysis. Some forms point to the Central Midlands rather than London. Cambridge, Trinity College MS O.1.77, dated 1460, is another manuscript of this group. It provides more material for comparison. The following forms are found in it:

(1)   *such, suche, mych, moche, eny, silf, silfe*
(2)   *þough, þorugh, thorugh, þorough, thourgh, bytwene, bytwen, bytwyxe, bitwyxte, bitwene, bitwixt, bytwyxen, bytwixte, togedir, yen, eyen*

The features in list (1) above include some Central Midland standard forms. List number (2) above has spellings not recorded in London, for example *þorugh* and *þorough*; only *þough* is recorded from London in *LALME*. The forms of 'between' are most revealing as they point to the East Midlands and surrounding areas. The *County Dictionary* of *LALME* shows that, for example, *bytwyxe* is found in Northamptonshire only, *bytwen* is found in Lancashire, Norfolk, and Staffordshire, and some of the forms (*bitwyxte, betwixt*, and *bytwixte*) are not in *LALME* at all.

(3)   The Midland Paradigm: The following third-person singular ind. pres. endings are found: *-ith, -iþ, -yþ, -eth, -yth*; *he goith, goiþ, goyþ, þis planete dwelliþ, ilke one haþ, fyghtiþ, destruyþ þe liyfly spirites*
        3rd p. pl. ind. pres. has *-en* and the reduced forms: *men fallen, planets mouen, they passe not, where þey gone þey caste hir yen unto þe erþe* (f. 126).

The paradigm of the 3rd p. pl. pronoun has both *th-* and *h-* forms: *they, þey, þei, hem, hir*. There are several items that show forms of common currency: *þese, these, thes, þes, dayes, daies*, etc. but there are also items with more provincial spellings and some of very limited currency. For example, *pepil* (f. 126) is a more northern form, *peple* (f. 128v) is more common elsewhere but not in London; *feyr* is recorded from Norfolk, Suffolk and some more southern locations. The form *dyȝe* 'die' has been recorded from Leicestershire, Norfolk, East Midlands and more north, *sythen* is East Midland and London, *þrydde* is East Midland and more to the north but not in London. *Sterris* is local in the area that includes the counties in focus (Buckinghamshire, Cambridgeshire, Derby, Isle of Ely, Huntingdonshire, Norfolk, Northamptonshire, Nottinghamshire, and Soke of Peterborough). There are many more examples of similar distributions, for example *fruytes, wirche, oon* (*LALME*, 3, dot map 857), *fleische, fleisch, ayr, aeyr, whiles, fourþe, chirche, renner, sterry heuen, neighnes* (*LALME*, 3, dot map 846), *lengþe, lyfe, ylke, er, nyȝe, ȝeuyþ*, and *tofore*. A great deal of variation is found in forms like *ben, ben, are, aren, if, ȝif, ȝit, ȝitte, fro, froo, from, from, euyl, yuel*, *iche, ech, eche, how, hou, passand oute* (f. 77), but also *-ing -yng.* An interesting *-iy-* spelling is found in *liyfly* (f. 74).

The above list of forms shows that the language of this codex has a very provincial character. Many of the forms listed above have limited distributions and show affinities with the Chauliac/*Rosarium* type of language. Several features are localisable in roughly the same area of East Midlands where the *Rosarium* was located (see McIntosh 1983). Yet there is external evidence that the manuscript was written in London *c.* 1460. There are differences as well, for example the paradigm of present indicative is in accordance with the Midland use.

9.10 Conclusions

This study shows that two different Midland types of language are found within medical writing. The Central Midland Standard type is one, the Chauliac/*Rosarium* type another, and both are found in several manuscripts. The Central Midland Standard, Samuels's Type I, has been connected with London, but its affinities with special scriptoria are still to be shown. The present survey points very clearly to a 'house-style' in Guy de Chauliac's surgical texts, but the features are present in varying degrees in other surgical manuscripts as well. The copies show variation, but on the whole they are so similar that they must have been produced under some kind of control (cf. McIntosh 1983; Waldron 1991 and 2004). The Delta Scribe provides a link to a London network of scribes, writing roughly a quarter of a century earlier than most of the scribes who wrote the manuscripts surveyed for this chapter. Scribe Delta's copying practices have been studied and he seems to vary from manuscript to manuscript (cf. Scribe D). He did not translate into his own type of language but followed the exemplars to the extent their repertoire was familiar. Several local forms from the East Midland dialect area are retained. Another important anchorage point is provided by the Sloane Group of manuscripts as their provenance has been defined on external evidence as London and the date is roughly contemporary with the Chauliac/*Rosarium* type of manuscripts (i.e. late for *LALME* localisations). The above survey of the linguistic features in one of the medical texts of the Sloane Group shows that provincial features were current in London manuscripts in scientific/medical register even in the middle of the fifteenth century.

All external evidence for a London location of the scriptorium writing in the Chauliac/*Rosarium* type of language is lacking, but the repertoire of linguistic features seems to fit in an urban environment. The innovative P-paradigm is basically a contact phenomenon. A metropolitan setting certainly provided plenty of opportunity for contact between people from different dialect areas. Other features like the co-occurrence of *hit* and *it* (*yt, itt*), *th-* and *h-* forms, with a preference for *h-*forms in the oblique cases, and the prefix *y-, i-* in past participle forms combine with features that suggest a much more northern origin, for example *thof (al)* and *atuix* in these texts. In the earlier literature, it has been suggested that unexpected combinations were a characteristic of metropolitan centres. Accordingly, the new metropolis with its immigration patterns and swiftly growing specialisation in the book trade may well provide a feasible explanation for the co-occurrence of such features. There are no records of a scribal centre with an output of learned medical texts in the East Midland area. The texts written in the Chauliac/*Rosarium* type of language may well have a connection with the capital. This assumption is supported by the likelihood of a discourse community of a high professional level in the capital rather than in the peripheral area indicated by Map 9.1. The motivations for the demand of learned texts in the vernacular, like Chauliac's treatises and the *Phlebotomy*, must have been in accordance with the ideology of vernacularisation in general and the desire to create a new prestige register of learned scientific writing in English (see Taavitsainen 2001b and Pahta and Taavitsainen in this volume). The language forms invite some further speculation. Some learned texts are written in the Central Midland Standard that has been located in London in earlier studies, but the more eastern type of language with its unexpected mixture of forms and no external evidence of provenance invites some speculation. It may be assumed that the translator/exemplar came from a provincial area, but the copies may have been multiplied in a metropolitan location, perhaps by scribes from the same parts or scribes whose linguistic repertoire encompassed the provincial features of the exemplar. This suggestion is in accordance with the view that the multiplication of Lollard manuscripts took place in the metropolis, and that the majority of Lollard books produced in the late fourteenth and early fifteenth centuries were London work (Doyle 1983: 169). Perhaps a comparison of forms of the scientific register with those of Lollard manuscripts produced in London would cast light on the issue. It is likely that we have 'house-styles' of specialised scriptoria here, and that the scribes' individual copying practices show in the linguistic repertoire of these texts. I shall pursue these issues in a further study. The conclusions here have been made on text internal evidence, but what we ultimately need to solve the problem is external evidence of the provenance of the manuscripts.

Notes

1. Scribal practices in medieval England have become an important object of study with the insight that written language operates in its own right. Thus, any consistently written Middle English text is capable of accurate localisation, and through regional language use it is possible to gain knowledge of the place where the scribe learned to write (*LALME* 1987: 4, 23). The present attitude rules out the word 'merely' from the above quotation by Bonaventura, and 'changing nothing' has long ago been found untenable (see below).

2. A rough estimate that social variation is reflected in the different traditions of writing does not hold as such, but applies perhaps more to the academic spectrum end of texts with Latinate models, whereas recipes and remedies were owned and read by a wide range of lay people as well as professional medical men, and the tradition was longer.

3. In addition, scientific register seems to have resisted the spread of the national standard for a fairly long time. This line of enquiry must, however, be left to future studies. The relation of medical language to the Wycliffite variety of Central Midland Standard is another major issue which requires further study, but it is beyond the scope of this chapter, as is the origins of the Central Midland Standard. The questions include whether Wycliffite manuscripts were made mostly in one centre or in several. The places mentioned in this connection include Oxford, London, Northampton, and Leicester (Doyle 1983: 169). The overlap with those mentioned as possible locations of medical manuscripts is striking, and even Oxford can be connected through Trevisa as a link (see Taavitsainen 2000b; see also Stenroos forthcoming).

4. In addition, there are texts with local features from different parts of the country. See *LALME*, 1, *Index of Sources*, with manuscript contents.

5. Dialect levelling is usually understood as the abolishment of most distinctive and provincial dialect features, taking place, for example, when speakers of different dialects come together. Studies on present-day materials focus on phonetic features and spoken language, see, for example, Trudgill (1986). The present material is different, and the question seems to be rather of dialect mixing than levelling. For a discussion of the various terms and processes in language contact, see Siegler (1985).

6. More external evidence of manuscripts written in London, scribal connections and practices will certainly cast new light on the issue. Linne Mooney is currently working on medieval scribes, and there is an ongoing project at York (see Pahta and Taavitsainen, p. 6 above)

7. The lunary text has been edited by Taavitsainen (1987).

8. The *Rosarium* is a Lollard text, an abbreviation of a longer compilation, made apparently to facilitate access to preachers of a handbook that they might find useful. The *Rosarium* supports Lollard viewpoints and helped to organise the structure of sermons. Concern for precision and accuracy is evident as accurate references are provided throughout, though the intended audience was far removed from the academic world (Hudson 1989: 128).

I am grateful to Dr Matti Peikola for providing me with an electronic copy of the text which I used to find the linguistic items under discussion in this study.

9. The Introduction of *LALME* notes special difficulties in connection with 'literary' manuscripts: the language of a manuscript may be Central Midland, but the local origin escapes identification: 'it appeared that little would be contributed to an understanding of the regional pattern by investigating yet more material of the same type. Accordingly, such writings were commonly passed over in the work that followed' *LALME*, 1: 40). The observation rests on a large number of witnesses, which are not, however, mentioned in more detail. *LALME* divides the materials into literary and documentary; medical writing is included in the former category, though these texts are usually classified as non-literary (confirmation from Benskin).

10. London, British Library, Sloane MS 505 seems to be an error, as it is, in fact, an Early Modern English manuscript on maritime journeys. It is not mentioned in *eVK*.

11. His works do not contain medical texts as such. He focused on vernacular poetry, particularly on the shorter poems of Chaucer and Lydgate, but the precise nature of his activities is not known and there are several divergent views (Connolly 1998: 1–5). He could have run some kind of a lending library and copied mainly literary manuscripts. Nearest to the scientific register in Shirley's manuscripts come tracts in

the *secreta secretum* tradition, occasional recipes included in his books (see *IMEP* 9 and 11), and the lunary poem under the false title 'A Dietary for Mans Heele' (*IMEV* 970; see Taavitsainen 1988). A regimen text printed in 1506? is also ascribed to Lydgate, but this is a false ascription as the text seems to be Mirfield's *Breviarium Bartholomei* (I owe this information to Glen Hanhingham).

12. A current research project lead by Teresa Tavormina aims at establishing facts and describing Cambridge, Trinity College MS R.14.52 in detail, and making more texts in it available to scholars (see Tavormina forthcoming b); some of the results influenced the chapters of this book as well.

13. Scribe D has been connected with the workshop of Herman Schierre or Skereuyeren, who copied Latin texts.

14. The following manuscripts form the core group: London, British Library, Sloane MSS 2320; 1118 (ff. 15–147a); 1313 (ff. 135–42); 2567 (ff. 4–10); 2948 (ff. 34–51 and 53–59); and Additional MS 19674 (ff. 1–72). Three manuscripts come fairly close to the core: Sloane 3566, Cambridge, Trinity College, MS O.1.77, and Boston, Medical Library manuscript, Ballard Catalogue No. 19, also known as Harvard medical MS. Two manuscripts, Cambridge, Gonville and Caius College, MS 336/725 and Tokyo, Takamiya MS 33, are from the 1480s or from the 1490s and can be regarded as descendants, and three further manuscripts, London, Wellcome Historical Medical Library MS 784, London, British Library, Additional MS 5467, and Oxford, Bodleian Library, Rawlinson MS C.815, also bear some resemblance to the group (Voigts 1990: 27; see the appendix of her article for further details). Several of these codices contain other manuscripts as well. For example, Sloane 1313 is a composite volume with several manuscripts bound together, but the other manuscripts in the codex may have no connection with the Sloane Group. A recipe collection has some interesting forms, for example *hed, mych, stede, aftyr, ich* 'each', *togedyr, thorow, self, ilkon, mykyll, qwhan, fyr*. The next English item is 'The mervelous & sothefast connyng' with nativities. It has the following forms: *fyre, heed, mykle, eny, aftyr, ʒouen, xall, brent, fyre, fyer ayen* 'again', *such, lyff, lyf* v., *hym sylff*. Some of the forms are in accordance with Samuels's core list (1989); but some point to more provincial areas, for example *xall* and *qwhan*.

15. The facts about the provenance have been discovered after Harley wrote her article. The contents made her conclude that 'the original handbook was compiled for a trained physician' and that 'the inclusion of these three pieces in Middle English testifies to the growth of informational works in the vernacular in the fifteenth century' (Harley 1982: 172). The latter part of the quotation holds, and becomes even more emphasised with the new knowledge of the commissioner. Her dialectal analysis is in accordance with the method developed by Meech, Moore, and Whitehall, and based on, for example, the following, most important criteria: the development of Old English *a*, *who-so*; the present indicative 3rd p. pl. ending in *-en, fallen*; consistent use of *sh* in *shall*, etc; Old English *a* before a nasal is unchanged, *mannys*; the oblique case of the 3rd p. pl. pronoun is 'them'; the present indicative 3rd p. sg. ending in *-ith, -yth*, or *-eth, behouyth, signifieth*; there is no voicing of Old English initial *f*; and the present participle ending is *-yng, asking* with *passand* as the single exception (Harvey 1982: 173). There is room for a reassessment.

16. The LP is made on the basis of the *Book of Quinte Essence*. I checked the other texts as well, and they seemed to be in the same kind of language, for example a herbal (Kyranides) contained the following forms: *togidere, myche, lijf, whiʒt wiyn, siche, sijk, aftir, siʒ* 'saw'. Recipes in various hands had *myche, sijknes, sijknesse, sikenesse, siknesse,*

hemsilf, hymsilf, ech, fier, togidere, siche, þoruȝ, yȝen, ȝeuen, etc., and the astrological tracts from f. 127v on had *sich, sijknessis, yȝen, myche, aftir, heed.*

17. The author index in *eVK* gives 29 items for Arderne manuscripts, but they occur in a fewer number of manuscripts, for example London, British Library, Sloane MS 76 contains eight items of Arderne; Cambridge, Trinity College MS O.2.49 four items; London, British Library, Additional MS 8093 three. My preliminary survey included London, British Library, Sloane MSS 6, 76, 277, 563, 776, British Library, Additional MS 8093, Cambridge, Trinity College MS O.9.37, Cambridge, Trinity College MS O.2.49. A more comprehensive survey remains to be carried out in the future.

18. For Roger Marshall and his manuscripts, see Voigts 1995a and b, and Jones in this volume.

Bibliography

Primary sources

(1) *The Corpus of Middle English Medical Texts (MEMT)*
(CD-ROM, forthcoming 2004, Amsterdam and Philadelphia: John
Benjamins)

Editions marked by an asterisk (*) have also been used in the study by Norri.

Asplund, Annika (ed.) 1970, *A Middle English Version of Lanfranc's* Chirurgia Parva:
The Surgical Part, Stockholm Theses in English 2, Stockholm University Press,
pp. 66–95.

Ayoub, Lois Jean (ed.) 1994, 'John Crophill's books: An edition of British Library ms.
Harley 1735', Ph.D. thesis, University of Toronto, pp. 182–93, 239–45, 256–7.

Barratt, Alexandra (ed.) 1992, *Women's Writing in Middle English*, London and New York:
Longman, pp. 29–39.

Beck, R. Theodore (ed.) 1974, *The Cutting Edge: The Early History of the Surgeons of
London*, London: Lund Humphries, pp. 106–19.

Benskin, Michael (ed.) 1985, 'For wound in the head: A late mediaeval view of the brain',
Neuphilologische Mitteilungen 86: 202–3.

Braekman, W. L. (ed.) 1986a, 'The alchemical waters of Saint Giles', in Braekman, W. L.
(ed.), *Studies on Alchemy, Diet, Medecine [sic] and Prognostication in Middle English*,
Scripta 22, Brussels: Omirel, pp. 26–37.

1986b, 'A collection of medicinal recipes and charms', in Braekman, W. L. (ed.), *Studies
on Alchemy, Diet, Medecine [sic] and Prognostication in Middle English*, Scripta 22,
Brussels: Omirel, pp. 125–45.

1986c, 'Queen Isabel's dietary and its context', in Braekman, W. L. (ed.), *Studies
on Alchemy, Diet, Medecine [sic] and Prognostication in Middle English*, Scripta 22,
Brussels: Omirel, pp. 67–76.

Brodin, Gösta (ed.) 1950, Agnus Castus: *A Middle English Herbal*, Essays and Studies on
English Language and Literature 6, Uppsala University Press, pp. 119–64.

Burton, T. L. (ed.) 1998–99, *Sidrak and Bokkus: A Parallel-text Edition from Bodleian
Library, MS Laud Misc. 559 and British Library, MS Lansdowne 793*, Early English
Text Society 311–312, 2 vols., Oxford University Press for the Early English Text
Society, pp. 155, 163, 167, 169–71, 193–5, 197–203, 209–15, 235–7, 239–41, 243,
249–51, 253–5, 285–7, 294, 295–305, 389–91, 397, 409–11, 425–7, 445–7, 459–63,

465–9, 475–7, 485, 489–93, 497–507, 517–21, 527–9, 559, 563, 579–81, 593, 599, 601–3, 605, 607, 613–17, 625–7, 639, 643, 651, 655, 669–71.

* Carrillo Linares, María José (ed.) 1993, 'An edition with an introduction, notes and a glossary of the Middle English translation of the Latin treatise *De humana natura*', Licentiate thesis, University of Seville, pp. 54–91.

1997, 'Edicíon de una versión en ingles medio del *Antidotarium Nicholai*', Ph.D. thesis, University of Seville.

Caxton, William 1491/1974, *Ars Moriendi: The Helthe of Mannes Sowle*, English Experience 639, Amsterdam and Norwood, NJ: Theatrum Orbis Terrarum and Walter J. Johnson, pp. AI–BIII.

* Dawson, Warren R. (ed.) 1934, *A Leechbook or Collection of Medical Recipes of the Fifteenth Century*, London: Macmillan, pp. 18–58.

Edmar, Désirée (ed.) 1967, 'Ms. Wellcome 405: A Middle English leech-book', Licenciate thesis, University of Stockholm, pp. 40–105.

Eldredge, L. M. (ed.) 1996, *Benvenutus Grassus:* The Wonderful Art of the Eye: *A Critical Edition of the Middle English Translation of his* De probatissima arte oculorum, East Lansing: Michigan State University Press, pp. 49–92.

* von Fleischhacker, Robert (ed.) 1894, *Lanfrank's* Science of Cirurgie, Part I, *Text*, Early English Text Society, O.S. 102, London: Kegan Paul, Trench, Trübner and Co. for the Early English Text Society, pp. 7–58, 106–57.

Fordyn, Patrick (ed.) 1983, *The* Experimentes of Cophon, the Leche of Salerne: *Middle English Medical Recipes*, Scripta 10, Brussels: Omirel, pp. 19–43.

Frisk, Gösta (ed.) 1949, *A Middle English Translation of* Macer Floridus de Viribus Herbarum, Essays and Studies on English Language and Literature 3, Uppsala University Press, pp. 57–105.

Furnivall, Frederick J. (ed.) 1866/1889, *The Book of Quinte Essence or the Fifth Being; that is to Say, Man's Heaven*, Early English Text Society, O.S. 16, London: Trübner and Co., pp. 1–26.

* Getz, Faye Marie (ed.) 1991, *Healing and Society in Medieval England: A Middle English Translation of the Pharmaceutical Writings of Gilbertus Anglicus*, Madison: University of Wisconsin Press, pp. 1–54.

Green, Monica (ed.) 1992, 'Obstetrical and gynecological texts in Middle English', *Studies in the Age of Chaucer* 14: 85–88.

* Grothé, Richard (ed.) 1982, 'Le ms. Wellcome 564: Deux traités de chirurgie en moyen-anglais', Ph.D. thesis, University of Montreal, pp. 1A–25A (*Chirurgie de 1392*), 275A–298A (Mondeville).

Hallaert, M.-R. (ed.) 1982, *The Sekenesse of Wymmen: A Middle English Treatise on Diseases in Women*, Scripta 8, Brussels: Omirel, pp. 27–55.

Halversen, Marguerite A. (ed.) 1998, 'The consideration of quintessence: An edition of a Middle English translation of John of Rupescissa's *Liber de consideratione de quintae essentiae omnium rerum* with introduction, notes and commentary', Ph.D. thesis, Michigan State University, pp. 101–254.

Hanna, Ralph III (ed.) 1994, 'Henry Daniel's *Liber uricrisiarum*', in Matheson, Lister M. (ed.), *Popular and Practical Science of Medieval England*, East Lansing: Colleagues Press, pp. 193–209.

Hargreaves, Henry (ed.) 1977, '*De spermate hominis*: A Middle English poem on human embryology', *Mediaeval Studies* 39: 507.

Harley, Martha Powell (ed.) 1982, 'The Middle English contents of a fifteenth-century medical handbook', *Mediaevalia* 8: 179–85.

Heffernan, Carol F. (ed.) 1993, '*The wyse boke of maystyr Peers of Salerne*: An edition and study of a fourteenth-century treatise of popular medicine', *Manuscripta* 37: 307–17.

* Heinrich, Fritz (ed.) 1896, *Ein Mittelenglisches Medizinbuch*, Halle: Niemeyer, pp. 64–89.

Henslow, George (ed.) 1899, *Medical Works of the Fourteenth Century Together with a List of Plants Recorded in Contemporary Writings, with their Identifications*, London: Chapman and Hall, pp. 79–83, 122–9, 132–9.

Jasin, Joanne (ed.) 1983, 'A critical edition of the Middle English *Liber uricrisiarum* in Wellcome Ms. 225', Ph.D. thesis, Tulane University, pp. 41–50, 119–57.

Keiser, George R. (ed.) 1994, 'Epilepsy: The Falling Evil', in Matheson, Lister M. (ed.), *Popular and Practical Science of Medieval England*, East Lansing: Colleagues Press, pp. 234–9.

Louis, Cameron (ed.) 1980, *The Commonplace Book of Robert Reynes of Acle: An Edition of Tanner Ms. 407*, Garland Medieval Texts 1, New York and London: Garland, pp. 157–61.

Mäkinen, Martti (ed.) 2002a, 'Henry Daniel's Rosemary in MS X.90 of the Royal Library, Stockholm', *Neuphilologische Mitteilungen* 103: 315–20.

Manzalaoui, Mahmoud A. (ed.) 1977a. 'The "Ashmole" version: *The Secrete of secretes*', in Manzalaoui, Mahmoud A. (ed.), Secretum Secretorum: *Nine English Versions*, Vol. 1, *Text*, Early English Text Society 276, Oxford University Press, pp. 48–68.

1977b, '*The booke of the gouernaunce of kinges and princes called the secreet of secreetes*', in Manzalaoui, Mahmoud A. (ed.), Secretum Secretorum: *Nine English Versions*, Vol. 1, *Text*, Early English Text Society 276, Oxford University Press, pp. 330–56.

1977c '*Þe priuyté of priuyteis*', in Manzalaoui, Mahmoud A. (ed.), Secretum Secretorum: *Nine English Versions*, Vol. 1, *Text*, Early English Text Society 276, Oxford University Press, pp. 142–73.

1977d '*Regimen Sanitatis: The Booke of Goode Governance and Guyding of Þe Body*', in Manzalaoui, Mahmoud A. (ed.), Secretum Secretorum: *Nine English Versions*, Vol. 1, *Text*, Early English Text Society 276, Oxford University Press, pp. 3–9.

Mayer, Claudius F. (ed.) 1939, 'Medieval English leechbook', *Bulletin of the History of Medicine* 7: 388–90.

Mooney, Linne R. (ed.) 1984, 'A Middle English verse compendium of astrological medicine', *Medical History* 28: 411–16.

1994, 'Diet and bloodletting: A monthly regimen', in Matheson, Lister M. (ed.), *Popular and Practical Science of Medieval England*, East Lansing: Colleagues Press, pp. 251–5.

Müller, Gottfried (ed.) 1929b, *Aus mittelenglischen Medizintexten: Die Prosarezepte des stockholmer Miszellankodex X.90*, Kölner Anglistische Arbeiten 10, Leipzig: Bernhard Tauchnitz, pp. 64–89.

* Ogden, Margaret S. (ed.) 1938/1969, *The* Liber de diversis medicinis, *in the Thornton Manuscript (Ms. Lincoln Cathedral A.5.2)*, Early English Text Society, O.S. 207, London: Oxford University Press, pp. 51–82.

* 1971, *The Cyrurgie of Guy de Chauliac*, Early English Text Society, O.S. 265, London, New York and Toronto: Oxford University Press, pp. 26–56.

Pahta, Päivi (ed.) 1998, *Medieval Embryology in the Vernacular: The Case of De spermate*, Mémoires de la Société Néophilologique de Helsinki 53, Helsinki: Société Néophilologique, pp. 161–255.

Pickett, J. P. (ed.) 1994, 'A translation of the *Canutus* plague treatise', in Matheson, Lister M. (ed.), *Popular and Practical Science of Medieval England*, East Lansing: Colleagues Press, pp. 270–81.

Power, D'Arcy (ed.) 1910, *Treatises of Fistula in Ano. Haemorrhoids, and Clysters by John Arderne*, Early English Text Society, O.S. 139, London: Kegan Paul, Trench, Trübner, pp. 1–37, 74–104.

Robbins, Rossell Hope (ed.) 1952, *Secular Lyrics of the XIVth and XVth Centuries: Practical Verse*, Oxford University Press, pp. 71–80.

Rowland, Beryl (ed.) 1981, *Medieval Woman's Guide to Health: The First English Gynecological Handbook*, Kent, OH: Kent State University Press, pp. 58–112.

* Schöffler, Herbert (ed.) 1919, *Beiträge zur mittelenglischen Medizinlitteratur*, Sachsische Forschungsinstitute in Leipzig 3, Anglistische Abteilung, Heft 1, Leipzig: Niemeyer, pp. 192–223.

* Seymour, M.C. *et al.* (eds.) 1975/1988, *On the Properties of Things: John Trevisa's Translation of Bartholomaeus Anglicus* De Proprietatibus Rerum, Vol. 1, Oxford University Press, pp. 129–96.

Stephens, George 1844, 'Extracts in prose and verse from an old English medical manuscript, preserved in the Royal Library at Stockholm', *Archaeologia* 30: 349–418.

Taavitsainen, Irma 1994c, 'A zodiacal lunary for medical professionals', in Matheson, Lister M. (ed.), *Popular and Practical Science of Medieval England*, East Lansing: Colleagues Press, pp. 293–300.

Voigts, Linda Ehrsam and McVaugh, Michael R. (eds.) 1984, *A Latin Technical Phlebotomy and its Middle English Translation*, Transactions of the American Philosophical Society 74, Part 2, Philadelphia: American Philosophical Society, pp. 37–53.

* Wallner, Björn (ed.) 1964b, *The Middle English Translation of Guy de Chauliac's Anatomy, With Guy's Essay on the History of Medicine*, Lund Universitets Årsskrift, N.F. Avd. 1, B.D. 56, Nr. 5, Lund: CWK Gleerup, pp. 114–42.

1976, *The Middle English Translation of Guy de Chauliac's Treatise on Wounds*, Part I, *Text. Book III of the Great Surgery*, Acta Universitatis Lundensis, Sectio 1 Theologica Juridica Humaniora 23, Lund: CWK Gleerup, pp. 3–51.

1982, *The Middle English Translation of Guy de Chauliac's Treatise on Ulcers*, Part I, *Text. Book IV of the Great Surgery*, Acta Universitatis Lundensis, Sectio 1 Theologica Juridica Humaniora 39, Stockholm: Almqvist and Wiksell International, pp. 3–40.

1995, *An Interpolated Middle English Version of the Anatomy of Guy de Chauliac*, Part I, *Text*, Skrifter utgivna av vetenskapssocieteten i Lund 87, Lund University Press, pp. 3–27.

Wright, Thomas and Halliwell, James Orchard (eds.) 1841–43, *Reliquæ Antiquæ: Scraps from Ancient Manuscripts, Illustrating Chiefly Early English Literature and the English Language*, 2 vols., London and Berlin: William Pickering and A. Asher, pp. 51–55, 163–4.

Zimmermann, E. L. (ed.) 1937, 'An early English manuscript on syphilis: A fragmentary translation from the second edition of Gaspar Torrella's *Tractatus cum consiliis contra pudendagram seu morbum gallicum*', *Bulletin of the Institute of the History of Medicine* 5: 461–71.

(2) Other editions

Barrat, Alexandra (ed.) 2001, *The Knowing of Woman's Kind in Childing: A Middle English Version of Material Derived from the Trotula and Other Sources*, Medieval Women, Texts and Contexts 4, Turnhout: Brepols, pp. 40–114.

Benson, Larry D. (ed.) 1987, *The Riverside Chaucer*, 3rd edn, Oxford and Boston: Oxford University Press and Houghton Mifflin.

Bitterling, Klaus (ed.) 1981, 'A ME treatise on angling from BL MS Sloane 1698', *English Studies* 62: 110–14.

Braekman, W. L. (ed.) 1986d, *Of Hawks and Horses: Four Late Middle English Prose Treatises*, Scripta 16, Brussels: Omirel.

Dawson, Warren R. (ed.) 1934b, *A Leechbook or Collection of Medical Recipes of the Fifteenth Century*, Appendix, London: Macmillan.

Erbe, Theodor (ed.) 1905, *Mirk's Festial*, Early English Text Society, E.S. 96, London: Kegan Paul, Trench and Trubner for the Early English Text Society.

Furnivall, Frederick J. (ed.) 1981, *Andrew Boorde's Introduction and Dyetary, with Barnes in the Defence of the Berde*, Millwood, NY: Kraus Reprint.

Furnivall, Frederick J. and Furnivall, Percy (eds.) 1930/1988, *The Anatomie of the Bodie of Man: The Edition of 1548 as Re-Issued by the Surgeons of St. Bartholomew's in 1577*, London: Oxford University Press.

Grattan, John Henry Grafton and Singer, Charles (eds.) 1952/1978, *Anglo-Saxon Magic and Medicine, Illustrated Specially from the Semi-Pagan Text* Lacnunga, Publications of the Wellcome Historical Medical Museum N.S. 3, London: Richard West.

Grewe, Rudolf (ed.) 1979, *Libre de Sent Sovi: Receptari de Cuina*, Els nostres classics, Col·lecció A, 115, Barcelona: Barcino.

Grymonprez, Pol (ed.) 1981, Here Men May Se the Vertues off Herbes: *A Middle English Herbal, c. 1450*, Scripta 3, Brussels: Omirel.

Hieatt, Constance B. and Butler, Sharon (eds.) 1985, *Curye on Inglysch: English Culinary Manuscripts of the Fourteenth Century (Including the* Forme of Cury*)*, Early English Text Society, S.S. 8, London: Oxford University Press for the Early English Text Society.

Hieatt, Constance B. and Jones, Robin F. (eds.) 1986, 'Two Anglo-Norman culinary collections edited from British Library manuscripts Additional 32085 and Royal 12.C.xii', *Speculum* 61: 859–82.

Keller, Henning (ed.) 1971, 'Die me. Rezepte des Ms. Harley 2253', *Archiv für das Studium der neueren Sprachen und Literaturen* 207: 94–100.

Larkey, Sandford V. and Pyles, Thomas (eds.) 1941, *An Herbal (1525): Facsimile Repr. of Richard Banckes' Herbal of 1525*, New York: Scholars' Facsimiles and Reprints.

McVaugh, Michael R. (ed.) 1997, *Guigonis de Caulhiaco (Guy de Chauliac): Inventarium sive Chirurgia Magna*, Vol. 1, *Text*, Leiden, New York and Cologne: Brill.

Miller, Elaine M. (ed.) 1978, '*In hoote somere*: A fifteenth-century medical manuscript', Ph.D. thesis, Princeton University, pp. 1–59.

Mory, Robert Nels (ed.) 1977, 'A medieval English anatomy', Ph.D. thesis, University of Michigan.

Pagel, Julius Leopold (ed.) 1892, *Die Chirurgie des Heinrich von Mondeville (Hermondaville): Nach Berliner, Erfurter und Pariser Codices*, Berlin: August Hirschwald.

Pettit, Edward (ed.) 2001, *Anglo-Saxon Remedies, Charms, and Prayers from British Library MS Harley 585, the* Lacnunga, Mellen Critical Editions and Translations 6, 2 vols., Lewiston, New York and Lampeter: E. Mellen.

Stanley, Eric G. (ed.) 1974, 'Directions for making many sorts of laces', in Rowland, Beryl (ed.), *Chaucer and Middle English Studies: In Honour of Rossell Hope Robbins*, London: George Allen and Unwin, pp. 89–103.

Svinhufvud, Anne Charlotte (ed.) 1978, *A Late Middle English Treatise on Horses: Edited from British Library MS Sloane 2584 ff. 102–117b*, Stockholm: Almqvist and Wiksell International.

Swaen, A. E. H. (ed.) 1943, '*The Booke of Hawkyng after Prince Edwarde Kyng of Englande* and its relation to the *Book of St. Albans*', *Studia Neophilologica* 16: 1–32.

Vallese, T. (ed.) 1940, *Un ignoto ricettario medico inglese del XIV secolo trovato nella biblioteca nazionale di Napoli*, Naples: A.G.D.A., pp. 19–53.

de Vriend, Hubert (ed.) 1984, *The Old English Herbarium and Medicina de Quadrupedibus*, Early English Text Society, O.S. 286, Oxford University Press for the Early English Text Society.

Wright, C. E. (ed.) 1955, *Bald's Leechbook: British Museum Royal Manuscript, 2. D. xvii*, Early English Manuscripts in Facsimile 5, Copenhagen: Rosenkilde and Bagger.

Zettersten, Arne 1967, *The Virtues of Herbs in the Loscombe Manuscript: A Contribution to Anglo-Irish Language and Literature*, Acta Universitatis Lundensis, Sectio 1, Theologica Juridica Humaniora 5, Lund: Gleerups.

(3) Early printed books

Boorde, Andrew 1547/1971, *The Breuiary of Helthe*, London: W. Myddleton. Facsimile edition: English Experience 362, Amsterdam and New York: Theatrum Orbis Terrarum and Da Capo Press.

von Braunschweig, Hieronymus 1525/1973, *The Noble Experyence of the Vertuous Handy Warke of Surgeri*, London: P. Treueris. Facsimile edition: English Experience 531, Amsterdam and New York: Theatrum Orbis Terrarum and Da Capo Press.

Elyot, Thomas 1541/1937, *The Castel of Helth Corrected and in Some Places Augmented, by the Fyrste Author Thereof*, London: T. Berthelet. Facsimile edition: New York: Scholars' Facsimiles and Reprints.

Guido's Questions 1579/1968, London: Thomas East. Facsimile edition: English Experience 35, Amsterdam and New York: Theatrum Orbis Terrarum and Da Capo Press.

Langton, Christopher 1547, *A Uery Brefe Treatise, Ordrely Declaring the Prīcipal Partes of Phisick*, London: E. Whitchurch.

Moulton, Thomas (bef.) 1531, *This is the Myrour or Glasse of Helthe, Necessary and Nedefull for Euery Person*, London: R. Wyre.

Prognostication Drawen out of the Bookes of Ipocras, Auicen, and Other Notable Auctours of Physycke, Shewynge the Daunger of Dyuers Syckenesses, that is to Say, Whether Peryll of Death Be in Them or Not, the Pleasure of Almyghtye God Reserued, 1530?/1554?, London: Robert Wyer?.

de Vigo, Joannes 1543/1968, *The Most Excellent Workes of Chirurgerye*, London: E. Whytchurch. Facsimile edition: English Experience 67, Amsterdam and New York: Theatrum Orbis Terrarum and Da Capo Press.

Secondary sources

Adams, J. N. 1980, 'Anatomical terminology in Latin epic', *Bulletin of the Institute of Classical Studies* (University of London) 27: 50–62.

Alonso Almeida, Francisco 2002, 'Estudio comparativo de los textos receta en español medieval y en inglés medieval', in Santana Henriquez and Santana Sanjurjo (eds.), pp. 649–76.

Amastae, Jon and Elías-Olivares, Lucía (eds.) 1982, *Spanish in the United States: Sociolinguistic Aspects*, Cambridge University Press.

Anderson, Douglas M., Jefferson, Keith and Novak, Patricia D. (eds.) 2000, *Dorland's Illustrated Medical Dictionary*, Philadelphia and London: W. B. Saunders.

André, Jacques 1991, *Le vocabulaire latin de l'anatomie*, Paris: Les Belles Lettres.

Arber, Agnes 1938/1986, *Herbals: Their Origin and Evolution, A Chapter in the History of Botany 1470–1670*, 3rd edn, Cambridge University Press.

Atkinson, Dwight 1999, *Scientific Discourse in Sociohistorical Context:* The Philosophical Transactions *of the Royal Society of London, 1675–1975*, Mahwah, NJ: Lawrence Erlbaum.

Auer, Peter (ed.) 1998, *Code-switching in Conversation: Language, Interaction and Identity*, London: Routledge.

Ayoub, Lois Jean (ed.) 1994, 'John Crophill's books: An edition of British Library ms. Harley 1735', Ph.D. thesis, University of Toronto.

Bailey, Benjamin 2000, 'Social/interactional functions of code switching among Dominican Americans', *Pragmatics* 10: 165–93.

Bailey, Richard W. (ed.) 1978, *Additions and Antedatings to the Record of English Vocabulary 1475–1700*, Hildesheim and New York: Georg Olms Verlag.

Barlow, Frank 1980, 'The King's evil', *English Historical Review* 95: 3–27.

Barratt, Alexandra (ed.) 2001, *The Knowing of Woman's Kind in Childing: A Middle English Version of Material Derived from the Trotula and Other Sources*, Medieval Women, Texts and Contexts 4, Turnhout: Brepols.

Barton, David 1994, *Literacy: An Introduction to the Ecology of Written Language*, Oxford: Blackwell.

Barton, David and Hamilton, Mary 2000, 'Literacy practices' in Barton *et al.* (eds.), pp. 7–15.

Barton, David, Hamilton, Mary and Ivanic, Roz (eds.) 2000, *Situated Literacies: Reading and Writing in Context*, Literacies Series, London: Routledge.

Bates, Don (ed.) 1995, *Knowledge and the Scholarly Medical Traditions*, Cambridge University Press.

Baugh, Albert C. and Cable, Thomas 1993, *A History of the English Language*, London: Routledge.

Beadle, Richard 1991, 'Prolegomena to a literary geography of later medieval Norfolk', in Riddy (ed.), pp. 89–108.

Beadle, Richard and Piper, A. J. (eds.) 1995, *New Science Out of Old Books*, Aldershot: Scolar Press.

Becela-Deller, Christine 1998, Ruta graveolens L.: *Eine Heilpflanze in Kunst– und Kulturhistorischer Bedeutung*, Würzburger medizinhistorische Forschungen 65, Würzburg: Königshausen und Neumann.

Beck, R. Theodore 1974, *The Cutting Edge: The Early History of the Surgeons of London*, London: Lund Humphries.

Bennett, Henry Stanley 1944/1969, *English Books and Readers*, Vol. 1, *1475–1557*, Cambridge University Press.

Benskin, Michael 1981, 'A linguistic atlas for late mediaeval English', *Mediaeval English Studies Newsletter* 4: 5–13.

1992, 'Some new perspectives on the origins of standard written English', in Leuven-steijn and Berns (eds.), pp. 71–105.

1997, 'Texts from an English township in late mediaeval Ireland', *Collegium Medievale* 10: 91–174.

Benson, Larry D. (ed.) 1987, *The Riverside Chaucer*, 3rd edn, Oxford and Boston: Oxford University Press and Houghton Mifflin.

Bergner, Heinz 1995, 'The openness of medieval texts', in Jucker (ed.), pp. 37–54.

Besson, Alain (ed.) 1990, *Thornton's Medical Books, Libraries and Collectors: A Study of Bibliography and the Book Trade in Relation to the Medical Sciences*, Aldershot: Gower.

Bex, T. 1996, *Variety in Written English: Texts in Society: Societies in Text*, Interface Series, London: Routledge.

Biber, Douglas 1988, *Variation across Speech and Writing*, Cambridge University Press.

Biber, Douglas, Johansson, Stig, Leech, Geoffrey, Conrad, Susan and Finegan, Edward (eds.) 1999, *Longman Grammar of Spoken and Written English*, London: Longman.

Biller, Peter and Hudson, Ann (eds.) 1994, *Heresy and Literacy, 1000–1530*, Cambridge Studies in Medieval Literature, Cambridge University Press.

Bitterling, Klaus (ed.) 1981, 'A ME treatise on angling from BL MS Sloane 1698', *English Studies* 62: 110–14.

Blake, Norman F. 1974, '*The Form of Living* in prose and poetry', *Archiv für das Studium der neueren Sprachen und Literaturen* 211: 300–8.

1996, *A History of the English Language*, Basingstoke and London: Macmillan.

Bonser, Wilfrid 1963, *The Medical Background of Anglo-Saxon England*, London: Wellcome.

Boyd, Sally, Andersson, Paula and Thornell, Christina 1997, 'Patterns of incorporation of lexemes in language contact: Language typology or sociolinguistics?' in Guy *et al.* (eds.), pp. 259–84.

Bracke, W. and Deumens, H. (eds.) 2000, *Medical Latin from the Late Middle Ages to the Eighteenth Century*, Brussels: Koninklijke Academie voor Geneeskunde van België.

Braswell, Laurel 1984, 'Utilitarian and scientific prose', in Edwards (ed.), pp. 337–87.

Brodin, Gösta (ed.) 1950, Agnus castus: *A Middle English Herbal*, Essays and Studies on English Language and Literature 6, Uppsala University Press.

Bullough, V. L. 1959, 'Training of nonuniversity-educated medical practitioners in the later Middle Ages', *Journal of the History of Medicine* 14: 446–58.

Burke, Peter and Porter, Roy (eds.) 1987, *The Social History of Language*, Cambridge University Press.

Burnett, Charles and Jacquart, Danielle 1994, *Constantine the African and ʿAlī ibn-al-ʿAbbās al-Maǧūsī: The Pantegni and Related Texts*, Leiden, New York and Cologne: Brill.

Burnley, David 2001, 'French and Frenches in fourteenth-century London', in Kastovsky and Mettinger (eds.), pp. 17–34.

Burrow, J. A. 1986, *The Ages of Man: A Study in Medieval Writing and Thought*, Oxford: Clarendon Press.

Burton, T. L. (ed.) 1998–99, *Sidrak and Bokkus: A Parallel-text Edition from Bodleian Library, MS Laud Misc. 559 and British Library, MS Lansdowne 793*, Early English Text Society 311–12, Oxford University Press for the Early English Text Society.

Bylebyl, J. J. 1979, 'The school of Padua: Humanistic medicine in the sixteenth century', in Webster (ed.), pp. 335–70.

Cabré, M. Teresa 1999, *Terminology: Theory, Methods and Applications*, Amsterdam and Philadelphia: Benjamins.

Cadden, Joan 1993, *Meanings of Sex Difference in the Middle Ages: Medicine, Science and Culture*, Cambridge University Press.

Cameron, Malcolm Laurence 1983a, 'Bald's *Leechbook*: Its sources and their use in its compilation', *Anglo-Saxon England* 12: 153–82.

1983b, 'The sources of medical knowledge in Anglo-Saxon England', *Anglo-Saxon England* 11: 135–55.

1993, *Anglo-Saxon Medicine*, Cambridge Studies in Anglo-Saxon England 7, Cambridge University Press.

Carey, Hilary M. 1992, *Courting Disaster: Astrology at the English Court and University in the Later Middle Ages*, New York: Saint Martin's Press.

Carrillo Linares, María José 1993, 'An edition with an introduction, notes and a glossary of the M.E. translation of the Latin treatise *De Humana Natura*', Licenciate thesis, University of Seville.

Carrillo Linares, María José (ed.) forthcoming, '*De Humana Natura (Liber Cerebri)*', in Tavormina (ed.) forthcoming b.

Carroll, Ruth 1999, 'The Middle English recipe as a text-type', *Neuphilologische Mitteilungen* 100: 27–42.

forthcoming, '*Recipes for Laces*: An example of a Middle English discourse colony', in Hiltunen and Skaffari (eds.).

Cassidy, Brendan (ed.) 1993, *Iconography at the Crossroads*, Princeton University Press.

Cavanaugh, Susan H. 1980, 'A study of books privately owned in England, 1300–1450', Ph.D. thesis, University of Pennsylvania.

Christianson, C. Paul 1987, *Memorials of the Book Trade in Medieval London: The Archives of Old London Bridge*, Manuscript Studies 3, Cambridge: D. S. Brewer.

1989a, *A Directory of London Stationers and Book Artisans 1300–1500*, New York: Bibliographical Society of America.

1989b, 'Evidence for the study of London's late medieval manuscript-book trade', in Griffiths and Pearsall (eds.), pp. 87–108.

Ciancaspro, Mauro, Cavallo, Guglielmo and Touwaide, Alain (eds.) 1998, *Dioscurides* De Materia Medica: Codex neapolitanus graecus 1 *of the National Library of Naples*, Miletos.

Clanchy, M. T. 1993, *From Memory to Written Record: England 1066–1307*, 2nd edn, Oxford: Blackwell.

Coleman, Julie 1995, 'The chronology of French and Latin loan words in English', *Transactions of the Philological Society* 93: 95–124.

Collins, Minta 2000, *Medieval Herbals: The Illustrative Traditions*, London: British Library.

Connolly, Margaret 1998, *John Shirley: Book Production and the Noble Household of Fifteenth-century England*, Aldershot, Brookfield, Singapore and Sydney: Ashgate.

Copeland, Rita 1991, *Rhetoric, Hermeneutics and Translation in the Middle Ages: Academic Traditions and Vernacular Texts*, Cambridge University Press.

Crisciani, Chiara 1990, 'History, novelty, and progress in scholastic medicine', *Osiris* 6: 118–39.

2000, 'Teachers and learners in scholastic medicine: Some images and metaphors', *History of Universities* 15: 75–101.

Croft, William 2000, *Explaining Language Change: An Evolutionary Approach*, London and New York: Longman.

Crombie, Alistair Cameron 1994, *Styles of Scientific Thinking in the European Tradition*, 3 vols., London: Duckworth.

1995, 'Commitments and styles of European scientific thinking', *History of Science* 33: 225–38.

Crossgrove, William 1998, 'Introduction', *Early Science and Medicine* 3: 81–7.

Curtius, Ernst Robert 1990, *European Literature and the Latin Middle Ages*, Princeton University Press.

Daiches, David and Thorlby, Anthony (eds.) 1973, *Literature and Western Civilization: The Medieval World*, London: Aldus.

Davis, Norman (ed.) 1971, *Paston Letters and Papers of the Fifteenth Century*, 2 vols., Oxford: Clarendon Press.

Dawson, Warren R. (ed.) 1934a, *A Leechbook or Collection of Medical Recipes of the Fifteenth Century*, London: Macmillan.

Demaitre, Luke E. 1975, 'Theory and practice in medical education at the University of Montpellier in the thirteenth and fourteenth centuries', *Journal of the History of Medicine and Allied Sciences* 30: 103–23.

1976, 'Scholasticism in compendia of practical medicine, 1250–1450', *Manuscripta* 20: 81–95.

1980, *Doctor Bernard de Gordon: Professor and Practitioner*, Toronto: Pontifical Institute of Mediaeval Studies.

1998, 'Medical writing in transition: Between *Ars* and *Vulgus*', *Early Science and Medicine* 3: 88–102.

van Dijk, Teun A. (ed.) 1997, *Discourse as Structure and Process*, London: Sage.

Diller, Hans-Jürgen 2001, '*Genre* in linguistic and related discourses', in Diller and Görlach (eds.), pp. 3–43.

Diller, Hans-Jürgen and Görlach, Manfred (eds.) 2001, *Towards a History of English as a History of Genres*, Anglistische Forschungen 298, Heidelberg: C. Winter,

Dirckx, John H. 1983, *The Language of Medicine: Its Evolution, Structure, and Dynamics*, New York: Praeger.

DML = *Dictionary of Medieval Latin from British Sources* 1975–, Latham, R. E. and Howlett, D. R. (eds.), Oxford University Press.

Dobson, Eric John 1968, *English Pronunciation 1500–1700*, Vol. 2, Oxford: Clarendon Press.

Dictionary of Old English 1988, edited by Amos, Ashley Crandell *et al.*, Pontifical Institute of Medieval Studies for the Dictionary of Old English Project, Centre for Medieval Studies, University of Toronto, online at http://www.doe.utoronto.ca.

Doyle, A. I. 1983, 'English books in and out of court from Edward III to Henry VII', in Scattergood and Sherborne (eds.), pp. 163–81.

Doyle, A. I. and Parkes, Malcolm B. 1978, 'The production of copies of the *Canterbury Tales* and the *Confessio Amantis* in the early fifteenth century', in Parkes and Watson (eds.), pp. 163–210.

Eamon, William (ed.) 1982, *Studies on Medieval Fachliteratur*, Scripta 6, Brussels: Omirel.

Eastman, Carol M. 1992, 'Code-switching as an urban language-contact phenomenon', *Journal of Multilingual and Multicultural Development* 13: 1–17.

1995, 'Codeswitching', in Verschueren *et al.* (eds.), pp. 1–23.

Edwards, A. S. G. (ed.) 1984, *Middle English Prose: A Critical Guide to Major Authors and Genres*, New Brunswick, NJ: Rutgers University Press.

Edwards, A. S. G. and Pearsall, Derek (eds.) 1981, *Middle English Prose: Essays on Bibliographic Problems*, New York: Garland.

Eggins, Suzanne and Martin, J. R. 1997, 'Genres and registers of discourse', in van Dijk (ed.), pp. 230–56.

Ekwall, Eilert 1956, *Studies on the Population of Medieval London*, Kungl. Vitterhets-, historie- och antikvitetsakademiens handlingar, Filologisk-filosofiska serien 2, Stockholm: Almqvist & Wiksell.

Eldredge, Lawrence M. 1992, *The Index of Middle English Prose, Handlist 9: A Handlist of Manuscripts Containing Middle English Prose in the Ashmolean Collection, Bodleian Library, Oxford*, Cambridge: D. S. Brewer.

Eldredge, Lawrence M. (ed.) 1996, *Benvenutus Grassus*, The Wonderful Art of the Eye: *A Critical Edition of the Middle English Translation of his* De probatissima arte oculorum, East Lansing: Michigan State University Press.

Ellenberger, Bengt 1974, 'On Middle English *mots savants*', *Studia Neophilologica* 46: 142–50.

Emden, A. B. 1957–59, 'Wallingford, Richard of', *A Biographical Register of the University of Oxford to A.D. 1500*, 3 vols., Oxford: Clarendon.

Evans, Ruth, Taylor, Andrew, Watson, Nicholas and Wogan-Browne, Jocelyn 1999, 'The notion of vernacular theory', in Wogan-Browne *et al.* (eds.), pp. 314–30.

eVK = Scientific and Medical Writings in Old and Middle English: An Electronic Reference, Voigts, Linda Ehrsam and Kurtz, Patricia Deery (compilers), CD-ROM, Ann Arbor: University of Michigan Press.

Fanego, Teresa, Méndez-Naya, Belén and Seoane, Elena (eds.) 2002, *Sounds, Words, Texts, Change: Selected Papers from the Eleventh International Conference on English Historical Linguistics*, Amsterdam and Philadelphia: Benjamins.

Fernandez, Francisco, Fuster, Miguel and Calvo, Juan José (eds.) 1994, *English Historical Linguistics 1992*, Amsterdam: Benjamins.

Fisher, John 1992, 'A language policy for Lancastrian England', *PMLA* 107: 1168–80.

Fishman, J. A. 1972/1979, 'The relationship between micro- and macro-sociolinguistics in the study of who speaks what language to whom and when', in Pride and Holmes (eds.), pp. 15–32.

Fisiak, Jacek (ed.) 1996, *Middle English Miscellany*, Poznan: Motivex.

Fisiak, Jacek and Trudgill, Peter (eds.) 2001, *East Anglian English*, Cambridge: D. S. Brewer.

von Fleischhacker, Robert (ed.) 1894, *Lanfrank's "Science of Cirurgie." Part I, Text*, Early English Text Society, O.S. 102, London: Kegan Paul, Trench, Trübner and Co. for the Early English Text Society.

Fonahn, Adolf Mauritz 1922, *Arabic and Latin Anatomical Terminology: Chiefly from the Middle Ages*, Kristiania: Videnskapselskapet i Kristiania.

Franceschini, Rita 1998, 'Code-switching and the notion of code in linguistics: Proposals for a dual focus model', in Auer (ed.), pp. 51–72.

French, Roger 1979, '*De Juvamentis Membrorum* and the reception of Galenic physiological anatomy', *Isis* 70: 96–109.

1994, 'Astrology in medical practice', in García-Ballester *et al.* (eds.), pp. 30–59; reprinted in French 2002, ch. 6.

2001, *Canonical Medicine: Gentile da Foligno and Scholasticism*, Leiden: Brill.

2002, *Ancients and Moderns in the Medical Sciences*, Variorum Collected Studies Series, Aldershot: Ashgate.

French, Roger and Cunningham, Andrew 1996, *Before Science: The Invention of the Friar's Natural Philosophy*, Aldershot: Scolar Press.

French, Roger, Arrizabalaga, Jon, Cunningham, Andrew and García-Ballester, Luis (eds.) 1998, *Medicine from the Black Death to the French Disease*, History of Medicine in Context Series, Aldershot: Ashgate.

Frisk, Gösta (ed.) 1949, *A Middle English Translation of* Macer Floridus de Viribus Herbarum, Essays and Studies on English Language and Literature 3, Uppsala: Almqvist & Wiksells.

Furnivall, Frederick J. (ed.) 1981, *Andrew Boorde's Introduction and Dyetary, with Barnes in the Defence of the Berde*, Millwood, NY: Kraus Reprint.

García-Ballester, Luis 1994, 'Introduction: Practical medicine from Salerno to the Black Death', in García-Ballester *et al.* (eds.), pp. 1–29.

García-Ballester, Luis, French, Roger, Arrizabalaga, Jon and Cunningham, Andrew 1994 (eds.), *Practical Medicine from Salerno to the Black Death*, Cambridge and New York: Cambridge University Press.

Getz, Faye Marie 1990a, 'Charity, translation, and the language of medical learning in medieval England', *Bulletin of the History of Medicine* 64: 1–17.

1990b, 'Medical practitioners in medieval England', *Social History of Medicine* 3: 245–83.

1992, 'The faculty of medicine 1500', in Catto and Evans (eds.), pp. 374–405.

Getz, Faye Marie (ed.) 1991, *Healing and Society in Medieval England: A Middle English Translation of the Pharmaceutical Writings of Gilbertus Anglicus*, Madison: University of Wisconsin Press.

Ghadessy, Mohsen (ed.) 1988, *Registers of Written English*, London: Pinter.

Görlach, Manfred 1991, 'Text types and the linguistic history of Modern English', in Uhlig and Zimmermann (eds.), pp. 195–215.

1992, 'Text-types and language history: The cookery recipe', in Rissanen *et al.* (eds.), pp. 736–61.

1993, *Introduction to Early Modern English*, Cambridge University Press.

Gotti, Maurizio and Dossena, Marina (eds.) 2001, *Modality in Specialized Texts: Selected Papers of the 1st CERLIS Conference*, Bern, Berlin, Brussels, Frankfurt am Main, New York, Oxford and Vienna: Peter Lang.

Graedler, Anne-Line 1999, 'Where English and Norwegian meet: Codeswitching in written texts', in Hasselgård and Oksefjell (eds.), pp. 327–43.

Graff, Harvey J. 1987, *The Legacies of Literacy: Continuities and Contradictions in Western Culture and Society*, Bloomington and Indianapolis: Indiana University Press.

Granovetter, M. 1973, 'The strength of weak ties', *American Journal of Sociology* 78: 1360–80.

Grant, Edward (ed.) 1974, *A Source Book in Medieval Science*, Cambridge, Mass.: Harvard University Press.

Gray, Douglas and Stanley, E. G. (eds.) 1983, *Middle English Studies Presented to Norman Davis*, Oxford: Clarendon Press.

Green, Monica H. 1992, 'Obstetrical and gynecological texts in Middle English', *Studies in the Age of Chaucer* 14: 53–88.

1996, 'A handlist of the Latin and vernacular manuscripts of the so-called *Trotula* texts. Part I: The Latin manuscripts', *Scriptorium* 50: 137–75.

1997, 'A handlist of the Latin and vernacular manuscripts of the so-called *Trotula* texts. Part II: The vernacular translations and Latin re-writings', *Scriptorium* 51: 80–104.

2000a, 'The possibilities of literacy and the limits of reading: Women and the gendering of medical literacy', in Green 2000b, ch. 7.

2000b, *Women's Healthcare in the Medieval West*, Variorum Collected Studies Series, Aldershot: Ashgate.

2001, *The* Trotula: *A Medieval Compendium of Women's Medicine*, Philadelphia: University of Pennsylvania Press.

Green, Monica H. and Mooney, Linne (eds.) forthcoming, '*Sickness of Women 2*', in Tavormina (ed.) forthcoming b.

Griffiths, Jeremy and Pearsall, Derek (eds.) 1989, *Book Production and Publishing in Britain, 1375–1475*, Cambridge University Press.

Grmek, Mirko D. (ed.) 1998, *Western Medical Thought from Antiquity to the Middle Ages*, Cambridge, Mass.: Harvard University Press.

Gross, Anthony 1996, *The Dissolution of the Lancastrian Kingship: Sir John Fortesque and the Crisis of Monarchy in Fifteenth-century England*, Stamford: Paul Watkins.

Grothé, Richard (ed.) 1982, 'Le ms. Wellcome 564: Deux traités de chirurgie en moyen-anglais', Ph.D. thesis, University of Montreal.

Grund, Peter 2002, 'In search of gold: Towards a text edition of an alchemical treatise', in Lucas and Lucas (eds.), pp. 265–79.

forthcoming, 'The golden formulas: Genre conventions of alchemical recipes in the Middle English period', *Neuphilologische Mitteilungen*.

Gumperz, John J. 1982, *Discourse Strategies*, Cambridge University Press.

Guy, Gregory R., Feagin, Crawford, Schriffrin, Deborah and Baugh, John (eds.) 1997, *Towards a Social Science of Language: Papers in Honour of William Labov*, Vol. 2, *Social Interaction and Discourse Structures*, Current Issues in Linguistic Theory 128, Amsterdam and Philadelphia: Benjamins.

Halliday, M. A. K. 1988/1993, 'On the language of physical science', in Ghadessy (ed.), pp. 162–78, reprinted in Halliday and Martin, pp. 54–85.

Halliday, M. A. K. and Martin, J. R. 1993, *Writing Science: Literacy and Discursive Power*, Pittsburgh Series in Composition, Literacy, and Culture, University of Pittsburgh Press.

Halmari, Helena 1997, *Government and Codeswitching: Explaining American Finnish*, Studies in Bilingualism 12, Amsterdam and Philadelphia: Benjamins.

Hanna, Ralph III 1997, *The Index of Middle English Prose, Handlist 12: Smaller Bodleian Collections*, Cambridge: D. S. Brewer.

Hargreaves, Henry 1981, 'Some problems in indexing Middle English recipes', in Edwards and Pearsall (eds.), pp. 91–113.

Harley, Martha Powell 1982, 'The Middle English contents of a fifteenth-century medical handbook', *Mediaevalia* 8: 171–88.

Hasselgård, Hilde and Oksefjell, Signe (eds.) 1999, *Out of Corpora: Studies in Honour of Stig Johansson*, Language and Computers: Studies in Practical Linguistics 26, Amsterdam and Atlanta: Rodopi.

Heath, Shirley Brice 1983, *Ways with Words: Language, Life, and Work in Communities and Classrooms*, Cambridge University Press.

Heinrich, Fritz (ed.) 1896, *Ein Mittelenglisches Medizinbuch*, Halle: Niemeyer, pp. 64–89.

Heller, Monika (ed.) 1988, *Codeswitching: Anthropological and Sociolinguistic Perspectives*, Berlin: Mouton de Gruyter.

Hellinga, Lotte and Trapp, J. B. (eds.) 1999, *The Cambridge History of the Book in Britain*, Vol. 3, *1400–1557*, Cambridge University Press.

The Helsinki Corpus of English Texts, Diachronic and Dialectal, Helsinki: Department of English, University of Helsinki.

Henslow, George (ed.) 1899, *Medical Works of the Fourteenth Century Together with a List of Plants Recorded in Contemporary Writings, with their Identifications*, London: Chapman and Hall.

Hibbott, Yvonne 1990, 'Medical books of the sixteenth century', in Besson (ed.), pp. 43–82.

Hickey, Raymond 2000, 'Processing corpora with *Corpus Presenter*', *ICAME Journal* 24: 65–84.

2003, *Corpus Presenter: Processing Software for Language Analysis*, Amsterdam: John Benjamins.

Hieatt, Constance B. and Butler, Sharon (eds.) 1985, *Curye on Inglysch: English Culinary Manuscripts of the Fourteenth Century (Including the* Forme of Cury*)*, Early English Text Society, S.S. 8, London: Oxford University Press for the Early English Text Society.

Hieatt, Constance B. and Jones, Robin F. (eds.) 1986, 'Two Anglo-Norman culinary collections edited from British Library manuscripts Additional 32085 and Royal 12.C.xii', *Speculum* 61: 859–82.

Hiltunen, Risto and Skaffari, Janne (eds.) forthcoming, *Discourse Perspectives on English: Medieval to Modern*, Amsterdam: John Benjamins.

Hoey, Michael 2001, *Textual Interaction: An Introduction to Written Discourse Analysis*, London and New York: Routledge.

Holbrook, Sue Ellen 1998, 'A medical scientific encyclopedia "Renewed by Goodly Printing": Wynkyn de Worde's English *De Proprietatibus Rerum*', in Crossgrove *et al.* (eds.), pp. 119–56.

Horn, Wilhelm and Lehnert, Martin 1954, *Laut und Lehre: Englische Lautgeschichte der neueren Zeit (1400–1950)*, Vol. 2, Berlin: Deutscher Verlag der Wissenschaften.

Hudson, Anne 1989, 'Lollard Book production', in Griffiths and Pearsall (eds.), 125–42.

Hunt, Tony 1990, *Popular Medicine in Thirteenth-Century England: Introduction and Texts*, Cambridge: D. S. Brewer.

2000, 'Code-switching in medical texts', in Trotter (ed.), pp. 131–47.

Hunt, Tony and Benskin, Michael (eds.) 2001, *Three Receptaria from Medieval England: The Languages of Medicine in the Fourteenth Century*, Medium Ævum Monographs, New Series 21, Oxford: The Society for the Study of Medieval Languages and Literature.

Hyltenstam, Kenneth and Obler, Loraine K. (eds.) 1989, *Bilingualism Across the Lifespan: Aspects of Acquisition, Maturity and Loss*, Cambridge University Press.

Hyrtl, Joseph 1879, *Das Arabische und Hebräische in der Anatomie*, Vienna: Wilhelm Braumüller.

IMEP = The Index of Middle English Prose, 1984 –, Vols. 1 –, Cambridge: D. S. Brewer.

The Index of Middle English Verse, 1943, Brown, Carleton and Robbins, Rossell Hope, New York: Columbia University Press.

The Index of Printed Middle English Prose 1985, Lewis, R. E., Blake, Norman F. and Edwards, A. S. G., Garland Reference Library of the Humanities 537, New York: Garland.

Jacquart, Danielle 1998, 'Medical scholasticism', in Grmek (ed.), pp. 197–240.

James, M. R. 1900–04, *The Western Manuscripts in the Library of Trinity College, Cambridge: A Descriptive Catalogue*, 4 vols., Cambridge University Press.

1907–08, *A Descriptive Catalogue of the Manuscripts in the Library of Gonville and Caius College*, 2 vols., Cambridge University Press.

Jasin, Joanne 1983, 'A critical edition of the Middle English *Liber uricrisiarum* in Wellcome Ms. 225', Ph.D. thesis, Tulane University.

1993, 'The transmission of learned medical literature in the Middle English *Liber uricrisiarum*', *Medical History* 37: 313–29.

Jespersen, Otto 1905/1972, *Growth and Structure of the English Language*, Oxford: Blackwell.

Jones, Claire 1998, 'Formula and formulation: "Efficacy phrases" in medieval English medical manuscripts', *Neuphilologische Mitteilungen* 99: 199–209.

2000, 'Vernacular literacy in late-medieval England: The example of East Anglian medical manuscripts', Ph.D. thesis, University of Glasgow.

2001, 'Elaboration in practice: The use of English in medieval East Anglian medicine', in Fisiak and Trudgill (eds.), pp. 163–78.

Jones, Peter Murray 1984, *Medieval Medical Miniatures*, London: British Library.

1989, 'Four Middle English translations of John Arderne', in Minnis (ed.), pp. 61–89.

1990, 'Medical books before the invention of printing', in Besson (ed.), pp. 1–29.

1994, 'John of Arderne and the Mediterranean tradition of scholastic surgery', in García-Ballester *et al.* (eds.), pp. 289–321.

1995, 'Harley MS 2558, a fifteenth-century medical commonplace book', in Schleissner (ed.), pp. 35–54.

1998a, *Medieval Medicine in Illuminated Manuscripts*, Noventa Padovana: The British Library and Centro Tibaldi.

1998b, 'Thomas Fayreford: An English fifteenth-century medical practitioner', in French *et al.* (eds.), pp. 156–83.

1999, 'Medicine and science', in Hellinga and Trapp (eds.), pp. 433–69.

2000, 'Medical libraries and medical Latin', in Bracke and Deumens (eds.), pp. 115–35.

Jordan, Mark D. and Emery, Jr., Kent (eds.) 1976, Ad Litteram: *Authoritative Texts and their Medieval Readers*, Notre Dame Conferences in Medieval Studies 3, University of Notre Dame Press.

Jucker, Andreas (ed.) 1995, *Historical Pragmatics: Pragmatic Developments in the History of English*, Pragmatics and Beyond, New Series 35, Amsterdam and Philadelphia: Benjamins.

Jucker, Andreas H., Fritz, Gerd and Lebsanft, Franz (eds.) 1999, *Historical Dialogue Analysis*, Pragmatics and Beyond, New Series 66, Amsterdam and Philadelphia: Benjamins.

Kahlas-Tarkka, Leena (ed.) 1987, *Neophilologica Fennica*, Mémoires de la Société Néophilologique de Helsinki 45, Helsinki: Société Néophilologique.

Kastovsky, Dieter (ed.) 1994, *Studies in Early Modern English*, Berlin and New York: Mouton de Gruyter.

Kastovsky, Dieter and Mettinger, Arthur (eds.) 2001, *Language Contact in the History of English*, Studies in English Medieval Language and Literature 1, Frankfurt am Main: Peter Lang.

Keen, Maurice 1990, *English Society in the Later Middle Ages: 1348–1500*, The Penguin Social History of Britain, Harmondsworth: Penguin Books.

Keene, Derek 2000, 'Metropolitan values: Migration, mobility and cultural norms, London 1100–1700', in Wright (ed.), pp. 93–114.

Keiser, George R. 1978, '*Epwort*: a ghost word in the Middle English Dictionary', *English Language Notes* 15: 163–4.

1996, 'Reconstructing Robert Thornton's herbal', *Medium Ævum* 65: 35–53.

1998, *A Manual of the Writings in Middle English 1050–1500*, Vol. 10, *Works of Science and Information*, New Haven: The Connecticut Academy of Arts and Sciences.

Keller, Henning (ed.) 1971, 'Die me. Rezepte des Ms. Harley 2253', *Archiv für das Studium der neueren Sprachen und Literaturen* 207: 94–100.

Kirk, John M. (ed.) 2000, *Corpora Galore: Analyses and Techniques in Describing English*, Language and Computers: Studies in Practical Linguistics 30, Amsterdam and Atlanta: Rodopi.

Kitson, Peter 1989, 'From Eastern learning to Western folklore: The transmission of some medico-magical ideas', in Scragg (ed.), pp. 57–71.

Knowles, Gerry 1997, *A Cultural History of the English Language*, London and New York: Arnold.

Kristeva, Julia 1986, 'Word, dialogue, and the novel', in Moi (ed.), pp. 35–61.

Laing, Margaret 1993, *Catalogue of Sources for a* Linguistic Atlas of Early Medieval English, Cambridge: D. S. Brewer.

LALME = A Linguistic Atlas of Late Mediaeval English 1986, McIntosh, Angus, Samuels, M. L., Benskin, Michael, with the assistance of Laing, Margaret and Williamson, Keith, 4 vols., Aberdeen University Press.

Lang, S. J. 1992, 'John Bradmore and his book *Philomena*', *Social History of Medicine* 5: 121–30.

Lawn, Brian 1963, *The Salernitan Questions: An Introduction to the History of Medieval and Renaissance Problem Literature*, Oxford: Clarendon Press.

1993, *The Rise and Decline of the Scholastic* Quaestio Disputata: *With Special Emphasis on its Use in the Teaching of Medicine and Science*. Leiden: Brill.

Lawn, Brian (ed.) 1979, *The Prose Salernitan Questions, Edited from a Bodleian Manuscript (Auct. F. 3. 10): An Anonymous Collection Dealing with Science and Medicine Written by an Englishman c. 1200, with an Appendix of Ten Related Collections*, London: Oxford University Press.

Lehrer, Adrienne 1974, *Semantic Fields and Lexical Structure*, Amsterdam and London: North-Holland.

Lerer, Seth 1985, *Boethius and Dialogue: Literary Method in* The Consolation of Philosophy, Princeton University Press.

Lester, G. A. 1987, 'The books of a fifteenth-century gentleman, Sir John Paston', *Neuphilologische Mitteilungen* 88: 200–17.

Leuvensteijn, J. A. and Berns, J. B. (eds.) 1992, *Dialect and Standard Language in the English, Dutch, German and Norwegian Language Area*, Amsterdam, Oxford, New York and Tokyo: North-Holland.

Levere, Trevor H. (ed.) 1982, *Editing Texts in the History of Science and Medicine: Papers given at the Seventeenth Annual Conference on Editorial Problems, University of Toronto, 6–7 November 1981*, New York and London: Garland.

Lipka, Leonhard 1990, *An Outline of English Lexicology*, Tübingen: Niemeyer.

Liuzza, Roy Michael 2001, 'Anglo-Saxon prognostics in context: A survey and handlist of manuscripts', *Anglo-Saxon England* 30: 181–230.

Lonie, Iain M. 1981, *The Hippocratic Treatises 'On Generation', 'On the Nature of the Child', 'Diseases IV': A Commentary*, Ars Medica, Abteilung 2, Band 7, Berlin and New York: Walter de Gruyter.

Louis, Cameron (ed.) 1980, *The Commonplace Book of Robert Reynes of Acle: An Edition of Tanner Ms. 407*, Garland Medieval Texts 1, New York and London: Garland.

Löweneck, Max (ed.) 1896, Peri Didaxeon: *Eine Sammlung von Rezepten in Englischer Sprache aus dem 11./12. Jahrhundert*, Erlanger Beiträge zur Englischen Philologie und Vergleichenden Litteraturgesichte 12, Erlangen: Fr. Junge.

Lucas, Angela M. and Lucas, Peter J. 2001, 'A description of Jesus College MS Q.G.23 containing Guy de Chauliac's *Chirurgie*: A supplement to M. R. James's *Catalogue*', *Transactions of the Cambridge Bibliographical Society* 21: 132–44.

Lucas, Peter and Lucas, Angela M. (eds.) 2002, *Middle English from Tongue to Text*, Studies in English Medieval Language and Literature 4, Frankfurt am Main: Peter Lang.

Machan, Tim William 2003, *English in the Middle Ages*, Oxford University Press.

MacKinney, Loren C. 1936, 'Dynamidia in medieval medical literature', *Isis* 24: 400–14.

Mäkinen, Martti 2002a, 'Henry Daniel's Rosemary in MS X.90 of the Royal Library, Stockholm', *Neuphilologische Mitteilungen* 103: 305–27.

   2002b, 'On interaction in herbals from ME to EModE', *Journal of Historical Pragmatics* 3: 229–51.

   2002c, 'Virtual recipes – virtues as a text type in early herbals', in Raumolin-Brunberg *et al.* (eds.), pp. 271–86.

Manzalaoui, Mahmoud (ed.) 1977e, Secretum Secretorum: *Nine English Versions*, Vol. 1, *Text*, Early English Text Society 276, Oxford University Press.

Marchand, Hans 1969, *The Categories and Types of Present-Day English Word-Formation: A Synchronic-Diachronic Approach*, Munich: C. H. Beck.

Matheson, Lister M. (ed.) 1994, *Popular and Practical Science of Medieval England*, East Lansing: Colleagues Press.

McConchie, Roderick W. 1997, *Lexicography and Physicke: The Record of Sixteenth-Century English Medical Terminology*, Oxford: Clarendon Press.

McIntosh, Angus 1983, 'Present indicative plural forms in the later Middle English of the North Midlands', in Gray and Stanley (eds.), pp. 235–44.

McIntosh, Angus, Samuels, M. L. and Laing, Margaret 1989, *Middle English Dialectology: Essays on Some Principles and Problems*, edited by Laing, Margaret, Aberdeen University Press.

McLean, Ian 1980, *The Renaissance Notion of Woman: A Study in the Fortunes of Scholasticism and Medical Science in European Intellectual Life*, Cambridge University Press.

McVaugh, Michael R. (ed.) 1997, *Guigonis de Caulhiaco (Guy de Chauliac): Inventarium sive Chirurgia Magna*, Vol. 1, *Text*, Leiden, New York and Cologne: Brill.

McVaugh, Michael R. and Ogden, Margaret S. 1997, *Guigonis de Caulhiaco (Guy de Chauliac): Inventarium sive Chirurgia Magna*, Vol. 2, *Commentary*, Leiden, New York and Cologne: Brill.

McVaugh, Michael R. and Siraisi, Nancy (eds.) 1990, *Renaissance Medical Learning: Evolution of a Tradition*, Osiris 2nd series 6, Philadelphia: University of Pennsylvania Press.

MED = *Middle English Dictionary* 1956–2001, Kurath, Hans, Kuhn, Sherman M. and Lewis, Robert E. (eds.), Ann Arbor: University of Michigan Press, online at http://ets.umdl.umich.edu/m/med/.

Meech, S. B., Moore, S. and Whitehall, H. 1935, 'Middle English dialect characteristics and dialect boundaries', in *Essays and Studies in English and Comparative Literature*, University of Michigan Publications, Language and Literature 13, Ann Arbor: University of Michigan Press.

Meeuwis, Michael and Blommaert, Jan 1998, 'A monolectal view of code-switching: Layered code-switching among Zairians in Belgium', in Auer (ed.), pp. 76–98.

Middle English Compendium, online at http://ets.umdl.umich.edu/m/mec.

Michler, Markwart 1961, 'Zur metaphorischen und etymologischen Deutung des Wortes Πεδίου in der anatomischen Nomenklatur', *Sudhoffs Archiv für Geschichte der Medizin* 45: 216–24.

Milroy, James 1992, *Linguistic Variation and Change: On the Historical Sociolinguistics of English*, Oxford: Blackwell.

Milroy, Lesley 1987, *Language and Social Networks*, 2nd edn, Oxford: Blackwell.

Milroy, Lesley and Muysken, Pieter (eds.) 1995, *One Speaker, Two Languages: Cross-disciplinary Perspectives on Code-switching*, Cambridge University Press.

Minkova, Donka and Stockwell, Robert P. (eds.) 2002, *Studies in the History of the English Language: A Millennial Perspective*, Topics in English Linguistics 39, Berlin and New York: Mouton de Gruyter.

Minnis, Alastair J. 1979, 'Late medieval discussions of *compilatio* and the rôle of the *compilator*', *Beiträge zur Geschichte der Deutschen Sprache und Literatur* 101: 385–421.

1984, *Medieval Theory of Authorship: Scholastic Literary Attitudes in the Later Middle Ages*, London: Scolar Press.

1987, '"Glosynge is a glorious thing": Chaucer at work on the *Boece*', in Minnis (ed.), pp. 106–24.

Minnis, Alastair J. (ed.) 1987, *The Medieval Boethius: Studies in the Vernacular Translations of* De Consolatione Philosophiae, Cambridge: D. S. Brewer.

1989, *Latin and Vernacular: Studies in Late-Medieval Texts and Manuscripts*, Cambridge: D. S. Brewer.

Minnis, Alastair J., Scott, A. B. and Wallace, David (eds.) 1988, *Medieval Literary Theory and Criticism c. 1100–c.1375: The Commentary Tradition*, Rev. edn, Oxford: Clarendon Press.

MNW = *Middelnederlandsch woordenboek* 1885–1941, Verwijs, Eelco and Verdam, Jakob, The Hague: Martinus Nijhoff.

Moi, Toril (ed.) 1986, *The Kristeva Reader*, New York: Columbia University Press.

Mooney, Linne R. 1995, *The Index of Middle English Prose, Handlist 11: Manuscripts in the Library of Trinity College, Cambridge*, Cambridge: D. S. Brewer.

2000, 'Professional scribes? Identifying English scribes who had a hand in more than one manuscript', in Pearsall (ed.), pp. 131–41.

Morton, A. G. 1981, *History of Botanical Science*, London and New York: Academic Press.

Mory, Robert Nels (ed.) 1977, 'A medieval English anatomy', Ph.D. thesis, University of Michigan.

Müller, Gottfried 1929a, 'Wortkundliches aus mittelenglischen Medizinbüchern', *Britannica*: 145–54.

Müller, Gottfried (ed.) 1929b, *Aus mittelenglischen Medizintexten: Die Prosarezepte des stockholmer Miszellankodex X.90*, Kölner Anglistische Arbeiten 10, Leipzig: Bernhard Tauchnitz.

Murdoch, John 1984, *Album of Science, Antiquity and the Middle Ages*, New York: Scribner.

Muysken, Pieter 2000, *Bilingual Speech: A Typology of Code-mixing*, Cambridge University Press.

Myers-Scotton, Carol 1993, 'Common and uncommon ground: Social and structural factors in codeswitching', *Language in Society* 22: 475–503.

1997, *Duelling Languages: Grammatical Structure in Code-switching*, 2nd edn, Oxford: Clarendon Press.

2002, *Contact Linguistics: Bilingual Encounters and Grammatical Outcomes*, Oxford and New York: Oxford University Press.

Myers-Scotton, Carol (ed.) 1998, *Codes and Consequences: Choosing Linguistic Varieties*, New York: Oxford University Press.

Nevalainen, Terttu and Kahlas-Tarkka, Leena (eds.) 1997, *To Explain the Present: Studies in the Changing English Language in Honour of Matti Rissanen*, Mémoires de la Société Néophilologique 52, Helsinki: Société Néophilologique.

von Nolcken, Christina 1979, *The Middle English Translation of the Rosarium Theologie*, Middle English Texts 10, Heidelberg: Carl Winter.

Norri, Juhani 1988a, 'A note on the entry *rede-wale* in the *Middle English Dictionary*', *Notes and Queries* 233: 11–12.

1988b, 'Notes on some corrupt passages in fifteenth-century medical manuscripts', *Neuphilologische Mitteilungen* 89: 320–3.

1992, *Names of Sicknesses in English, 1400–1550: An Exploration of the Lexical Field* (Diss.), Annales Academiae Scientiarum Fennicae, Dissertationes Humanarum Litterarum 63, Helsinki: Academia Scientiarum Fennicae.

1998, *Names of Body Parts in English, 1400–1550*, Annales Academiae Scientiarum Fennicae, Humaniora 291, Helsinki: Academia Scientiarum Fennicae.

North, John 1990. 'Richard of Wallingford', *Dictionary of Scientific Biography*, edited by Charles Gillispie, New York: Scribner.

North, John (ed.) 1976, *Richard of Wallingford: An Edition of His Writings*, 3 vols., Oxford: Clarendon Press.

Nurmi, Arja and Pahta, Päivi forthcoming, 'Social stratification and patterns of code-switching in early English correspondence', *Multilingua*.

OED = *The Oxford English Dictionary* 1989, Murray, James A. H., Bradley, Henry, Craigie, W. A. and Onions, C. T. (eds.), 2nd edn, Oxford: Clarendon Press, on-line at http://www.oed.com/.

Ogden, Margaret S. (ed.) 1938/1969, *The* Liber de diversis medicinis, *in the Thornton Manuscript (Ms. Lincoln Cathedral A.5.2)*, Early English Text Society, O.S. 207, London: Oxford University Press.

1971, *The Cyrurgie of Guy de Chauliac*, Early English Text Society, O.S. 265, London, New York and Toronto: Oxford University Press.

OLD = *Oxford Latin Dictionary* 1985, Glare, P. W. G. (ed.) Oxford: Clarendon Press.

O'Neill, Ynez Violé 1993, 'Diagrams of the medieval brain: A study in cerebral localization', in Cassidy (ed.), pp. 91–105.

Ong, Walter J. 1958, *Ramus: Method, and the Decay of Dialogue*, Cambridge, Mass.: Harvard University Press.

Orme, Nicholas 1983, 'The education of the courtier', in Scattergood and Sherborne (eds.), pp. 63–85.

Ormerod, Fiona and Ivanic, Roz 2000, 'Texts in practices: Interpreting the physical characteristics of children's project work', in Barton *et al.* (eds.), pp. 91–107.

Ottosson, Per-Gunnar 1984, *Scholastic Medicine and Philosophy: A Study of Commentaries of Galen's Tegni (ca. 1300–1450)*, Naples: Bibliopolis.

Pagel, Julius Leopold (ed.) 1892, *Die Chirurgie des Heinrich von Mondeville (Hermondaville): Nach Berliner, Erfurter und Pariser Codices*, Berlin: August Hirschwald.

Pahta, Päivi 1998, *Medieval Embryology in the Vernacular: The Case of De spermate* (Diss.) Mémoires de la Société Néophilologique de Helsinki 53, Helsinki: Société Néophilologique.

2001, 'Creating a new genre: Contextual dimensions in the production and transmission of early scientific writing', *EJES* 5: 205–20.

2003, 'On structures of code-switching in medical texts from medieval England', *Neuphilologische Mitteilungen* 104: 197–210.

forthcoming, 'Description of the manuscript', in Tavormina (ed.) forthcoming b.

Pahta, Päivi and Carrillo Linares, María José forthcoming, 'Translation strategies in *De spermate* and *De humana natura*', in Tavormina (ed.) forthcoming b.

Pahta, Päivi and Nevanlinna, Saara 1997, 'Re-phrasing in early English: The use of expository apposition with an explicit marker from 1350 to 1710', in Rissanen *et al.* (eds.), pp. 121–83.

Pahta, Päivi and Taavitsainen, Irma 1999, 'Noun phrase structures in scientific language 1375–1550', A paper presented at ICAME 20, Freiburg.

Palmer, Frank Robert 1981, *Semantics*, 2nd edn, Cambridge University Press.

Palmer, Leonard Robert 1936, *An Introduction to Modern Linguistics*, London: Macmillan.

Parkes, Malcolm B. 1973, 'The literacy of the laity', in Daiches and Thorlby (eds.), pp. 555–77.

1976, 'The influence of concepts of *Ordinatio* and *Compilatio* on the development of the book', in Jordan and Emery (eds.), pp. 113–34.

Parkes, Malcolm B. and Watson, Andrew G. (eds.) 1978, *Medieval Scribes, Manuscripts and Libraries: Essays Presented to N. R. Ker*, London: Scolar Press.

Pearsall, Derek 1989, 'Introduction', in Griffiths and Pearsall (eds.), pp. 1–10.

Pearsall, Derek (ed.) 2000, *New Directions in Later Medieval Manuscript Studies: Essays from the 1998 Harvard Conference*, York Medieval Press.

Pearson, David 1994, *Provenance Research in Book History*, The British Library Studies in the History of the Book, London: The British Library.

Plett, Heinrich, 1991, 'Intertextualities', in Plett (ed.), pp. 3–29.

Plett, Heinrich (ed.) 1991, *Intertextuality*, Research in Text Theory 15, Berlin and New York: Walter de Gruyter.

Pollington, Stephen 2000, *Leechcraft: Early English Charms, Plantlore and Healing*, Hockwold-cum-Wilton: Anglo-Saxon Books.

Pope, M. K. 1966, *From Latin to Modern French with Especial Consideration of Anglo-Norman*, Manchester University Press.

Poplack, Shana 1982, 'Sometimes I'll start a sentence in Spanish *y termino en español*: Toward a typology of code-switching', in Amastae and Elías-Olivares (eds.), pp. 230–63.

Poplack, Shana, Wheeler, S. and Westwood, A. 1989, 'Distinguishing language contact phenomena: Evidence from Finnish-English bilingualism', in Hyltenstam and Obler (eds.), pp. 132–54.

Porter, Roy (ed.) 1992, *The Popularization of Medicine, 1650–1850*, The Wellcome Institute Series in the History of Medicine, London and New York: Routledge.

Power, D'Arcy (ed.) 1910, *Treatises of Fistula in Ano. Haemorrhoids, and Clysters by John Arderne*, Early English Text Society, O.S. 139, London: Kegan Paul, Trench, Trübner.

Pride, J. B. and Holmes, Janet (eds.) 1972/1979, *Sociolinguistics: Selected Readings*, Harmondsworth: Penguin.

Rand Schmidt, Kari Anne 1994, '*The Index of Middle English Prose* and late medieval English recipes', *English Studies* 5: 423–29.

  2001, *The Index of Middle English Prose, Handlist 17: Manuscripts in the Library of Gonville and Caius College, Cambridge*, Cambridge: D. S. Brewer.

Raumolin-Brunberg, Helena, Nevala, Minna, Nurmi, Arja and Rissanen, Matti (eds.) 2002, *Variation Past and Present: VARIENG Studies on English for Terttu Nevalainen*, Mémoires de la Société Néophilologique de Helsinki 61, Helsinki: Société Néophilologique.

Rawcliffe, Carole 1995, *Medicine and Society in Later Medieval England*, Stroud: Alan Sutton.

Reimer, Stephen R. 1998, 'Palaeography sample: William Herebert, OFM', *Manuscript Studies: Medieval and Early Modern* (Web-page), http://www.ualberta.ca/~sreimer/ms-course/course/herebert.htm, 17 November 2002.

Rhodes, Dennis E. 1956, 'Provost Argentine of King's and his books', *Transactions of the Cambridge Bibliographical Society* 2: 205–12.

Richter, Michael 1979, *Sprache und Gesellschaft im Mittelalter: Untersuchungen zur mündlichen Kommunikation in England von der Mitte des elften bis zum Beginn des vierzehnten Jahrhunderts*, Monographien zur Geschicte des Mittelalters 18, Stuttgart: Hiersemann.

  2000, 'Collecting miracles along the Anglo-Welsh border in the early fourteenth century', in Trotter (ed.), pp. 53–60.

Riddy, Felicity (ed.) 1991, *Regionalism in Late Medieval Manuscripts and Texts: Essays Celebrating the Publication of* A Linguistic Atlas of Late Mediaeval English, Cambridge: D. S. Brewer.

Rissanen, Matti, Ihalainen, Ossi, Nevalainen, Terttu and Taavitsainen, Irma (eds.) 1992, *History of Englishes: New Methods and Interpretations in Historical Linguistics*, Berlin and New York: Mouton de Gruyter.

Rissanen, Matti, Kytö, Merja and Palander-Collin, Minna (eds.) 1993, *Early English in the Computer Age: Explorations through the Helsinki Corpus*, Topics in English Linguistics 11, Berlin and New York: Mouton de Gruyter.

Rissanen, Matti, Kytö, Merja and Heikkonen, Kirsi (eds.) 1997, *English in Transition: Corpus-based Studies in Linguistic Variation and Genre Styles*, Topics in English Linguistics 23, Berlin and New York: Mouton de Gruyter.

RMLW = Revised Medieval Latin Word-list from British and Irish Sources, with Supplement 1989, Latham, R. E. (ed.), Oxford University Press.

Robbins, Rossell Hope 1970, 'Medical manuscripts in Middle English', *Speculum* 45: 393–415.

Robbins, Rossell Hope (ed.) 1952, *Secular Lyrics of the XIVth and XVth Centuries: Practical Verse*, Oxford University Press.

Roeder, Helen 1955, *Saints and Their Attributes: With a Guide to Localities and Patronage*, London: Longmans, Green and Co.

Rohde, Eleanour S. 1922/1971, *The Old English Herbals*, New York: Dover.

Romaine, Suzanne 1995, *Bilingualism*, 2nd edn, Oxford: Blackwell.

Rothwell, William 1991, 'The missing link in English etymology: Anglo French', *Medium Ævum* 60: 173–96.

2000, 'Aspects of lexical and morphosyntactical mixing in the languages of medieval England', in Trotter (ed.), pp. 213–32.

Rotuli Parliamentorum.

Rubin, Stanley 1974, *Medieval English Medicine*, Newton Abbot: David and Charles.

Sager, Juan C. 1990, *A Practical Course in Terminology Processing*, Amsterdam and Philadelphia: Benjamins.

Sager, Juan C., Dungworth, David and McDonald, Peter F. 1980, *English Special Language: Principles and Practice in Science and Technology*, Wiesbaden: Oscar Brandstetter.

Samuels, Michael L. 1963/1989, 'Some applications of Middle English dialectology', *English Studies* 44: 81–94, reprinted in McIntosh *et al.*, pp. 64–80.

1972, *Linguistic Evolution, with Special Reference to English*, Cambridge University Press.

1988, 'The scribe of the Hengwrt and Ellesmere manuscripts of *The Canterbury Tales*', in Smith (ed.), pp. 38–50.

Samuels, Michael L. and Smith, Jeremy J. 1981, 'The language of Gower', *Neuphilologische Mitteilungen* 82: 294–304.

Sánchez-Roura, Teresa 2001, 'The medieval English culinary recipe today', A paper presented at the 6th Cardiff Conference on the Theory and Practice of Translation in the Middle Ages, Santiago de Compostela.

Santana Henriquez, Germán and Santana Sanjurjo, Victoriano (eds.) 2002, *Studia Humanitatis in Honorem Antonio Cabrera Perera*, Servicio de Publicaciones de la Universidad de Las Palmas de Gran Canaria.

Sass, Lorna J. 1981, 'Religion, medicine, politics and spices', *Appetite* 1: 7–13.

Scattergood, Vincent John and Sherborne, James W. (eds.) 1983, *English Court Culture in the Later Middle Ages*, London: Duckworth.

Schäfer, Jürgen 1989a, *Early Modern English Lexicography*, Vol. 1, *A Survey of Monolingual Printed Glossaries and Dictionaries 1475–1640*, Oxford: Clarendon Press.

1989b, *Early Modern English Lexicography*, Vol. 2, *Additions and Corrections to the OED*, Oxford: Clarendon Press.

Schendl, Herbert 2000a, 'Linguistic aspects of code-switching in medieval English texts', in Trotter (ed.), pp. 77–92.

2000b, 'Syntactic constraints on code-switching in medieval texts', in Taavitsainen *et al.* (eds.), pp. 67–86.

2002a, 'Code-choice and code-switching in some early fifteenth-century letters', in Lucas and Lucas (eds.), pp. 247–262.

2002b, 'Mixed language texts as data and evidence for English historical linguistics', in Minkova and Stockwell (eds.), pp. 51–78.

Schleissner, Margaret R. (ed.) 1995, *Manuscript Sources of Medieval Medicine: A Book of Essays*, Garland Medieval Casebooks 8, New York and London: Garland.

Schöffler, Herbert (ed.) 1919, *Beiträge zur mittelenglischen Medizinlitteratur*, III Anglistische Abteilung, Heft 1, Leipzig: Niemeyer.

Scragg, D. G. (ed.) 1989, *Superstition and Popular Medicine in Anglo-Saxon England*, Manchester Centre for Anglo-Saxon Studies.

Scully, Terence 1995, 'Tempering medieval food', in Weiss Adamson (ed.), pp. 3–23.

Searle, John R. 1985, *Expression and Meaning: Studies in the Theory of Speech Acts*, Cambridge University Press.

Serjeantson, Mary S. 1935, *A History of Foreign Words in English*, London: Kegan Paul, Trench, Trübner & Co.

Seymour, Michael C. *et al.* (eds.) 1975/1988, *On the Properties of Things: John Trevisa's Translation of Bartholomaeus Anglicus De Proprietatibus Rerum*, Vol. 1, Oxford University Press.

Seymour, Michael C. *et al.* 1992, *Bartholomaeus Anglicus and his Encyclopaedia*, London: Ashgate.

Shank, Michael H. (ed.) 2000, *The Scientific Enterprise in Antiquity and the Middle Ages*, University of Chicago Press.

Short, Ian 1980, 'On bilingualism in Anglo-Norman England', *Romance Philology* 33: 467–79.

Siegler, Jeff 1985, 'Koines and koineization', *Language in Society* 14: 357–78.

Sigurs, G. 1964, 'Le vocabulaire médical français aux XIVe–XVIe siècles: Sa formation et son développement', *Revue des langues romanes* 76: 63–74.

1965, 'La langue médicale française: Nouvelles datations', *Le français moderne* 33: 199–218.

Singer, Charles 1927, 'The herbal in antiquity and its transmission to later ages', *The Journal of Hellenistic Studies* 47: 1–52.

1948, 'Galen's elementary course on bones', *Proceedings of the Royal Society of Medicine* 41, Section of the History of Medicine, pp. 767–76.

1959, 'The strange histories of some anatomical terms', *Medical History* 3: 1–7.

Singer, Dorothea W. 1919, 'Survey of the medical manuscripts in the British Isles dating from before the sixteenth century', *Proceedings of the Royal Society of Medicine* 12, Section of the History of Medicine, pp. 96–107.

Siraisi, Nancy 1984, 'Some current trends in the study of Renaissance medicine', *Renaissance Quarterly* 37: 585–600.

1990, *Medieval and Early Renaissance Medicine: An Introduction to Knowledge and Practice*, Chicago and London: University of Chicago Press.

1994, 'How to write a Latin book on surgery: Organizing principles and authorial devices in Guglielmo da Saliceto and Dino del Garbo', in García-Ballester *et al.* (eds.), pp. 88–109.

2001, *Medicine and the Italian Universities, 1250–1600*, Leiden: Brill.

Skaffari, Janne, Peikola, Matti, Carroll, Ruth, Hiltunen, Risto and Wårvik, Brita (eds.) forthcoming, *Opening Windows on Texts and Discourses of the Past*.

Skinner, Henry Alan 1949, *The Origin of Medical Terms*, Baltimore: Williams and Wilkins.

Slack, Paul 1979, 'Mirrors of health and treasures of poor men: The uses of vernacular medical literature of Tudor England', in Webster (ed.), pp. 237–73.

Sloane Catalogue = *Catalogus librorum manuscriptorum bibliothecae Sloaniane* 1837–40, London: British Museum.

Smiley, Timothy 1995, *Philosophical Dialogues: Plato, Hume, Wittgenstein*, Proceedings of the British Academy 85, Oxford University Press for the British Academy.

Smith, Jeremy J. 1988, 'The Trinity Gower D-scribe and his work on two early *Canterbury Tales* manuscripts', in Smith (ed.), pp. 38–50.

1996, *An Historical Study of English: Function, Form and Change*, London: Routledge.

Smith, Jeremy J. (ed.) 1988, *The English of Chaucer and his Contemporaries*, Aberdeen University Press.

Sournia, J.-C. 1976, 'Remarques sur quelques termes d'anatomie', *Histoire des Sciences Médicales* 10: 102–5.

Staczek, John 1996, '*Đin* in Late Middle English and its contemporary reflex in instructional settings', in Fisiak (ed.), pp. 245–52.

Stannard, Jerry 1982, 'Rezeptliteratur as Fachliteratur', in Eamon (ed.), pp. 59–73.

STC = *A Short-Title Catalogue of Books Printed in England, Scotland, and Ireland and of English Books Printed Abroad 1475–1640*, 1976/1986, Pollard, A. W. and Redgrave, G. R., Oxford University Press.

Stenroos, Merja forthcoming, 'Middle English dialects: A variationist approach'.

Stephen, Leslie and Lee, Sidney (eds.) 1885–1900, *Dictionary of National Biography*, London: Smith, Elder and Co.

Stephens, George 1844, 'Extracts in prose and verse from an old English medical manuscript, preserved in the Royal Library at Stockholm', *Archaeologia* 30: 395.

Stølen, Marianne 1990, 'Harmonien: An ethnohistorical sociolinguistic analysis of a Danish-American organization', Ph.D. thesis, University of Washington.

1992, 'Code-switching for humour and ethnic identity: Written Danish-American occasional songs', *Journal of Multilingual and Multicultural Development* 31: 215–28.

Street, Brian V. 1995, *Social Literacies*, Real Language Series, London: Longman.

Sudhoff, Karl 1910, 'Planta noctis', *Archiv für Geschichte der Medizin* 3: 352.

1914, 'Beiträge zur Geschichte der Chirurgie im Mittelalter, Erster Teil', *Studien zur Geschichte der Medizin* 10: 214–16.

Svinhufvud, Anne Charlotte (ed.) 1978, *A Late Middle English Treatise on Horses: Edited from British Library MS Sloane 2584 ff. 102–117b*, Stockholm: Almqvist and Wiksell International.

Swales, John M. 1990, *Genre Analysis: English in Academic and Research Settings*, Cambridge Applied Linguistics Series, Cambridge University Press.

1993, 'Genre and Engagement', *Revue Belge de Philologie et d'Histoire*, 71 (3): 687–98.

Taavitsainen, Irma 1987, '*Storia Lune* and its paraphrase in prose: Two versions of a Middle English lunary', in Kahlas-Tarkka (ed.), 521–55.

1988, *Middle English Lunaries: A Study of the Genre* (Diss.), Mémoires de la Société Néophilologique de Helsinki 47, Helsinki: Société Néophilologique.

1994a, 'On the evolution of scientific writings from 1375 to 1675: Repertoire of emotive features', in Fernandez *et al.* (eds.), pp. 329–42.

1994b, *The Index of Middle English Prose, Handlist 10: Manuscripts in Scandinavian Collections*, Cambridge: D. S. Brewer.

1994c, 'A zodiacal lunary for medical professionals', in Matheson (ed.), pp. 283–300.

1999, 'Dialogues in late medieval and Early Modern English medical writing', in Jucker *et al.* (eds.), pp. 243–68.

2000a, 'Metadiscursive practices and the evolution of early English medical writing 1375–1550', in Kirk (ed.), pp. 191–207.

2000b, 'Scientific language and spelling standardisation 1375–1550', in Wright (ed.), pp. 131–54.

2001a. 'Evidentiality and scientific thought-styles: English medical writing in Late Middle English and Early Modern English', in Gotti and Dossena (eds.), pp. 21–52.

2001b, 'Language history and the scientific register', in Diller and Görlach (eds.), pp. 185–202.

2001c, 'Middle English recipes: Genre characteristics, text type features and underlying traditions of writing', *Journal of Historical Pragmatics* 2: 85–113.

2002, 'Historical discourse analysis: Scientific language and changing thought-styles', in Fanego *et al.* (eds.), pp. 201–26.

forthcoming, 'Genres and the appropriation of science: *loci communes* in English literature in the late medieval and early modern period', in Skaffari *et al.* (eds.).

Taavitsainen, Irma, Nevalainen, Terttu, Pahta, Päivi and Rissanen, Matti (eds.) 2000, *Placing Middle English in Context*, Topics in English Linguistics 35, Berlin and New York: Mouton de Gruyter.

Taavitsainen, Irma and Pahta, Päivi 1995, 'Scientific "thought-styles" in discourse structure: Changing patterns in a historical perspective', in Wårvik *et al.* (eds.), pp. 519–29.

1997, 'The Corpus of Early English Medical Writing: Linguistic variation and prescriptive collocations in scholastic style', in Nevalainen and Kahlas-Tarkka (eds.), pp. 209–25.

1998, 'Vernacularisation of medical writing in English: A corpus-based study of scholasticism', *Early Science and Medicine* 3: 157–85.

2001, 'Transferring classical discourse forms into vernacular: Commentaries in early English medical writing', A paper presented at the 36th Medieval Studies Conference, Kalamazoo, Michigan.

Taavitsainen, Irma, Pahta, Päivi, Leskinen, Noora, Ratia, Maura and Suhr, Carla 2002, 'Analysing scientific thought-styles: What can linguistic research reveal about the history of science?', in Raumolin-Brunberg *et al.* (eds.), pp. 251–70.

Talbert, E. W. 1942, 'The notebook of a fifteenth-century practising physician', *Texas Studies in English* 21: 5–30.

Talbot, Charles Hugh and Hammond, Eugene Ashby 1965, *The Medical Practitioners in Medieval England: A Biographical Register*, London: Wellcome Historical Medical Library.

Tavormina, M. Teresa (ed.) forthcoming a, 'Commentary of the Hippocratic *Prognostics*', in Tavormina (ed.) forthcoming b.

forthcoming b, *Sex, Aging, and Death in a Medieval Medical Compendium: Trinity College Cambridge R.14.52, Its Language, Scribe, and Texts*, Medieval and Renaissance Texts and Studies, Tempe: Arizona Center for Medieval and Renaissance Studies.

Thorndike, Lynn 1955/2000, 'The true place of astrology in the history of science', *Isis* 46: 273–8, reprinted in Shank (ed.), pp. 239–44.

Thurston, Herbert S. J. and Attwater, Donald (eds.) 1956, *Butler's Lives of the Saints*, 4 vols., New York: P. J. Kennedy and Sons.

TK = Thorndike, Lynn and Kibre, Pearl 1963, *A Catalogue of Incipits of Mediaeval Scientific Writings in Latin*, Rev. edn, Cambridge, Mass.: Mediaeval Academy of America.

Touwaide, Alain 1998, 'Dioskurides: *De materia medica*', in Ciancaspro *et al.*, pp. 37–55.

Trotter, D. A. (ed.) 2000, *Multilingualism in Later Medieval Britain*, Cambridge: D. S. Brewer.

Trudgill, Peter 1986, *Dialects in Contact*, Oxford and New York: Blackwell.

Uhlig, Claus and Zimmermann, Rüdiger (eds.) 1991, *Anglistentag 1990 Marburg: Proceedings*, Tübingen: Max Niemeyer,

Ullmann, Stephen 1977, *Semantics: An Introduction to the Science of Meaning*, Oxford: Blackwell.

Verschueren, Jef, Östman, Jan-Ola and Blommaert, Jan (eds.) 1995, *Handbook of Pragmatics 1995*, Amsterdam and Philadelphia: Benjamins.

Voigts, Linda Ehrsam 1979, 'Anglo-Saxon plant remedies and the Anglo-Saxons', *Isis* 70: 250–68.

    1982, 'Editing Middle English medical texts: Needs and issues', in Levere (ed.), pp. 39–68.

    1984, 'Medical prose', in Edwards (ed.), pp. 315–35.

    1989a, 'The character of the *carecter*: Ambiguous sigils in scientific and medical texts', in Minnis (ed.), pp. 91–109.

    1989b, 'Scientific and medical books', in Griffiths and Pearsall (eds.), pp. 345–402.

    1990, 'The "Sloane Group": Related scientific and medical manuscripts from the fifteenth century in the Sloane Collection', *The British Library Journal* 16: 26–57.

    1995a, 'A doctor and his books: The manuscripts of Roger Marchall (d. 1477)', in Beadle and Piper (eds.), pp. 249–314.

    1995b, 'Multitudes of Middle English medical manuscripts, or the English of science and medicine', in Schleissner (ed.), pp. 183–95.

    1996, 'What's the word? Bilingualism in late-medieval England', *Speculum* 71: 813–26.

Voigts, Linda Ehrsam and McVaugh, Michael R. (eds.) 1984, *A Latin Technical Phlebotomy and its Middle English Translation*, Transactions of the American Philosophical Society 74, Part 2, Philadelphia: American Philosophical Society.

de Vriend, Hubert (ed.) 1984, *The Old English Herbarium and* Medicina de Quadrupedibus, Early English Text Society, O.S. 286, Oxford University Press for the Early English Text Society.

de Vries, Ad 1974, *Dictionary of Symbols and Imagery*, Amsterdam: North-Holland.

Waldron, Ronald 1991, 'Dialect aspect of manuscripts of Trevisa's translation of the *Polychronicon*', in Riddy (ed.), pp. 67–87.

Waldron, Ronald (ed.) 2004, *John Trevisa's Translation of the Polychronicon of Ranulph Higden, Book VI*, Middle English Texts 35, Heidelberg: Universitätsverlag C. Winter.

Wales, Katie 1996, *Pronouns in Present-day English*, Cambridge University Press.

Wallis, Faith 1995, 'The experience of the book: Manuscripts, texts, and the role of epistemology in early medieval medicine', in Bates (ed.), pp. 101–26.

Wallner, Björn 1964a, 'Lexical matter in the Middle English translation of Guy de Chauliac', *English Studies* 45 (Supplement): 151–6.

    1969, 'A note on some Middle English medical terms', *English Studies* 50: 499–503.

    1987, 'On the .i. periphrasis in the N.Y. Chauliac', *Neuphilologische Mitteilungen* 88: 286–94.

1991, 'A newly discovered Guy de Chauliac manuscript', *Notes and Queries* 38: 159.

Wallner, Björn (ed.) 1964b, *The Middle English Translation of Guy de Chauliac's Anatomy, With Guy's Essay on the History of Medicine*, Lund Universitets Årsskrift, N.F. Avd. 1, B.D. 56, Nr. 5, Lund: CWK Gleerup.

Warner, George and Gilson, Julius 1921, *Catalogue of Western Manuscripts in the Old Royal and King's Collections in the British Museum*, 4 vols., London: British Museum.

Wårvik, Brita, Tanskanen, Sanna-Kaisa and Hiltunen, Risto (eds.) 1995, *Organization in Discourse: Proceedings from the Turku Conference*, Anglicana Turkuensia 14, University of Turku.

Wear, Andrew 1992, 'The popularization of medicine in early modern England', in Porter (ed.), pp. 17–41; reprinted in Wear 1998, ch. 9.

1998, *Health and Healing in Early Modern England*, Variorum Collected Studies Series, Aldershot: Ashgate.

Webster, Charles 1975, *The Great Instauration: Science, Medicine and Reform 1626–1660*, London: Duckworth.

Webster, Charles (ed.) 1979, *Health, Medicine and Mortality in the Sixteenth Century*, Cambridge University Press.

Weisheipl, James A. 1965, 'Classification of the sciences in medieval thought', *Mediaeval Studies* 27: 54–90.

Weiss Adamson, Melitta (ed.) 1995, *Food in the Middle Ages: A Book of Essays*, New York and London: Garland.

Werlich, Egon 1976, *A Text Grammar of English*, Heidelberg: Quelle and Meyer.

Wogan-Brown, Jocelyn, Watson, Nicholas, Taylor, Andrew and Evans, Ruth (eds.) 1999, *The Idea of the Vernacular: An Anthology of Middle English Literary Theory, 1280–1520*, Exeter Medieval Texts and Studies, University of Exeter Press.

Wright, Laura 1994, 'Early Modern London business English', in Kastovsky (ed.), pp. 449–65.

2000, 'Bills, accounts, inventories: Everyday trilingual activities in the business world of later medieval England', in Trotter (ed.), pp. 149–56.

2001, 'Models of language mixing: Code-switching versus semicommunication in medieval Latin and Middle English accounts', in Kastovsky and Mettinger (eds.), pp. 363–76.

Wright, Laura (ed.) 2000, *The Development of Standard English: Theories, Descriptions, Conflicts*, Cambridge University Press.

Wright, Thomas and Halliwell, James Orchard (eds.) 1841–43, Reliquœ Antiquœ: *Scraps from Ancient Manuscripts, Illustrating chiefly Early English Literature and the English Language*, 2 vols., London and Berlin: William Pickering and A. Asher.

Index of manuscripts

General index

tautology 136
Tegni 47, 70, 151
Teodorico Borgognoni of Lucca 101, 122, 139
terminology 10, 12, 35, 48, 81, 95, 100, 101, 106, 108, 110–112, 119, 122, 128, 137, 138, 183, 187, 190
terms, *see also* medical 10, 15, 17, 48, 67, 76, 79–84, 96, 97, 101, 104–107, 109–113, 115, 118–121, 123, 124, 126, 127, 129–131, 133–138, 140–142, 187, 204
  anatomical 116, 121, 133, 136
  foreign 102, 106, 107
Testament 52, 70
textbook 15, 46, 48, 61, 67, 70
text categories 15, 75, 93
text production 2, 11, 12, 58, 73, 80, 97, 210
text-type 3, 146, 148, 174, 176, 178–181, 183, 185, 188–190
text-organising device 86, 90, 95, 191
textual 3, 6, 10, 73, 90, 91, 93, 144
textual transmission 9, 11–14, 26, 28–29, 32, 39, 40, 42, 49, 61, 62, 67, 150–152, 163, 170, 200
  abbreviating 91
  abridging 10
  adapting 10–12, 14, 37, 43, 48, 49, 61, 66
  amalgamating 14
  amplifying 86
  assimilating 12
  blending 13
  borrowing 79–84, 103, 106, 129, 170
  commenting 12, 58, 69, 87
  conflating 12
  editing 3, 4, 14, 152
  embedding 79, 88, 90
  excerpting 12, 13
  extracting 12
  imitating 14
  modifying 38, 44, 45, 206
  paraphrasing 12, 13, 86, 152
  rearranging 13
  standardising 40, 189
  translating 11–13, 30, 38, 42, 49, 67, 73, 86, 97, 136, 174, 176, 177, 180–182, 184, 197–207, 236
  vernacularising 174, 189
Themistius 47
Theodoric, Bishop of Cervia 102, 177
theology 10, 44, 63

Theophrastos 149, 151
theoretical 2, 7, 9, 12, 23, 68, 77, 111
theory 1, 2, 4, 10, 12, 13, 23, 24, 28, 36, 39, 41, 51, 57, 65, 68, 70, 72, 79
therapeutic 181
things natural 105
third-person 58, 59, 67, 222, 223, 225–233, 235, 239
Thomas Cantimprensis 10
Thornton, Robert 103
Timaeus 40
token 180, 185, 187
Toledan tables, *see* Alfonsine tables
Torrigiano 47
tradition 1, 3, 7, 8, 13–15, 41–43, 45–48, 57–58, 73–75, 81, 82, 84, 85, 94, 97, 98, 103, 145, 149, 151,v 152, 169, 170, 174, 176, 197–207, 237, 239
  academic 15, 57, 177, 183
  commentary 14, 40, 41, 47, 52, 56, 85
  remedybook 9, 11, 177, 189
  Wycliffite 214
Traheron, Bartholomew 102
translation 9–11, 13, 14, 27, 29–31, 34, 36, 38, 43, 46–48, 51–59, 61, 67, 69, 84, 93, 97, 98, 101, 102, 107–109, 113, 114, 117, 121, 122, 124, 125, 127–129, 135, 136, 140, 151–152, 156, 163, 179, 182, 186, 187, 199, 200, 204–206, 211, 212, 216, 217, 219
  techniques 4, 10, 13, 14, 52, 70, 97, 131, 179, 206
  translators 10, 13, 14, 17, 41, 50, 52, 54, 58, 59, 67, 100, 102, 107, 108, 110, 111, 122, 123, 129, 133–135, 137, 138, 144, 179, 237
transmission, *see* textual transmission
Treatise on the Astrolabe 4
Trevisa, John 14, 59, 69, 70, 84, 87, 102, 109, 135, 212, 215, 217, 238
trigonometry, *see also* instrument 197–207
trilingual 11, 12, 74–76
Trota 10, 11
Trotula 10, 76

Uery Brefe Treatise 102, 104
universe, *see also* macrocosm 59
university, *see also* medical practitioners 9, 10, 12, 15, 16, 23, 26–31, 38, 39, 44, 47, 49, 51–69, 102
  curricula 9, 40, 44
  faculty 70, 197

Milton Keynes UK
Ingram Content Group UK Ltd.
UKHW041519181024
449640UK00003B/11